AF664495

INDIAN VETERINARY PHARMACEUTICAL INDEX

THE AUTHOR

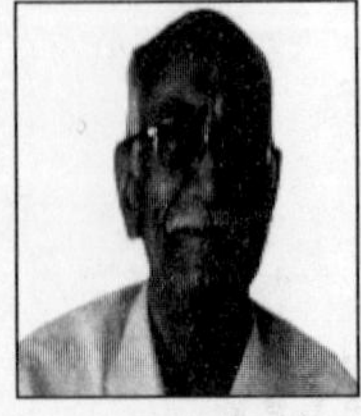

Dr. V.K. Narula is a Veterinary Graduate of 1968 batch from prestigious College of Veterinary Sciences, Hisar under Punjab Agriculture University, Ludhiana with a Diploma in Business Management and a condensed course from ASCI (Administrative Staff College of India), Hyderabad. He has 45 years of experience in Sales, Marketing and Product Management apart from Operational and Technical expertise. Dr. Narula has made out standing contribution in Veterinary Pharma, Education and Management. He has been the author of large number of books, monographs, resource inventories and technical articles. He also worked as editor in magazine Pharma Pramarsh (Monthly). Presently focusing on Technical Advisory to companies, promoter-professional vet pharma consultancy, trainer-sales executives and managers, online service provider to pet owners, guide to a group of Goshalas located in different states of country and seminars on self development.

IVPI-2023

INDIAN VETERINARY PHARMACEUTICAL INDEX

The Reference Volume Only for Veterinary Practitioners

— *Compiled by* —

Dr. V. K. Narula

2023

Daya Publishing House®

A Division of

Astral International Pvt. Ltd.

New Delhi – 110 002

Disclaimer:

The product profile published in Astral IVPI has been taken by the Editor through marketing companies in form of their Broachers, information booklets and promotional material submitted by them.

Publisher and Editor do not take any responsibility for any error in publishing various features of their products. Composition, Dose, administration and Presentation have been added in classified form as per their informative indication. For any difference of opinion regarding these can be enquired directly from these organisations listed. Any query for this will not be entertained by Publisher, Printer or Editor as these are entirely copied from their information.

ISBN: 978-93-5461-662-4

Publisher's Note:

Every possible effort has been made to ensure that the information contained in this book is accurate at the time of going to press, and the publisher and author cannot accept responsibility for any errors or omissions, however caused. No responsibility for loss or damage occasioned to any person acting, or refraining from action, as a result of the material in this publication can be accepted by the editor, the publisher or the author. The Publisher is not associated with any product or vendor mentioned in the book. The contents of this work are intended to further general scientific research, understanding and discussion only. Readers should consult with a specialist where appropriate.

Every effort has been made to trace the owners of copyright material used in this book, if any. The author and the publisher will be grateful for any omission brought to their notice for acknowledgement in the future editions of the book.

Published by : **Daya Publishing House®**
A Division of
Astral International Pvt. Ltd.
– ISO 9001:2015 Certified Company –
4736/23, Ansari Road, Darya Ganj,
New Delhi-110 002
Ph. 011-43549197, 8130496929
E-mail: info@astralint.com
Website: www.astralint.com

PREFACE

Astral IVPI 2023 provides ready access to key information on the selection, prescribing, dispensing and administration of products. Formulations, generally prescribed across India are included. Basic information is drawn from the marketer's product literature given in their Product Information Booklets, broachers or brief sent by their personal communique to the Publishers. Many individuals contributed towards the preparation of this edition of IVPI 2023.

This reference index is designed as a digest for rapid reference and it may not always include all the information necessary for prescribing and dispensing. IVPI 2023 is intended to be interpreted in the light of professional knowledge and it should be supplemented as necessary by specialized publication of the company's literature.

Astral Publishers of IVPI 2023 welcomes comments from veterinary Professional. Such comments help to ensure that the IVPI remains relevant to practice. Comments and constructive criticism should be sent to editor or publisher. This IVPI 2023 will be updated every year. We assure to take your suggestion/comments in affirmative way and add in coming edition. It is neither a textbook nor a Veterinarian's guide as information provided is in brief.

Since many marketing organizations have come up throughout the country operating around their town or Taluka. We have tried to include only the companies with good turn over and those operating in more than 4-5 states. We have also included those also which had been previously included in any such book by any eminent author.

We sincerely thank each individual who contributed directly or indirectly to bring IVPI 2023 in your hands.

Dr. V.K. Narula

CONTENTS

CANINE SECTION

Abbreviations used in IVPI

Administration	Adm.	Large Animal	LA
As much as desired	ad lib	Liquid	Liq.
Availability	Ava.	Meter	M
Body Weight	B.Wt.	Minimum inhibitory concentration	MIC
British Vety. Codex &Supplement	B Vet C	Microgram	μg
British Pharmacopoela	BP	Milligram	mg
Brand	Brd.	Hydrogen Ion concentration	pH
By mouth	Po.	Once a day	OD
Calories	Cal.	Parts per million	ppm
Capsule	Cap.	Percent	%
Composition	Com.	Powder	Pd.
Dosage by Company	Dos.	Presentation	Pre.
Dose rate	@	Quantity Sufficient	qs
For example	e.g.	Red Blood Cells	RBC
Four times a day	qid	Six hourly	qid
Gastro – Intestinal	GI	Small Animal	SA
Gram	g	Solution	Sol.
Haemoglobin	Hb.	Special Instruction by Company	SIC
Hour	Hr.	Special Precaution	SPC
Indications	Ind.	Sub cutaneous	SC
Indian Pharmacopia	IP	Suspension	Sus.
International Units	I.U.	Tablet	Tab
Intramammary	Im	Tea Spoonful	Tsf.
Intramuscular	IM	That is	i.e.
Intrauterine	IU	Three times a day	tid
Intravenous	IV	Twice a day	bid
Kilocalories	Kcal	Weight	Wt.
Kilogram	Kg	When needed	SOS

Understanding and Using Drugs

What are Drugs?

Drug refers to medicine—substances that can cure or arrest disease, relieve symptoms, ease pain and provide other benefits. Also includes Vitamins and minerals given to correct deficiencies.

Source of Drugs?

Drugs were earlier substances extracted from herbs and animals. Now all are virtually developed in laboratories, manufactured through chemical processes; derived from plants and organisms. Some are synthetic chemical analogues. Some are still extracted from natural source. Some are now genetically engineered.

Classification of drugs:

(*a*) **Generic Name:** Official medical name of basic active susbstance.

(*b*) **Brand Name:** Chosen by manufacturer, can be easily pronounced, recongnised and remembered. It may be of some brand with ingredient C by different manufacturer). Difference may be slight in brands related to absorption, convenience and digestibility.

(c) **Chemical Names:** Is technical description of drug and is not used as brand or generic name.

Action of drugs:

1. Replacing chemicals that are deficient e.g. Vitamin & mineral formulation.
2. Interfering with cell functions—these change the way cells work. These decrease or increase the normal activity. These bring different changes in different cells.
3. Action against invading organism or abnormal cells.

Effect of drugs:

A veterinarian selects a drug for positive results and / or for the relief from symptoms. As all drugs are potentially harmful, he has to consider the benefits and risk by administering a drug like:

1. Action time— Some act rapidly with immediate relief. Some take long time.
2. Adverse effect- Undesirable effects on tissue, organ or body of the animal also known as side effects.
3. Benefits versus adverse effect- Therapeutic benefits to the sick animal against possible adverse effect are taken into consideration.

Interaction of drugs:

When 2 different drugs are taken together or in combination with some food, produce different effect when drug given alone. Sometimes these are given to increase the effectiveness of a drug. Their action can be:

(*a*) After absorption— Absorption is slowed

(b) Enzymic effect- Increase production of enzymes in liver to break down the drugs.

(c) Excretion – May reduce or increase excretion in urine.

(d) Reception effect

(e) Similar or opposite effect

(f) Reduced protein binding.

Administration of Drugs

1. Oral
2. Local
3. Rectal
4. Parertal/ Injection IM/ IV/ SC/Others
5. Topical

(Slow Release or Rapid action)

Form of Drugs

I Tablets

II Bolus

III Capsule

IV Liquid

V Mixture

VI Elxir

VII Empulsion

VIII Syrups

IX Topical creams

X Ointments

XI Lotion

XII Injectable Sol

XIII Eye drops

XIV Ear drops

XV Intramammary

XVI Intrauterine

XVII Pessaries

XVIII Suppositories

Constituents of Drugs

1. Drugs
2. Diluent
3. Granulating agent
4. Binding agent

5. Disintegrating agent
6. Coating
7. Colouring
8. Preservative

Availability of Drugs

(*a*) Over the counter Drugs OTC

(*b*) Prescription Drug

Storing Drugs

(*a*) In a cool dry place

(*b*) Away from direct sunlight

(*c*) Away from source of heat

(*d*) A few in refrigerator

(*e*) Out of children's reach

(*f*) Caps or lids closed after use

(*g*) If kept in other container or loose label it

When to Dispose off the Drugs

* Expiry date is reached
* Vinegar smell
* Tablets chipped, cracked, discoloured, soften or stuck together
* Liquids thickened, discoloured different smell or taste
* Any visibility of foreign material in drug
* Tubes when cracked or leaky
* Ointment/ cream- when change of appearance, colour or odour and hardened without refrigeration

While Purchasing Drugs

* Match the name
* Look at expiry
* Look at Batch No.
* Take the bill

While Administering Drugs

* Read the PIL/ Label
* Read the prescription
* Use as per advice
* Administer after advised duration
* Complete the course of medication
* Discontinue on veterinarians advice.

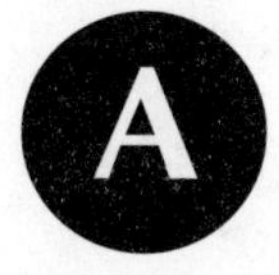

Alimentary System

Terms and Diseases related to Alimentary System

Acidosis: Increase in pH towards acidosis/ acidic

Anorexia: Complete absence of appetite

Aphagia: (Also Anophagia) decreased food intake.

Appetite: Conditional reflex and expresses the degree of hunger.

Bloat: Overdistension of rumen, reticulum with gases of fermentation.

Chelitis: Inflammation of lips.

Cholecystitis: Inflammation of gall bladder.

Choleliths: Stones in gall bladder.

Colic: Abdominal pain.

Constipation: Faeces are dry, hard and small bulk passed at infrequent intervals.

Defaecation: Passing of dung.

Diarrhoea: Increase in frequency of defaecation and normal dung is soft.

Distension: Increased enlarged abdomen which causes pain.

Dysphagia: Difficulty in eating or swallowing.

Enteritis: Inflammation of intestinal mucosa.

Flatulence: Distended abdomen due to Presence of gas in stomach.

Gastric dyspepsia: Abomasum becomes impacted with syndrome of indigestion.

Gastritis: Inflammation of stomach.

Gingivitis: Inflammation of gums.

Glossitis: Inflammation of tongue.

Hepatitis: Inflammation of liver.

Hypermotility: Increased movement.

Hyperorexia: Increased appetite.

Hypomotility: Decreased movement.

Impaction: Moderate abdominal pain with constipation and general depression with anorexia and complete ruminal stasis.

Inappetance: Partial absence of appetite.

Indigestion: Caused by atony of forestomach characterised by anorexia lack of ruminal movement and constipation.

Jaundice: It is a clinical sign as a result of accumulation of bilirubin.

Mastication: Cutting of feedstuff in pieces by teeth.

Oseophagitis: Inflammation of oseophagus.

Palatitis: Inflammation of palate.

Pancreatitis: Swelling of pancreas with abdominal pain and vomiting.

Parotitis: Inflammation of any salivary gland.

Peritonitis: Inflammation of peritoneum.

Pharyngitis: Inflammation of pharynx.

Polyphagia: Increased food intake.

Scours: Passage of soft, fluid faeces varying from yellow to green colour.

Spasmodic Colic: Abdominal pain which is characterised by short spasms.

Starvation: Complete deprivation of food.

Stomatitis: Inflammation of oral mucosa.

Swallowing: Comple act by creation of pressure to force the bolus/food into oesophagus from mouth.

Thirst: Increased desire for water.

Tympany: Distension of abdomen with severe abdominal pain.

Vomiting: Removing excessive quantities of ingesta or toxic material from stomach.

Antacids

Aluminium Hydroxide/ Combination

Cures acidity its action is to neutralize hydrochloric acid in the gastric fluid. Aluminium Hydroxide is an effective adsorbent and decreases intestinal motility and may lead to constipation.

Disogel Susp	Concept
Comp	5ml contains: Aluminium Hydroxide 250 mg, Simethicone 40 mg, Milk of Magnesium 250 mg
Adm.	Oral
@	LA 25-30 ml tid SA 5-7ml tid
Pres.	175 ml, 450 ml

Anti-diarrhoeal

Diarrhea and dysentery are symptoms usually caused by enteritis due to many factors viz bacteria, virus, protozoa, parasite or even food.

Antimicrobials – Also known as antibiotics. They kill the invading bacteria.

Amoxicyllin (Amoxycycline)	
Amoxirum Bol	**Virbac**
Com	Amoxicycline trihydrate 750 mg, 1.5 G
Adm	Oral
@	10mg/kg B.wt 1 Bol/200 kg B.wt
Pres	Blister of 2

Symoxyl calf Bol	Zydus
Com	Amoxicycline trihydrate 750 mg, 1.5 G
Adm	Oral
@	10mg/kg B.wt,1 Bol/200 kg B.wt
Pres	Strip of 4

Chloramphenicol	
Vetnicol Bol	**Vets Farma**
Comp	Chloramphenicol 500 mg
Adm.	Oral
@	2-6 Bol for LA 3-5 d ½ -1 Bol SA
Pres.	50 Bol

Furazolidone

Neftin Tab	Zydus (Pfizer)
Comp	Furazolidone 200 mg
Adm.	Oral
@	1 Tab/20 kg B.wt for 3 days
Pres.	12 Tab strip

Scorid Tab	Vets Farma
Comp	Furazolidone 500 mg
Adm.	Oral
@	1 Tab/50 kg B.wt for 3 days
Pres.	10 Tab strip

Furaltadons

Solfural Pow.	Sterling
Comp	Furaltadone 20%
Adm.	Oral
@	1g/20 kg B.wt
Pres.	20g sachet

Neomycin

Unimycin Bol	Cargill (unichem)
Comp	Neomycin Sulphate 500mg
Adm.	Oral
@	2.5-5 mg/ kg B.wt
Pres.	Strip of 10

Halquinol

3 Care Bol	Cargill (Vetcare)
Comp	Halquinol 1.5 g
Adm.	Oral
@	L.A. 1-2 Bol SA ½ -1 Bol bid
Pres.	Strip of 10 Boli

Quixalin Bol	Zydus (sarabhai)
Comp	Halquinol 1.5 g
Adm.	Oral
@	30-60 mg/kg B.wt bid
Pres.	Bottle containting 25 boluses

Multicare Bol.	Neospark
Comp	Halquinol 1.5 g
Adm.	Oral
@	LA 1-2 Bol bid SA ½ -1 Bol bid
Pres.	Strip of 10 Bol

Metronidazole	
Anarohin	Cargill
Comp	Metronidazole 5 mg/ml
Adm.	Oral
@	4ml/kg B.wt
Pres.	50 ml

Combinations

Furazolidone + Metronidazole	
Diamet Bol	**Novartis**
Comp	Metroridazole 1000 mg + Furazolidone 200 mg
Adm.	Oral
@	1 Bol/50 kg B.wt
Pres.	4 Bol Strip

Fazole Bol	Cargill (unichem)
Comp	Metroridazole 1000 mg + Furazolidone 200 mg
Adm.	Oral
@	1 Bol/50 kg B.wt
Pres.	Strip of 4 Bol

Nildir Bol	Pranav
Comp	Metroridazole 1000 mg + Furazolidone 200 mg
Adm.	Oral
@	1 Bol/50 kg B.wt
Pres.	Strip of 4 Bol

Neomycin + Doxcyclin	
Mega Dox N Sol. Pow	**Neospark**
Comp	Each gm contain Neomycin sulphate 100 mg+ Doxyclin 100 mg
Adm.	Oral
@	1g/25 kg Body wt.
Pres.	50 g

Gastina Tab	**Virbac**
Comp	Eact tab contain Streptomycin Sulphate 250 mg Neomycin Sulphate 100 mg
Adm.	Oral
@	LA 4-5 tab bid for 3 days SA 2 tab bid for 3 day New born 1 tab bid
Pres.	Pack of 10 tab

Miscellaneous

Pesulin Bol	**Cardila Pharma**
Comp	Each Bol contains Phthalysyphathiazole 1 mg Kaolin 3 g Pectin 75 mg Potassium chloride 15.6 mg Sodium chloride 31.8 mg Potassium citrate 67.8 mg Sodium acid phosphate 26.4 mg
Adm.	Oral
@	LA 4-8 Bol SA 2-4 Bol bid
Pres.	Strip of 4 Bol

Pesulin Syp	**Cadila**
Comp	Each 15 ml contains Phthalysyphathiazole 1 g Kaolin 3 g Pectin 150 mg
Adm.	Oral
@	LA 100-150 ml bid SA 50-60 ml bid
Pres.	100 ml, IL

Swifta Liq.	**Zydus (Sarabhai)**	
Comp	Each 15 ml contains	
	Phthalysyphathiazole	1 mg
	Kaolin	3 g
	Pectin	75 mg
	Potassium chloride	15.6 mg
	Sodium chloride	31.8 mg
	Potassium citrate	67.8 mg
	Sodium acid phosphate	26.4 mg
Adm.	Oral	
@	LA 100 ml bid SA 50 ml lid	
Pres.	100 ml	

Enterokap Bol	**Neospark**	
Comp	Each 15ml contains	
	Phthalysyphathiazole	1 mg
	Kaolin	3 g
	Pectin	75 mg
	Potassium chloride	15.6 mg
	Sodium chloride	31.8 mg
	Potassium citrate	67.8 mg
	Sodium acid phosphate	26.4 mg
Adm.	Oral	
@	LA 4-8 Bol bid SA 2-4 Bol bid	
Pres.	Strip of 4 Bol	

Centrogyl LM Bol	**Century**	
Comp	Each Bol contains	
	Metronidazole	1 g
	Furazolidon	500 mg
	Loperamide hydrochloride	7.5 mg
Adm.	Oral	
@	LA 4-6 Bol/ day SA 1-2 Bol/ day	
Pres.	Strip of 4 Bol	

Furagyl Bol	**Vest Pharma**	
Comp	Each Bol contains	
	Metronidazole	1 g
	Furazolidon	500 mg
	Loperamide hydrochloride	7.5 mg
Adm.	Oral	
@	LA 4-6 Bol/ day SA 1-2 Bol/ day	
Pres.	Strip of 4 Bol	

Metrofural Bol	**Alembic**
Comp	Each Bol contains Metronidazole 1 g Furazolidon 500 mg Loperamide hydrochloride 7.5 mg
Adm.	Oral
@	LA 4-6 Bol/ day SA 1-2 Bol/ day
Pres.	Strip of 4 Bol

Ciptas TZ Liq	**Intas**
Comp	Ciproflaxacin 125 mg + Tinidazole 150 mg/5ml
Adm.	Oral
@	LA 10-15 ml SA 5-7 ml bid
Pres.	50 ml

Qdiar	**Phoenix**
Comp	1 Bolus contains Oflaxacin 900 mg Ornidazole 2500 mg Dicyclomine 50 mg Dimethicone 75 mg
Adm.	Oral
@	LA 2Bol bid SA ½ Bol bid
Pres.	4 Bol strip

Mekodiar Bol	**Carevet Pharma**
Comp	Bolus contains Quinodochlor 1000 mg Furazolidons 500 mg Atropine sulphate 0.5 mg
Adm.	Oral
@	LA 1 Bol bid
Pres.	Stip of 2 Bol

DD Rok Bolus	**Nicosia**
Comp	Bolus contains Metronidazole 1 g Furazolidone 500 mg Atropine sulphate 0.5 mg
Adm.	Oral
@	1 Bol tid
Pres.	Strip of 4

Vetfur TL Bol	**Boehringer Ingelheim**
Comp	Metronidazole 1000 mg Furazolidone 500 mg Loperamide 75 mg Tinidazol 5 mg
Adm.	Oral
@	4-6 Bol od for 3-5 days
Pres.	Strip of 4

Reptoban Bol	**Herstel**
Comp	Bolus contains Furazolidone 500 mg Quinodochlor 1000 mg Atropin sulphate 0.5 mg Zinc 400 mg Kaolin q.s
Adm.	Oral
@	4 Bol od
Pres.	4 Bol strip

Diaroak Powder **Ayurvet**

Indications: DiarrhaeaDysentry

- ❖ Checks diarrhea of variable etiology.
- ❖ Minimizes the loss of water and nutrients.
- ❖ Repairs the damaged G% mucosa, restoring effective absorption.
- ❖ Optimizes intestinal peristalsis.

Composition:

Polygonum aviculare	Tinospora cordifolia	Holarrhenaantidysenterica
Cyperusrotundus	Zingiber officinale	Acacia catechu
Aeglemarmelos	Punicagranatum	Woodfordia fruticosa
Berbislycium	Symplocos racemosus	Salmalia malabarica
Andrographis paniculata		

Adm. Oral

Dosage: 30 gm twice daily orally in severe cases repeat dose 6 hours interval.

Catorrhoea Pow/Tab **Cattle Remedies**

Indications: Diarrhoea, Dysentry

Composition: 100 g contains

Aeglemarmelos	24.5 g	Zingiber officianale	15 g
Acacia catechu	5 g	Berberis aristla	7 g
Baykumbha	7 g	Aluminium Sulphate	6 g
Copper Sulphate	4 g	Calcium Carbonate	24.5 g
Helicterisis oralina	7 g		

Adm.	Oral
@	25-50 q mor 3-4 tab. thrice daily for 3-4 days.
Pres.	100 g, 200 g 1 kg 8 × 6 tab.

Diardon				**Vets Farma**
Indications: Diarrhoea, Dysentry, Calfscous				
Composition:	Acasia catechu	10%	Khaira	20%
	Berberis aristata	3%	Creta paraeparata	20%
	Aeglemarmelos	10%	Base	qs
	Panicagranatum	25%		
Adm.		Oral		
@		50 g twice a day		
Pres.		150 g 1 kg		

Neblon Pow.	**Indian Herbs**
Indications:	Dysentry, Diarrhoea
Comp	Not given
@	40-80 g two hourly
Pres.	100 g

Desenta Pow.	**Arosol Herbal**
Indications:	Diarrhoea, Dysentry
Comp	Not given
@	50 g twice daily
Pres.	100 gm, 1 kg

Diarextablet	**Himalya**
Indications:	Diarrhoea, Bloat
Comp	Not given
@	16-20 tab thrice daily
Pres.	100 tablet

Miscellaneous

Diacure Pow	Rakesh Pharma			
Comp	Acacia catechu	5%	Holarrhoea antidysenterice	7%
	Spriphal ghanstva	11%	Dadin	6%
	Dhatki ghanstva	5.5%	Amritvallary	8%
	Pitta	3.5%	Brihat patra	5%
	Kathani	32%	Gundra	6.5%
	Mochras	1%	Nagar	1.5%
	Ajwar	2%	Kapardak bhasm	6%
Adm.	Oral			
@	LA 30-40 g bid SA 10-15 g bid			
Pres.	30 g, 100 g, 1k g			

Becknor Bol	Natural Remedies
Comp	Not given
Adm.	Oral
@	LA one bolus bid SA ½ bolus bid
Pres.	Strip of 6 bol

Gutlyte GS Pow	Indian Herbs
Comp	Not given
Adm.	Oral
@	LA 20g (in bloody dysentery)
Pres.	20g

Antizymotic/Antiflatulent

Diamethicone or Simethicons.

Its action is surfactant and antiflatulant. It's a mixture of liquid dimethyl polysiloxanes with antifoaming and water repellent property. It prevents gas formations in GI.tract. It is indicated in Tympany and bloat in ruminants.

Bloat Care sus.	**Neospark**
Comp	1% Susp. Of Silica in Diemthicone
Adm.	Oral
@	LA 100 ml SA 20 ml
Pres.	100 ml

Gasonil sus.	**Pranav**
Comp	1% Susp. Of Silica in Dimethicone
Adm.	Oral
@	LA 100 ml SA 20 ml
Pres.	100 ml

Blonil Antibloat Liq	**Sterling**
Comp	1% Susp. Of Silica in Dimethicone Archild oil 0.5%
Adm.	Oral
@	LA 100 ml SA 20 ml
Pres.	100 ml

Blotosil sus.	**Merial Wockhardt**
Comp	1% Susp. Of Silica in Dimethicone
Adm.	Oral
@	LA 100 ml SA 20 ml
Pres.	100 ml

Tymfree sys.	**Zydus**
Comp	Simethicone 1%, Dil oil 0.5%

Adm.	Oral
@	100 ml
Pres.	100 ml bottle

Simethicone combination

Gastina Susp	Virbac
Comp	1% Susp. Of Silica in Dimethicone 0.5 Dil oil
Adm.	Oral
@	LA 100 ml SA 20 ml
Pres.	100 ml

Blotyn Susp	Unjha Formulation
Comp	1% Susp. Of Silica in Dimethicone Archild oil 0.5%
Adm.	Oral
@	LA 100 ml SA 20 ml
Pres.	100 ml

Bloatochina Susp	Sequent
Comp	1% Susp. Of Silica in Dimethicone Archild oil 0.5%
Adm.	Oral
@	LA 100 ml SA 20 ml
Pres.	100ml

Brisil Susp	Brihans Labs
Comp	1% Susp. Of Silica in Dimethicone 0.5% Dil oil
Adm.	Oral
@	LA 50-100 ml SA 20 ml
Pres.	100 ml

Nobloat Susp	Cipla
Comp	1% Susp. Of Silica in Dimethicone 0.5% Dil oil
Adm.	Oral
@	LA 50-100 ml SA 20 ml
Pres.	100 ml

Tympex Susp	**Vet Farma**
Comp	1% Susp. Of Silica in Dimethicone 0.5% Dil oil
Adm.	Oral
@	LA 50-100 ml SA 20 ml
Pres.	100 ml

Miscellaneous

Afanil Liq	**Ayurvet**		
Comp	Ricinus communis	Pinus longifolia	Eucalyptus globules
	Acorus calamus	Trachyspermum ammi	Anethum sowa
	Terminalia chebula	Balanites roxburghii	Eclipta alba
	Azadirachta indica	Terminalia belerica	Andrographis paniculata
	Boerrhavia diffuse	Plumbago zoylanica	Tinospora cordifolia
	Woodfordia fruticosa		
Adm.	Oral		
@	50 ml twice daily for 2 days		
Pres.	100 ml		

Blotinox Liq.	**Cattle Remedies**	
Comp	Mallotus philpensis	1.5 g
	Sulphur sublimatum	0.5 g
	Ferula asfoetida	1.0 g
	Oleum pinus roxburghii	48 ml
Adm.	Oral	
@	LA 100 ml SA 50m can be given intra-ruminal	
Pres.		

Inpacdon Pow.	**Vets Farma**			
Comp	Terminalia chebula	10%	Pipminella anisum	4%
	Rheum emodi	10%	Krishan lavan	10%
	Cassia angustifolia	5%	Julabi namak	50%
	Strychnos nuxvomica	2%	Zingiber officinale	4%
Adm.	Oral			
@	LA 100-200 g bid SA 20-50 g bid			
Pres.	200 g, 1k g			

Impacnil Pow	**Rajshree**
Comp	Not given
Adm.	Oral
@	LA 100 g bid SA 25 g bid
Pres.	100 g

Timpanimol Pow	Arosol
Comp	Not given
Adm.	Oral
@	LA 70-80 g SA 20-40 g (in lukewarm water)
Pres.	100 g 1k g

Timpol Pow	Indian Herbs
Comp	Not given
Adm.	Oral
@	LA 80 g at 3-4 internal SA 40 g
Pres.	100 g, 1 kg

Tyrel Liq	Natural Remedies
Comp	Not given
Adm.	Oral
@	LA 100 ml SA 50 ml
Pres.	100 ml

Bloatnil Liq.	Argano
Comp	Not given
Adm.	Oral
@	LA 100 ml SA 50 ml
Pres.	100 ml

D Bloat Liq	Indian Herbs
Comp	Not given
Adm.	Oral
@	LA 100 ml
Pres.	100 Ml

Himbloat Liq	Himalya
Comp	Not given
Adm.	Oral
@	LA 100ml
Pres.	100ml

Antispasmodics

Atropine Sulphate

It causes relaxation of G.I. muscles to reduce gastric secretions and salivation. It is also used as antidote to organo phosphorous compund as well as antemetic.

Atropine Sulphate Inj.	**Morvel**
Comp	0.6 mg/ml
Adm.	IM
@	LA 0.25 mg 1kg B.wt SA 0.05 mg/kg B.wt
Pres.	10ml

Atropine Sulphate Inj.	**Cipla**
Comp	0.6 mg/ml
Adm.	IM
@	LA 0.25 mg 1 kg B.wt SA 0.05 mg/kg B.wt
Pres.	10 ml

Metoclopramide

It has Dopamine antagonistic action which induce emesis, increases gastric motility. Indicated in gastric stasis, vomiting.

Metin Inj	**Vets Farma**
Comp	Each ml contains 5 mg of Metoclopramide hydrochloride
Adm.	IM
@	LA 10 ml SA 3 ml
Pres.	10 ml

Dicyclomine

Antispasmodic drug acts on GI tract, bilary tract. It reduces pain without proding antisecretory effect. It has also relaxant action on smooth muscles. It's indicated in abdominal and intestinal colic.

Spasmovet Inj	**Merial (wockhardt)**
Comp	10 mg/ml Dicyclo hydrochloride
Adm.	IM Inj
@	0.5 mg 1 kg B.wt LA 10-15 ml SA 1-2 ml bid
Pres.	30 ml

Spas inj	**G. Loucatos**
Comp	10 mg/ml Dicyclo hydrochloride
Adm.	IM Inj
@	0.5 mg 1 kg B.wt LA 10-15 ml SA 1-2 ml bid
Pres.	30 ml

Jospas inj	**Animax Healthcare**
Comp	Dicyclomine hydrochloride 10 mg/ml
Adm.	IM
@	1 ml/10-15 kg B.wt
Pres.	30 ml, 100 ml

Other Combination

Spas Bol	**G. Loucatos**
Comp	Each ml contains Dicyclo hydrochloride 100 mg Diclo fenac 250 mg Paracetamol 1500 mg
Adm.	Oral
@	LA 1-2 bol SA ½ -1 bol
Pres.	Strip of 4

Ridalpin Inj	**KAPL**
Comp	Each ml contains Analgin 500mg Pitofenon hydrochloride 0.02mg
Adm.	IM or IV
@	LA 20-60 ml SA 5-15 ml
Pres.	10 ml, 30 ml, 100 ml

Libragen Bol	**Libra**
Comp	Dicyclomine and Mefenamic acid
Adm.	Oral
@.	2-4 Bolus od
Pres.	4 Bol strip

Baralgan Vet Inj	**Novartis**	
Comp	Each ml contains Analgin Pitofenon hydrochloride	 500 mg 0.02 mg
Adm.	IM or IV	
@	LA 20-60 ml SA 5-1 5ml	
Pres.	10 ml, 30 ml, 100 ml	

Valginate Vet Inj	**TTK**	
Comp	Each ml contains Valethamate bromide Analgin Chlorbutol	 2 mg 500 mg 0.4%
Adm.	IM	
@	LA 20-60 ml SA 5-15 ml	
Pres.	10 ml, 30 ml,	

Pecorex Bol	**Pranav**	
Comp	Each ml contains Dicyclo hydrochloride Diclo fenac Paracetamol	 100 mg 250 mg 1500 mg
Adm.	Oral	
@	LA 1-2 bol SA ½ -1 bol	
Pres.	Strip of 4	

Appetite- Stimulants

Anorexon Bolus	**Zydus (Pfizer)**	
Comp	Each Bolus contains Cobalt sulfate B vet C Dried Ferrous sulphate IP Thiamine hydrochloride IP Vitamin B12 Choline bitarate NF	 100 mg 200 mg 50 mg 40 mcg 18.2 mg
Adm.	Oral	
@	LA 2 Bol bid	
Pres.	Strip of 2 Bol	

Rumen Bolus	**Alembic**	
Comp	Each Bolus contains	
	Ferrous sulphate	1 g
	Cobalt chloride	200 mg
	Copper sulphate	50 mg
	Vitamin B12	20 mg
	Vitamin B1	25 mg
	Yeast	300 mg
Adm.	Oral	
@	2 Bol bid	
Pres.	Strip of 4 Bol	

Anrocare Bol	**Neospark**	
Comp	Each Bolus contains	
	Cobalt sulfate B vet C	100 mg
	Dried Ferrous sulphate IP	200 mg
	Thiamine hydrochloride IP	50 mg
	Vitamin B12	40 mcg
	Choline bitaratrate NF	18.2 mg
Adm.	Oral	
@	LA 2 Bol bid	
Pres.	Strip of 2 Bol	

Cadfeed Bolus	**Zydus**	
Comp	Each Bolus contains	
	Nicotinamide	100 mg
	Piper nigrum	100 mg
	Copper sulphate	250 mg
	Zingiber officinale	20 mg
	Cobalt chloride	40 mg
	Andrographis paniculata	220 mg
	Ferrous sulphate	500 mg
	Apium graveolens	100 mg
	Dibasic sod phosphate	100 mg
	Dried yeast	700 mg
	Sodium bicarbonate	600 mg
	Lysine	20 mg
	Magnesium trisilicate	800 mg
	Methionine	20 mg
	Dextrose	500 mg
Adm.	Oral	
@	LA 4 Bol daily bid SA 1 Bol	
Pres.	Strip of 4 Bol	

Floratone Bol	**Concept**	
Comp	Each Bolus contains	
	Methionine	40 mg
	Gentian powder	220 mg
	Cobalt sulphate	0.88 mg
	Ginger	44 mg
	Copper sulphate	0.44 mg
	Vit B1	145 mg
	Sodium phosphate	100 mg
	Nicotinamide	165 mg
	Sodium bicarbonate	660 mg
	Dried yeast	700 mg
	Magnesium trisilicate	1 g
	Dextrose	500 mg
Adm.	Oral	
@	LA 4 Bol daily bid SA 1 Bol	
Pres.	Strip of 4	

Onfeed Bol	**Cadila Pharma**	
Comp	Each Bolus contains	
	Methionine	20 mg
	Nicotinamide	100 mg
	Piper nigrum	100 mg
	Copper sulphate	250 mg
	Zingiber officinale	20 mg
	Cobalt chloride	40 mg
	Andrographis paniculata	220 mg
	Ferrous sulphate	500 mg
	Apium graveolens	100 mg
	Dibasic sod phosphate	100 mg
	Dried yeast	700 mg
	Sodium Bicarbonate	600 mg
	Lysine	20 mg
	Magnesium Trisilicate	800 mg
	Dextrose	500 mg
Adm.	Oral	
@	LA 4 Bol daily SA 1 Bol	
Pres.	Strip of 4	

Rumicare Pow	**Novartis (Intervet)**	
Comp	125 gm packet contains	
	Calcium propionate	60 g
	Vitamin B6	40 mg
	Methionine	5 g
	Dextrose anhydras	53.5 g
	Cobalt gluconate	40 mg
	Picorrhiza dry extract	250 mg
Adm.	Oral	
@	1 Sachet	
Pres.	125 g sachet	

Feedon Bol	**Virbac (Glaxo)**	
Comp	Each Bolus contains	
	Cobalt aulphate	100 mg
	Thiamine mononitrate	50 mg
	Ferrous aulphate	200 mg
	B 12	40 mcg
	Choline bitartrate	18.2 mg
Adm.	Oral	
@	LA 1-2 Bol SA ½ Bol	
Pres.	Strip of 4	

Digest forte Pow	**Anmark**	
Comp	125 g contains	
	Calcium	60 g
	Methinonine	5 g
	Cobalt	40 mg
	Picorrhiza	250 mg
	Dextrose	53.5 g
	B6	40 mg
Adm.	Oral	
@	LA 125 g bid SA 15 g bidl	
Pres.	125 g, 500 g	

Rumalife Pow.	**Macnor Lifescince**	
Comp	Each 10 g contains	
	Probiotic blend	7 g
	Cobalt sulphate	100 mg
	MoS	1 g
	Phytase	25 mg
	Liver extact	50 mg
	Copper sulphate	100 mg
	Lysine	50 mg
	Ginger extract	5 mg
	Buffer	500 mg
Adm.	Oral	
@	LA 10 g bid SA 5 g h/d	
Pres.	10 g sachet	

Start Bol	**PAIL**	
Comp	Each Bolus contains	
	Live yeast culture	3 g
	Copper sulphate	5 mg
	Lactic acid bacillus CFU	20 million
	Magnesium trisilicate	100 mg
	Amino acid	2 g
	Calcium propionate	200 mg
	Ginger	10 mg
	Vitamin B1	50 mg
	Liver extract	5 mg
	Vitamin B12	20 mcg
Adm.	Oral	
@	LA 2 Bol bid SA 1Bol bid	
Pres.	2 Bol	

Ruchamax Pow	**Ayurvet**	
Comp	Phyllanthus emblica	Embelia ribes
	Eclipta alba	Piper longum
	Woodfordia fruticosa	Trigonella foenumgraecum
	Curcuma longa	Swertia chirata
	Andrographis paniculate	Commiphora mukul
	Piper nigrum	Balanites roxburghii
	Gardenia gummifera	Acorus calmus
	Centratherum anthelmenticum	Tinosphora cordifolia
	Calotropis procera	Allium sativum
	Semicarpus anacerdium	Zingiber officinale
	Azadirachta indica	Trachyspermum ammi

Adm.	Oral
@	LA 2 Bol bid SA 1Bol bid
Pres.	2 Bol

Shilpa Batisa	**Arosol**
Comp	Not given
Adm.	Oral
@	LA 40-50 g bid SA 10-20 g bid
Pres.	100 g, 200 g, 400 g, 1k g

Digestovet Pow	**Vets Farma**
Comp	Ptychotis ajowan 10% Pimpinella anisum 5% Illicium verum 5% Emblica officinalis 10% Krishan lavan 5% Terminalia belerica 10% Swertia chirata 5% Curcuma longa 1% Lavan 20% Zingiber officinale 3% Terimnalia chebula 9% Luffa amara 3% Strychnos nuxvomica 2% Mentha avensis 5% Rheum emodi 5% Carum carvi 1% Ferula jaeschkeana 1%
Adm.	Oral
@	LA 50 g bid SA 20 g bid
Pres.	100 g, 400 g, 1k g

Batisapro Pow	**Patanjali**
Comp	Not given
Adm.	Oral
@	25g bid
Pres.	100 g, 400 g, 1k g

Kepatite Bol	**Kepler**
Comp	Each Bolus contains Lactobacillus Live yeast Piper longum Zingiber officinale Sodium bicarbonate Cobalt sulphate Ferrous sulphate
Adm.	Oral
@	LA 2 Bol bid
Pres.	Strip of 4 Bol

Suruchi Pow/ Bol	KAPL		
Comp	Powder	5 g	1 Bolus
	Chitraka	2 g	1g
	Pippalli	200 mg	100 mg
	Mareecha	200 mg	100 mg
	Hing	350 mg	175 mg
	Ajwain	550 mg	375 mg
	Shankh bhasma	1500 mg	750 mg
	Sunthi	200 mg	100 mg
Adm.	Oral		
@	LA 1 Bol bid or 10 g bid		
Pres.	4's strip, 50 g, 250 g		

Anigest Pow	Sarabhai Zydus
Comp	Not given
Adm.	Oral
@	LA 15 g bid SA 25 g bid
Pres.	15 g, 100 g, 1k g

Appetone Pow	Himalya Drug
Comp	Not given
Adm.	Oral
@	LA 50 g bid SA 25 g bid
Pres.	100 gm, 1 kg

Appetone FortePow	Himalaya Drug
Comp	Not given
Adm.	Oral
@	LA 15 g bid SA 7-8 g bid
Pres.	100 gm, 1 kg

Catone	Cattle Remedies			
Comp	100 g contains			
	Swertia chirata	5 g	Aegle marmelos	5 g
	Operculina turpethum	5 g	Kuchla	5 g
	Centratherum anthelminiticum	5 g	Foeniculum vulgarae	4 g
	Tachyspermum amnilinn	5 g	Piper nigrum	5 g
	Emblica officinalis	5 g	Hellborous niger	5 g

	Terminalia chebula	5 g	Sodium bicarbonate	6 g
	Terminalia belerice	5 g	Black salt	5 g
			Ferrous sulphate	0.5g
			Copper sulphate	0.5g
			Sodium chloride	25 g
Adm.	Oral			
@	LA 40-50 g bid SA 10-50 g bid			
Pres.	100 g, 200 g, 400 g, 1k g			

Himalya Batisa	**Indian Herbs**
Comp	Not given
Adm.	Oral
@	LA 40-60 g SA 20-30 g
Pres.	100 g, 200 g, 400 g, 1k g

H B Strong	**Indian Herbs**
Comp	Not given
Adm.	Oral
@	LA 10 g
Pres.	10 g sachet

Promin Bolus	**Rajshree**
Comp	Not given
Adm.	Oral
@	LA 4 Bol bid SA 2 Bol bid
Pres.	20 Bol

Livroli Syp	**Libra Biotech**			
Comp	10ml contains			
	Surpunkha	375 mg	Kalmegh	250 mg
	Silymarin	375 mg	Makoi	250 mg
	Bhuiamla	350 mg	Punarva	250 mg
	Arjun	275 mg	Bhringraj	150 mg
	Neem	150 mg	Tulsi	150 mg
Adm.	Oral			
@	LA 50 ml bid SA 0 ml bid			
Pres.	500 ml, 1 L, 5 L			

Dig up strong Bol	**Animax Healthcare**			
Comp	Lactobacillus sporogenes	4 billion	Thermostable yeast culture	
	Lactobacillus acidophillus	4 billion	Sacharromyces cervisiae	350 mg
	Bacillus subtillis	4 billion	Sea flora	500 mg
	Bacillus amyloliqui facens	4 billion	Enzyme mixture	1000 mg
	Propionebacterium	4 billion	Nuxvomica	500 mg
Adm.	Oral			
@	LA 1-2 Bolus bid SA 1/2-1 Bol bid			
Pres.	4 Bol strip			

Florasac C Bol	**Phoenix**	
Comp	Each Bolus contains	
	Saccharomyces cerevisiae	25×10^9 CFU
	Zinc sulphate	100 mg
	Lactobacillus sporogenes	25×10^7 CFU
	Cobalt	200 mg
	Fructo oligosaccharide	150 mg
	Copper sulphate	50 mg
	Biotin	5 mg
	Enzymes	2.5 g
	Methionine	2 g
	Nuxvomica	500 mg
	Sodium bicarbonate	150 mg
	Choline chloride	300 mg
	Cannalus indica	250 mg
	Antimony potassium tartrate	100 mg
	Propionbacterium freussureichi	100 mg
Adm.	Oral	
@	LA 2 Bol bid SA 1 Bol bid 8 Bol in impacts	
Pres.	Strip of 4	

IND Forte Bol	**Macwell**	
Comp	Each Bol has	
	Saccharomyces cervisae	17.5 billions CFU
	Phytase	25 mg
	Liver ext.	5 mg
	Lactobacillus sporogenes	20 million CFU
	DL Methionine	1 g
	Seaweed ext.	1 g

	Aspergillus oryza 100 mg L Lysine 50 mg Cobalt sulphate 40 mg Copper sulphate 100 mg Cobalt chloride 250 mg Defaunation agent Amino acid 1 g Fungal diastase 50 mg Pepsin 10 mg
Adm.	Oral
@	2 Bolus bid
Pres.	12 Bol pack

Floraboon Bol	**Carevet Pharma**
Comp	Each Bol contains Live yeast culture 3 g Magnesium trisilicate 100 mg Amino acid 2 g Dicalcium phosphate 200 mg Copper sulphate 5 mg Vit B1 15 mg B12 20 mcg Ginger extract 10 mg Lactobacillus millions spores 30 Liver extract 5 mcg
Adm.	Oral
@	2 Bol bid
Pres.	Strip of 4 Bol

Agiboost Bol	**Agilis**
Comp	Each Bolus contains Live yeast culture 3 g Lactobacillus sporogenes culture 20 millions CFU Llysine 2.25 g DL methionine 0.75 g Liver extract 5 mg Rumen stable enzyme 100 mg Fructo-oligosacharide 1250 mg
Adm.	Oral
@	1-2 Bolus od
Pres.	Strip of 6 Boli

Natural Batisa Pow	**Natural Remedies**
Comp	Selective herbs
Adm.	Oral
@	50 g od for 3-5 day
Pres.	50g, 1 kg

Herbobatisa Pow	**IHC (International Health Care)**
Comp	Herbal
Adm.	Oral
@	LA 50 g od SA 20 g od
Pres.	200 g, 500 g, 1 kg

Probiotics

Addon Bol	**Virbac (Glaxo)**
Comp	Each Bol. Contains 2.5 g yeast powder
Adm.	Oral
@	2 Bol od
Pres.	Strip of 4 Bol

Bioboost Bol/Pow	**Sequent (Lyka)**		
Comp	Live yeast culture	Each Bol contains 3 g	25 g
	Live Lactobacillus spore	20 Million	200 Million
	Amino acids	2 g	25 g
	Liver Ext	5 mg	500 mg
	Each 100 g contains		
Adm.	Oral		
@	LA 1-2 Bol od SA ½ Bol od LA 10 g od SA 5 g od		
Pres.	Strip of 4 Bol, Pow 1kg		

Boost up Bol/Pow	**Merial (Dosch)**		
Comp		Bolus	100 g pow.
	Live yeast culture	3 g	25 g
	Live Lactobacillus spore	20 Million	200 Million
	Amino acids	2 g	25 g
	Liver Ext	5 mg	500 mg
Adm.	Oral		
@	LA 1-2 Bol od SA ½ Bol od LA 10 g od SA 5 g od		
Pres.	Strip of 4 Bol, Pow 1kg		

Biotone Bol/Pow	**KAPL**
Comp	Each Bol 500 g powder Lactobacillus 30 Million coagulanes 500 g 30 Million Live yeast 3 g 30 g Amino acid (Lysine+Methonine) 2 g 20 g
Adm.	Oral
@	LA 2-3 Bol od SA ½ Bol od Pow LA 50 g od SA 25 od
Pres.	Strip of 4, Pow 500g

Biovet Plus Bol	**Merial (Wockharctt)**
Comp	Each Bol Live yeast 3 g Liver extract 5 g Amino acid 1 g Lactobacillus 20 Million Alpha amylase 10 mg Essential trace minerals 1 g
Adm.	Oral
@	LA 2-4 Bol bid SA 1-2 Bol bid
Pres.	Strip of 4

Yeasacc Bol	**Cargil (Vetcare)**
Comp	Each Bol Culture of Saccharomyces cerevisiae 25 Billion CFU per Bol
Adm.	Oral
@	LA 2-4 Bol od SA ½ -1 Bol bid
Pres.	Strip of 4

Amyst Bolus	**Tineta**
Comp	Each Bolus contains Live yeast culture 17.5 Billion CFU Aspergillus oryzae 100 mg Sea flora 1g
Adm.	Oral
@	LA 1-2 Bol od SA ½ -1 Bol od
Pres.	Strip of 4

Neoboost bolus	**Novartis**			
Comp	Each Bolus contains Live yeast culture Lactobacillus Fungl diastase	 3 g 20 Million 50 g	 Amino acid Liver extract	 2 g 5 g
Adm.	Oral			
@	LA 1-2 Bol od SA 1 Bol od			
Pres.	Strip of 4			

Rumobuf Pow	**Merial (Dosch)**
Comp	Balanced rumen buffers fortified with live yeast culture
Adm.	Oral
@	LA 50 g bid SA 25 g bid
Pres.	200 g

Apifast Bolus	**Wellcon**	
Comp	Probiotic cocktail Metabolic restorer Chelated mineral	Vitamins NPN Ph Regulator
Adm.	Oral	
@	LA 2 Bol bid SA 1 Bol bid	
Pres.	Strip of 4 Bol	

Vetyboost Forte Pow	**Avivet Pharma**	
Comp	Live Yeast Lactobacillus Saccharomyces	Bacillus subtillis Sea flora
Adm.	Oral	
@	LA 20-30g bid	
Pres.	300g	

Appevet Bolus	Rakesh Pharma			
Comp	Each Bol contains			
	Piper nigrum	100 mg	Zingiber officinale	100 mg
	Sodium choride	200 mg	Terminalia beleria	300 mg
	Cuminum cyminum	50 mg	Saussurealappa	50 mg
	Aristolocania bracteates	50 mg	Asfetida compound	50 mg
	Sindhar	200 mg	Emblica officinalia	300 mg
	Coriandrum sativum	150 mg	Kasish	150 mg
	Piper longum	30 mg	Terminalia chebula	300 mg
	Piperimul	50 mg	Acorus calamus	70 mg
	Cinnamomum zeylanicum	150 mg	Black salt	300 mg
	Alpina galonga	350 mg	Cinnamomum tamala	150 mg
	Sombhurlun	150 mg	Carryopmgphyllus aromaticus	150 mg
	Melia azadirachta	150 mg	Papadi khar	100 mg
	Trachyspermum ammi	150 mg	Swertia chirata	50 mg
	Embella ribes	150 mg	Sajikhar	200 mg
Adm.	Oral			
@	LA 4-6 Bol bid SA 2-4 Bol bid			
Pres.	10 Bol, 100 Bol pack			

Levucell SB Pow	Venky's
Comp	(Saccharomyces cerevisiae boulardii 2x109 (live cell) per g
Adm.	Oral
@	LA 6-10g od
Pres.	100g

Bovifur Pow	Phoenix	
Comp	100 g contains	
	Saccharomyces cerevisiae	60 x 109 CFU
	Nonprotein nitrogen	1.788 g
	Saccharomyces boulardii	20 x 109 CFU
	Bypass fat	4.4 g
	Propionibacterium freusenreichii	20 x 108 CFU
	Bypass protein	2.0 g
	Bacillus licheniformis	20 x 108 CFU
	Cyproheptadine	100 mg
	Lactobacillus acidophillis	20 x 108 CFU
Adm.	Oral	
@	LA 50-100 g bid SA 25 g bid	
Pres.	100 g	

Amlyga Pow	**Cadila Pharma**
Comp	Buffer neutralizer Metabolic enhancer Probiotic and digestive herbs
Adm.	Oral
@	50 g bid x 5 days
Pres.	250 g

Quikrumi	**Zydus**
Comp	Sodium butyrate lactic acid and bacillus
Adm.	Oral
@	1.5 g od
Pres.	200 g, 500 g

Buffboost Pow	**Zydus**
Comp	1 kg contains MHA, HMT Bg and Antioxidant factor S
Adm.	Oral
@	40 g od in bulfaloes
Pres.	1 kg, 5 kg

Actisaf Pow	**Boehringer Ingelheim**
Comp	Saccharomyces cervisiae SC 47 1 x 1010 CFU/g
Adm.	Oral
@	LA 5 g SA 2 g od
Pres.	150 g, 1 kg, 25 kg

Boost Bolus	**IHC (International Health Care)**
Comp	Enzymes and Amino acids
Adm.	Oral
@	2-4 Bolus od
Pres.	4 Bol blister

Bafarin Pow	**Alivira**
Comp	Combination of Rumen buffer fortified and yeast
Adm.	Oral
@	100 g
Pres.	200 g

Ruchamax Pow.	**Ayurvet**
Indications: ❖ Products prompt and complete relief from tympany and bloat. ❖ Brings back normalcy. ❖ Reduces the slime-producing bacteria responsible for froath formation.	
Composition: Phyllanthus emblica, Calotropis procera, Balanites roxburghji Eclipta alba, Semecarpus anacardium, Acorus calamus Woodfordia fruitcosa, Commiphora mukul, Tinospora cordifolia Curcuma longa, Terminalia chebula, Picrorrhiza kurroa Andrographis paniculata, Swertia chirata, Allium sativum Piper nigrum, Trigonella foenumgraecum, Azadirachta indica Gardenia gummifera, Piper longum, Zingiber officinale Centratherum anthelmenticum, Embelia ribes, Trachyspermumammi	
Adm	Oral
A	15 g orally twice daily for 3-5 days.
Pres.	15 & 60 gm regular pack, 225 gm dairy pack 1 kg economy pack.

Catone	**Cattle Remedies**
Indications: Appetiser, Digestive tonic	

Composition:

Each 100 g	5 g	Swertia chirata	5 g
Operculina turpethum	5 g	Centratherum anthelminticum	5 g
Tachyspermum ammilinn	5 g	Embica officinalis	5 g
Terminalia chebula	5 g	Terminaliabaleria	5 g
Aeagle marmelos	5 g	Kuchla	5 g
Zinziber officinale	4 g	Foeniculumvulgare	5 g
Piper nigrum	5 g	Hellborusniger	6 g
Sodium bicarbonate	6 g	Blacksalt	5 g
Ferrous sulphate	0.5	Copper sulphate	0.5
Sodium chloride	25 g		

Admn	Oral
@	40-50 g twice daily
Pres.	100 g, 200 g, 400 g, 1 kg

Appetonic Forte Powder	**Himalya**
Indi.	Indigestion, Anorexia
Comp.	Not given
@	2 Bol. Twice a day or 50 gm twice a day
Pres.	Strip of 4 Bol., 100 gm, 1 kg

Appevet Bol. — **Rakesh Pharma**

Indications: Digestive, Casminative, Appetizer

Composition: Each Bol. contains

Piper nigrum	100 mg	Zingiher officinale	100 mg
Terminalia beleria	300 mg	Cuminum cyminum	100 mg
Aristolochia bracteate	50 mg	Asfoetida compound	50 mg
Emblica officinalia	300 mg	Coriandrun sativum	150 mg
Piper longum	30 mg	Terminalia chebula	300 mg
Acorus calamus	70 mg	Cinnamomum zeylanicum	150 mg
Alpina galanga	350 mg	Sodium chloride	200 mg
Carryophyllus aromatias	150 mg	Saussurealappa	50 mg
Trachyspermium ammi	150 mg	Cinnamomum tamala	150 mg
Sindhav	200 mg	Kaghis	150 mg
Pipermul	50 mg	Sajikhar	200 mg
Blacksalt	300 mg	Sombhurlun	150 mg
Sunertia chirata	50 mg	PapadiKhar	100 mg
Embella ribes	150 mg	Melia azadirachta	150 mg

@	4-6 Bol. daily
Pres.	10 Bol. 100 Bol. Pack

Batisa Pro. Pow.	**Patanjali**
Indi.	Appetite Stimulating, Digestive
Comp.	Not given
@	25 gm twice daily
Pres.	100 g, 400 g, 1 kg

Laxatives and Purgatives

Paraffin Liquid

Its high lubricant laxative. It softens the fecal mass.

Agarol	**Generic**
Comp	Liquid Paraffin
Adm.	Oral
@	LA 200 ml od
Pres.	450 ml

Mag Sulphate

A purgative and increases peristaltic movement

Mag Sulphate Pow	**Ranbaxy**
Comp	Magnesium sulphate
Adm.	Oral with water dissolution
@	LA 150-200 g SA 25-30 g
Pres.	450 g

Castor Oil

It acts promptly and evacuates whole intestine acting irritant purgative.

Castrol	**Generic**
Comp	Castor oil pure
Adm.	Oral
@	LA 75-100 ml SA 5-10 ml
Pres.	100 ml, 450 ml

Rumenotorics and Stomachics

These effect rumen. These include ingredients to stimulate rumen motility, maintain pH, rumen microflora, fermentation process and vitamin B synthesis. Thus these set the rumen to function actively for optimum digestion.

Antimony potassium tartrate/ Combinations Bolus

Bovirex Bol	**Marc**	
Comp	Each Bolus contains	
	Antimony potassium tartrate	2 g
	Ferrous sulphate	2 g
	Copper sulphate	50 mg
	Cobalt chloride	100 mg

Adm.	Oral
@	LA 3-4 Bol in divided dose
Pres.	Strip of 4

Bovirum Bol	**Zydus (Sarabhai)**	
Comp	Each Bolus contains	
	Antimony potassium tartrate	2 g
	Ferrous sulphate	2 g
	Copper sulphate	50 mg
	Cobalt chloride	100 mg
Adm.	Oral	
@	LA 3-4 Bol in divided dose	
Pres.	Strip of 4	

RumentonBol	**Zydus (Pfizer)**	
Comp	Each Bolus contains	
	Antimony potassium tartrate	2 g
	Ferrous sulphate	2 g
	Copper sulphate	50 mg
	Cobalt chloride	100 mg
Adm.	Oral	
@	LA 3-4 Bol in divided dose	
Pres.	Strip of 4	

Rumentas Bol	**Intas**	
Comp	Each Bolus contains	
	Antimony potassium tartrate	2 g
	Ferrous sulphate	2 g
	Copper sulphate	50 mg
	Cobalt chloride	100 mg
Adm.	Oral	
@	LA 3-4 Bol in divided dose	
Pres.	Strip of 4	

Apeton Cap	**Parnav**	
Comp	Each Cap 800mg contains	
	Antimony potassium tartrate	32 mg
	Ferrous sulphate	32 mg
	Chitrak	160 mg
	Live yeast 10000 million CFU/g	576 mg

Adm.	Oral
@	LA 8-16 Cap bid SA 4-8 Cap bid
Pres.	Pack of 16

Rumioton Bol	**Century**
Comp	Each Bolus contains Antimony potassium tartrate 2 g Ferrous sulphate 2 g Copper sulphate 50 mg Cobalt chloride 100 mg
Adm.	Oral
@	LA 3-4 Bol in divided dose
Pres.	Strip of 4

Antic K inj	**Libra**
Comp	Antimony potassium tartrate
Adm.	IV
@.	30 ml, 3-5 days od
Pres.	30 ml

Rumen Bol	**Alembic**
Comp	Each Bolus contains Ferrous sulphate 1 g, Vit B1 25 mg Cobalt chloride 200 g, Yeast 300 mg Copper sulphate 50 g Vit B12 20 mcg
Adm.	Oral
@	LA 2 Bolus bid
Pres.	Strip of 4

Probiotics

Rumiquick Pow	**Libra**
Comp	22 g sache provides Saccharomyces 200 billion CFU Bacillus subtalis 1.5 billion CFU Aspergillus oryzal 1000mg

	Bacillus amylo liqvefaciens 1.5 billion CFU Ginger extract 100mg Propionibacterium frendenerichii 11.5 billion CFU
Adm.	Oral
@.	LA 1 sachet bid Sa ½ bid
Pres.	Sachet of 22 g

Rumisaac Bol	Zydus
Comp	Each Bolus contains 4 Probiotic 4 Enzymes 6 Aminoacids Liver extract Ginger Rumen buffer with prebiotic
Adm.	Oral
@	2-4 Bol for 3-5 days
Pres.	Strip of 4 bol

Other Combination

Anigest	Zydus
Comp	Not given
Adm.	Oral
@	LA 15 g bid SA 5 g bid
Pres.	100 g, 200, 400 g, 1 kg

Rumbion	Natural Remedies
Comp	Not given
Adm.	Oral
@	LA 2 Bol bid
Pres.	Strip of 4

Rumec Pow	Rakesh Pharma			
Comp	100 g contains			
	Piper nigrum	2%	Curcuma longa	9.0%
	Asfoetida	0.05%		
	Zingihber officiniale	3%	Trigonella foenum	1.0%
	Melia azdirachta	2.5%		
	Trachyspermum ammi	4%	Copper sulphate	0.2%
	Sodium chloride	9.5%		
	Coriandum sativum	3%	Foeniculum vulgare	1.0%
	Acorus calamus	0.55%		
	Holarrhena antidysenterica	5%	Cuminum cyminum	1.0%
	Black salt	9.5%		

	Cinnamomum graveoleus	3%	Tinosphora cordifolia	2.5%
	Carsia fistula	0.5%		
	Peucadanum graveoleus	3%		
	Cernonia anthelmintica	1.5%	Suertia chirata	2%
	Terminalia chebula	8.7%	Terminalia belerica	8.7%
	Aegla marmeloso	5%	Alpinja calanga	9.8%
	Embica officinalis	4.0%	Sodium bicarbonate	4.5%
	Embelia ribes	2.5%		
Adm.	Oral			
@	LA 80-100 g od SA 25-30 g od			
Pres.	200 g, 400 g, 1 kg			

Rumigest	**Alembic**			
Comp	100 g contains			
	Sindhuj	5 g	Raktpushpak	5 g
	Keshraj	5 g	Kuruvinda	5 g
	Abhaya	5 g	Plihari	20 g
	Karan	5 g	Karshaphal	5 g
	Karvi	5 g	Avartini	5 g
	Manthapak	5 g	Kharmanjri	5 g
	Subhras	7.5 g	Ikshurarsar	7.5g
	Sriphal	5 g	Rasayni	5 g
Adm.	Oral			
@	LA 40 g bid			
Pres.	100 g, 200 g, 500 g			

Rumiset	**Herbotrend**
Comp	Not given
Adm.	Oral
@	LA 25-50 g bid
Pres.	100 g, 250 g, 400 g

Bembem Bolus	**Herstel**
Comp	Not given
Adm.	Oral
@	LA 2 Bol bid
Pres.	Strip of 4

Pachoplus Bol	**Ayurvet**	
Comp	Boerrhavia diffuse Eclipta alba Zingiber officinale Picrorhiza kurroa Piper longum Commiphore mukul Andrographis paniculata Embelia ribes	Cuminum cyrnium Balanites roxburghii Piper nigrum Acrous calamus Terminalia chebula Allium sativa Tachyspermum ammi
Adm.	Oral	
@	2 Bolus bid for 2-3 days	
Pres.	Strip of 4	

Bovifur Pow	**Phoenix**	
Comp	100 g contains	
	Saccharomyces cerevisae	60×10^9 CFU
	Saccharomyces boulardii	20×10^9 CFU
	Propionibacterium freudenreichii	20×10^8 CFU
	Bacillus bicheniformis	20×10^8 CFU
	Lactobacillus acidophllis	20 x 10 CFU
	Nonprotein nitroxgen	1.7888 g
	Bypass fat	4.4 g
	Bypass protein	2.0 g
	Cyproheptadine	100 mg
Adm.	Oral	
@	50-100 g bid	
Pres.	100 g pouch	

IND Forte Bol	**Macwell**			
Comp	Saccharomyces cerevisiae (Live yeast culture SC 47)	17.5 billion CFU	Amino acid	1 g
	Lactobacillus sporogene	20 million CFU	Phytase	25 mg
	Amylase alpha	100 mg	Pepsin	10 mg
	Fungal diastase	50 mg	Seaweed extract	1 g
	Defaunation agent	500 mg	D.L.Methionine	1 g
	Cabalt sulphate	40 mg	L.Lysine	50 mg
	Copper sulphate	100 mg	Choline chloride	250 mg
	Liver extract	5 mg		
Adm.	Oral			
@	2 Bol 0 D for 3 days			
Pres.	Pack of 12 Bol			

Suruchi Pow/Bolus	KAPL		
Comp		Pow 5 g	1 Bolus
	Chitrak	2 g	1 g
	Pipalli	200 mg	100 mg
	Sunti	200 mg	100 mg
	Mareeche	200 mg	100 mg
	Hing	350 mg	175 mg
	Ajwain	550 mg	375 mg
	Shankh bhasm	1500 mg	750 mg
Adm.	Oral		
@	10 g or 1 Bol bid		
Pres.	Strip of 4, 50 g, 250 g		

Livroli Syp.	Libra Biotech			
Comp	100 ml contains			
	Surpunkha	375 mg	Arjun	275 mg
	Bhringraj	150 mg	Silymarin	375 mg
	Kalmegh	250 mg	Neem	150 mg
	Bhui amla	370 mg	Makoi	250 mg
	Tulsi	150 mg	Punarva	250 mg
Adm.	Oral			
@	50 ml bid			
Pres.	500 ml, 1 L, 5 L			

Bonnisan Liq.	Himalya
Comp	Not given
Adm.	Oral
@	50 ml bid
Pres.	120 ml

Digest Forte Pow.	Anmarks Pharma			
Comp	125 g contains			
	Calcium propionate	60 g	Picrorrhiza dry Ext.	250 mg
	Methionine USP	5 g	Vit. B6 IP	40 mg
	Cobalt gluconate	40 mg	Dextrose anhydras	53.5 g
Adm.	Oral			
@	25 g bid			
Pres.	125 g pouch			

Rumiprotec Gold Pow	**Argano**
Comp	Not given
Adm.	Oral
@	Not given
Pres.	Not given

Sequboost Pow	**Alvira**
Comp	Not given
Adm.	Oral
@	Not given
Pres.	Not given

Rumivet Bolus	**Unjha**	
Comp	Each Bolus contains	
	Antimony potassium tartrate	2 g
	Ferrous sulphate	2 g
Adm.	Oral	
@	2 Bolus bid	
Pres.	Strip of 4 Pack of 50	

Rumicell Bolus	**Bovian**	
Comp	Each bol of 10 g contains	
	Saccharomyces cerevisiase	25 x 10^9 CFU
	Biotin	5 mg
	Zinc sulphate	100 mg
	Lactobacillus sporogenes	25 x 10^9 CFU
	DL Methionine	2 g
	Fructooligo Sachharide	250 mg
	Aspergillus oryzae	25 x 10^9 CFU
	Cobalt sulphate	20 mg
	Copper sulphate	50 mg
Adm.	Oral	
@	LA 2 Bolus bid for 3-4 days	
Pres.	Strip of 4	

Digest Bol.	**Anmark Pharma**
Comp	Each Bol contains
	Copper sulphate 50 mg Ferrous sulphate 200 mg

	Ext. sarponkha	50 mg	Ext. picororrhiza	50 mg
	Pulv ginger	100 mg	Cobalt sulphate	50 mg
	Ext. shringrraj	100 mg		
Adm.	Oral			
@	2-3 Bol bid			
Pres.	Strip of 4			

Start Bol	**PAIL**			
Comp	Each Bolus contains			
	Cobalt chloride	50 mg	Vit B1	15 mg
	Copper sulphate	5 mg	Vit B12	20 mcg
	Ginger extract	10 mg	Amino acids	2 g
	Magnesium trisilicate	100 mg	Live yeast culture	3 g
	Dicalcium phosphate	200 mg	Lactobacillus Sporogenes	20 million CFU
			Liver extract	5 mg
Adm.	Oral			
@	LA 2 Bolus bid SA 4 Bol bid			
Pres.	Strip of 4			

Rumistrong	**Cadila Pharma**		
Comp	Sunthi	Amruta	Atmagupta
	Sauvarchal	Bahula	Dhanyak
	Ashwabala	Yashthi	madhu
	Jirak	Shatpushpa	Yavani
	Amalki	Marich	Dev Kusum
	Saindhav	Haridra	
Adm.	Oral		
@	10 g bid		
Pres.	10 g, 100 g		

Rumentonic Pow. or Rumec			**Rakesh Pharma**
Indications: Digestive, Carminative, Laxative			
Composition: 100 g contain			
Piper nigrum	2%	Curcuma longa	9%
Zingiber officinale	3%	Trigonella foenum	1%
Trachyspermum ammi	4%	Copper Sulphate	0.2%
Coriandrum sativum	3%	Foeniculum vulgare	1%

Holarrhena antidysenterica	0.5%	Cuminum cyminum	1%
Cinnamomum graveolens	3%	Tinospara cordifolia	2.5%
Peucadanum graveolens	3%	Asfoetida compound	0.05%
Termmalia chebula	8.7%	Vernonia anthelmintica	1.5%
Alpinia galanga	9.8%	Melia azdirachta	2.5%
Cassia fistula	0.5%	Swerita chirata	2%
Soda bi carb	4.5%	Aegle marmelos	0.5%
Emoelica officinalis	4%	Acorus calanus	0.55%
Sodium Chloride	9.5%	Terminalia belerica	8.7%
Black Salt	9.5%		

Adm	Oral
@	80-100 g daily
Pres.	200 g, 400 g, 1 kg pack

Hepato Protective

These are remedies for acute and chronic liver disorders, hepatitis, Jaundice, fatty liver, cirrhosis, hepatotoxic condition. These are used for debility, anemia and stress of various etiology.

Injectable

Combination of vitamin B complex and Liver Extract

Belamyl inj	**Zydus (Sarabhai)**	
Comp	Each ml contains	
	Thiamine hydrocholoride	25 mg
	Riboflavin	3 mg
	Naicinamide	100 mg
	Vit B_{12}	10 mcg
	Crude Liver extract	0.66 ml
Adm.	IM inj	
@	LA 5 - 10 ml SA 0.25 - 0.5 ml	
Pres.	10 ml, 30 ml, 50 ml, 100 ml	

Beekom L inj	**Merial (Wockhardt)**	
Comp	Each ml contains	
	Thiamine hydrocholoride	25 mg
	Riboflavin	1.5 mg
	Naicinamide	50 mg

	Vit B_6	5 mg
	Vit B_{12}	50 mcg
	Choline Chloride	25 mg
	Crude Liver extract provides	2 mcg of B_{12}
Adm.	IM	
@	LA 5-10 ml SA 0.5-2 ml	
Pres.	30 ml	

Bivinal Forte inj	**Alembic**	
Comp	Each ml contains	
	Vitamin B_1	50 mg
	Riboflavin	5 mg
	Vitamin B_6	5 mg
	Niacinamide	100 mg
	DL Panthenol	10 mg
	Inositol	2 mg
	Methionine	5 mg
	Liver Extr. from 2 g of fresh liver B_{12} = 0.2 mcg	
Adm.	IM inj	
@	LA 5-10 ml Sa 0.5-2 ml	
Pres.	10 ml, 30 ml	

Bovoplex CC	**Indian Immunology**	
Comp	Each ml contains	
	Thiamine hydrocholoride	25 mg
	Riboflavin	1.5 mg
	Naicinamide	50 mg
	Vit B_6	5 mg
	Vit B_{12}	50 mcg
	Choline Chloride	25 mg
	Crude Liver extract provides	2 mcg of B_{12}
Adm.	IM inj	
@	LA 5-10 ml Sa 0.5-2 ml	
Pres.	10 ml, 30 ml	

Centroplex inj	**Century**	
Comp	Each ml contains	
	Thiamine hydrocholoride	25 mg
	Riboflavin	3 mg

	Naicinamide	100 mg
	Vit B_{12}	10 mcg
	Crude Liver extract	0.66 ml
Adm.	IM	
@	LA 5-10 ml SA 0.25-0.5 ml	
Pres.	30 ml	

Livamyl inj	**Cattle Remedies**	
Comp	Each ml contains	
	Thiamine hydrocholoride	25 mg
	Riboflavin	3 mg
	Naicinamide	100 mg
	Vit B_{12}	10 mcg
	Crude Liver extract	0.66 ml
Adm.	IM	
@	LA 5-10 ml SA 0.25-0.5 ml	
Pres.	10 ml, 30 ml	

Livoplex inj	**Pranav**	
Comp	Each ml contains	
	Vitamin B1	25 mg
	Riboflavin	1.37 mg
	Naicinamide	100 mg
	D panthenol	5 mg
	Vitamin B_6	5 mg
	Vitamin B_{12}	30 mcg
	Choline Chloride	15 mg
	Liver extract from 8 g of fresh liver	
	Lignocaine	1%
Adm.	IM	
@	LA 5-10 ml SA 0.25-0.5 ml	
Pres.	30ml	

Liverjet inj	**Cadila**	
Comp	Each ml contains	
	Liver extract from 8 g of liver having 2mcg of vit B_{12}	
	Lignocaine	1%
Adm.	IM	
@	LA 5-10 ml SA 0.25-0.5 ml	
Pres.	10 ml, 30 ml	

Liverubra inj	**Zydus**	
Comp	Each ml contains	
	Liver extract from 8 g of liver having 2 mcg of vit B_{12}	
	Lignocaine	1%
Adm.	IM	
@	LA 5-10ml SA 0.25-0.5ml	
Pres.	10 ml, 30 ml	

Livobex inj	**TTK**	
Comp	Each ml contains	
	Vitamin B_1	10 mg
	Vitamin B_6	5 mg
	Riboflavin	3 mg
	Niacinamide	100 mg
	Crude Liver extract	0.66 ml
Adm.	IM	
@	LA 5-10ml SA 0.5-2 ml	
Pres.	10 ml, 30 ml	

Livogen	**Virbac (Glaxo)**	
Comp	Each ml contains	
	Vitamin B_1	25 mg
	Panthenol	5 mg
	Vitamin B_2	1.37 mg
	Nicotinamide	100 mg
	Vitamin B_{12}	30 mcg
	Choline Chloride	15 mg
	Liver ext. from 8 g fresh liver with 2 mcg of B_{12}	
Adm.	IM	
@	LA 5-10 ml SA 0.5-2 ml	
Pres.	10 ml, 30 ml	

Livovet inj	**Marc**	
Comp	Each ml contains	
	Thiamine hydrocholoride	25 mg
	Riboflavin	3 mg
	Naicinamide	100 mg
	Vit B_{12}	10 mcg
	Crude Liver extract	0.66 ml
Adm.	IM	
@	LA 5-10 ml SA 0.25-0.5 ml	
Pres.	10 ml, 30 ml, 50 ml, 100 ml	

Supraplex L	**Neospark**	
Comp	Each ml contains	
	Vitamin B_1	25 mg
	Vitamin B_2	1.37 mg
	Vitamin B_6	5 mg
	Vitamin B_{12}	30 mcg
	Choline Chloride	15 mg
	D Pathenol	5 mg
	Nicotinamide	5 mg
	Liver ext. 8 g fresh liver with 2 mcg B_{12}	
Adm.	IM	
@	LA 5-10 ml SA 1-2 ml	
Pres.	10 ml, 30 ml	

Livoguard	**Carevet Pharma**	
Comp	Each ml contains	
	Vitamin B_1	25 mg
	Panthenol	5 mg
	Vitamin B_2	1.37 mg
	Nicotinamide	100 mg
	Vitamin B_{12}	30 mcg
	Choline Chloride	15 mg
	Liver ext. from 8 g fresh liver with 2 mcg of B_{12}	
	Lignocaine	1%
Adm.	IM	
@	LA 5-10 ml SA 0.5-2 ml	
Pres.	10 ml, 30 ml, 100 ml	

Becom Vet	**Sequent (Lyka)**	
Comp	Each ml contains	
	Vitamin B_1	25 mg
	Vitamin B_2	3 mg
	Vitamin B_{12}	12 mcg
	Liver exact providing 2 mcg B_{12}	
Adm.	IM	
@	LA 5-10 ml SA 0.5-2 ml	
Pres.	10 ml	

Hepaplex	**Cargill (Unichem)**	
Comp	Each ml contains	
	Vitamin B_1	25 mg
	Riboflavin	1.37 mg
	Nicotinamide	100 mg
	Vitamin B_6	5 mg
	Vitamin B_{12}	30 mcg
	Crude Liver oil with 2 mcg of B_1	
Adm.	IM	
@	LA 5-10 ml SA 0.5-2 ml	
Pres.	10 ml	

Nutriliv inj	**Vetcare**	
Comp	Each ml contains	
	Vitamin B_1	25 mg
	Riboflavin	1.37 mg
	Nicotinamide	100 mg
	Vitamin B_6	5 mg
	Vitamin B_{12}	30 mcg
	Crude Liver oil with 2 mcg of B_{12}	
Adm.	IM inj	
@	LA 5-10 ml SA 0.5-2 ml	
Pres.	10 ml	

Stronic inj	**Ranbaxy**	
Comp	Each ml contains	
	Vitamin B_1	25 mg
	Vitamin B_2	5 mg
	Vitamin B_{12}	50 mcg
	Niacinamide	50 mg
	Pyridoxine	5 mg
	Liver extract providing 2 mcg B_{12}	
Adm.	IM inj	
@	LA 10 ml SA 1-2 ml	
Pres.	10 ml, 30 ml	

Pinkojet inj	**Brihans**	
Comp	Each ml contains	
	Vitamin B_1	20 mg
	Vitamin B_2	1 mg

	Vitamin B_6	20 mg
	Vitamin B_{12}	200 mcg
	Nicotinamide	20 mg
	D Pathenol	10 mg
	Choline chloride	3 mg
Adm.	IM	
@	LA 5-10 ml SA 1-2 ml	
Pres.	10 ml, 30 ml	

Ripason inj	**TTK**
Comp	Each ml contains extract of liver 0.26 g
Adm.	IM
@	LA 10 ml SA 3-5 ml
Pres.	100 ml

Livron inj	**Vets Farma**	
Comp	Each ml contains	
	Thiamine hydrocholoride	25 mg
	Riboflavin	3 mg
	Naicinamide	100 mg
	Vit B_{12}	10 mcg
	Crude Liver extract	0.66 ml
Adm.	IM	
@	LA 5-10 ml SA 0.25-0.5 ml	
Pres.	10 ml, 30 ml, 50 ml, 100 ml	

Meritone inj	**Merial (Wockhardt)**	
Comp	Each ml contains	
	Vitamin B1	25 mg
	Riboflavin	1.37 mg
	Naicinamide	100 mg
	D panthenol	5 mg
	Vitamin B_6	5 mg
	Vitamin B_{12}	30 mcg
	Choline Chloride	15 mg
	Liver extract from 8 g of fresh liver	
	Lignocaine	1%
Adm.	IM	
@	LA 5-10 ml SA 0.25-0.5 ml	
Pres.	30 ml	

Bovilin Forte inj	Vest Farma
Comp	Each ml contains Vitamin B_1 50 mg Riboflavin 5 mg Vitamin B_6 5 mg Niacinamide 100 mg DL Panthenol 10 mg Inositol 2 mg Methionine 5 mg Liver Extr. from 2 g of fresh liver B_{12}= 0.2 mcg
Adm.	IM
@	LA 5-10 ml Sa 0.5-2 ml
Pres.	10 ml, 30 ml

B Pliv	Venky
Comp	Each ml contains Vitamin B_1 25 mg Panthenol 5 mg Vitamin B_2 1.37 mg Nicotinamide 100 mg Vitamin B_{12} 30 mcg Choline chloride 15 mg Liver ext. from 8 g fresh liver with 2 mcg of B_{12}
Adm.	IM
@	LA 5-10 ml SA 0.5-2 ml
Pres.	10 ml, 30 ml

Ciplamyl	Cipla
Comp	Each ml contains Thiamine hydrocholoride 25 mg Riboflavin 3 mg Naicinamide 100 mg Vit B_{12} 10 mcg Crude Liver extract 0.66 ml
Adm.	IM
@	LA 5-10 ml SA 0.25-0.5 ml
Pres.	10 ml, 30 ml

Pepsid inj	**Concept**
Comp	Each ml contains Vitamin B_1 100 mg Vitamin B_2 1 mg Vitamin B_6 5 mg Vitamin B_{12} 100 mcg Nicotinamide 100 mg D Panthenol 10 mg Crude liver 8 gm with 2 mcg B_{12}
Adm.	IM
@	LA 5-10 ml SA 0.5-2 ml
Pres.	10 ml, 30 ml

Reliver inj	**PAIL**
Comp	Each ml contains Vitamin B_1 10 mg Vitamin B_6 5 mg Riboflavin 3 mg Niacinamide 100 mg Crude liver 0.66 ml
Adm.	IM inj
@	LA 5-10 ml SA 0.5-2 ml
Pres.	10 ml, 30 ml

Cobiliv inj	**Sushima Pharma**
Comp	Each ml contains Thiamine hydrocholoride 25 mg Riboflavin 3 mg Naicinamide 100 mg Vit B_{12} 10 mcg Crude Liver extract 0.66 ml
Adm.	IM inj
@	LA 5-10ml SA 0.25-0.5 ml
Pres.	10 ml, 30 ml, 50 ml, 100 ml

Hipaliv inj	**Phoenix**
Comp	Each ml contains Thiamine hydrocholoride 25 mg Riboflavin 1.5 mg Naicinamide 50 mg Vit B_6 5 mg Vit B_{12} 50 mcg Choline Chloride 25 mg Crude Liver extract provides 2 mcg of B_{12}
Adm.	IM inj
@	LA 5-10 ml Sa 0.5-2 ml
Pres.	30 ml

Livirubra inj	**Cadila Healthcare**
Comp	Each ml contains Liver extract from 8 g of liver 25 mg having 2 mcg of vit B_{12} Lignocaine 1%
Adm.	IM
@	LA 5-10 ml
Pres.	30 ml

Yakrifit Liq/Bol	**Ayurvet**	
Comp	Emblica officinalis	Terminalia arjuna
	Fumaria indica	Eclipta albi
	Boerhavia diffusa	Solanum nigrum
	Terminalia chebula	Swertia chirata
	Phyllanthus niruri	Picrorhiza kurroa
	Embellia ribes	Boberis aristata
	Azadirachta indica	Aphunamixis polystachya
	Achyranthes aspere	Andographis paniculate
	Tinospora cardifolia	Ichnocarpus frutescens
Adm.	Oral	
@	50 ml or 2 Bol bid for 5-7 days	
Pres.	Strip of 4, 250 ml, IL	

Macliv DS	**Macwell**			
Comp	10 ml contains			
	Silybum marianum	400 mg	Emelia ribes	200 mg
	Androphis paniculata	200 mg	Picrorrhiza kurroa	300 mg
	Swertia chirata	200 mg	Piper longum	200 mg
	Rauwolfia serpentine	200 mg	Terminalia chebula	150 mg
	Ocimum sanctum	200 mg	Boerhaavia diffusa	300 mg
	Terminalia arjuna	200 mg	Eclipta alba	300 mg
	Rheum officinale	400 mg	Kuttu tandalwak	200 mg
Adm.	Oral			
@	100 ml od x 5 days			
Pres.	250 ml, 500 ml, IL, 5L			

Aviliv Liq	**Avivet**	
Comp	Not given	Fourteen herbs and kutkee
Adm.	Oral	
@	50 ml bid	
Pres.	500 ml, IL	

Malivetgrow	**National Vet Pharma**
Comp	Not given
Adm.	Oral
@	100 ml od x10 days
Pres.	500 ml, IL

Meboliv Liq	**Indian Herbs**			
Comp	Kutaki	12.5 mg	Shatavari	187.5 mg
	Vacha	125.0 mg	Bhumyamalaki	375.0 mg
	Ashwagandha	187.5 mg	Sariva	437.5 mg
	Rohitak	375.0 mg	Pippali	125.0 mg
	Bhringraj	375.0 mg	Punarnava	375.0 mg
	Marchica	125.0 mg	Shunthi	125.0 mg
	Trifla	750.0 mg	Yashthimadhu	750.0 mg
	Chitraka	125.0 mg	Sarapunkha	750.0 mg
Adm.	Oral			
@	20 ml bid			
Pres.	100 ml, 460 ml, 5L			

Hepatoprotactive Miscellaneous

Livoferol Liq	**Cargill (Unichem)**			
Comp	Each 30 ml contains			
	Ferrous gluconate	200 mg	Vitamin B1	5 mg
	Ferrous chloride	80 mg	Nicotinamide	45 mg
	Calcium lactate	300 mg		
	Liver ext from 3.75 g fresh liver			
Adm.	Oral			
@	LA 50 ml bid SA 25 ml bid			
Pres.	450 ml, 5L			

Boostup Pow	**Merial (Dosch)**	
Comp	Each Kg contains	
	Live lactobacillus spore	20 million CFU
	fungal diastase	5 g
	Liver extract	500 mg
	Amino Acids	25 g
Adm.	Oral	
@	10-15 g od	
Pres.	1 kg	

Brotone Liq.	Virbac
Comp	Each 10 ml contains Fresh Liver ext 1.2 5 g with 7.5 mcg B_{12}, yeast ext. 0.4 g Thiamine 2.5 mg Nicotinic acid 24 mg
Adm.	Oral
@	LA 40 ml od x 3 days SA 5-10 ml od x 3 days
Pres.	120 ml, 500 ml

Catliv	Cattle Remedies
Comp	Not given
Adm.	Oral
@	LA 20 ml bid SA 7.5-10 ml bid
Pres.	100 g, 250 g, IL

Miscellaneous/Hepatoprotective/Bolus/ Tablet

Livoma. Tablet	Rakesh Pharma
Comp	Each Tab Tinospora cordifolia 12 mg Terminalia arjuna 18 mg Kalmegh 18 mg Eclipte longum 12 mg Terminalia chebula 12 mg Embellia ribes 9 mg Cassia occidentalis 12 mg Picrorrhizia kurroa 15 mg Eclipta alba 15 mg Cichorium intybus 18 mg Tephrosia purpurus 9 mg Mondur bhasma 15 mg Solanum nigrum 15 mg Lawsonia alba 9 mg Aarogyavardhini rasa 3 mg Boerhaavia diffusa 18 mg Phyllanthus niruri 6 mg Ocimum sanctum 12 mg
Adm.	Oral
@	10 Tablets bid
Pres.	100 Tab, 1000 Tab

Livoboost / Liq. Bol.	Herbotrend
Comp	Not given
Adm.	Oral
@	2-4 Bol bid or 50-100 ml bid
Pres.	Strip of 4, IL

Liv 62 Powder	**Parnav**
Comp	Not given
Adm.	Oral
@	50 g od
Pres.	I kg

Liverolin Pow	**Zydus (Ranbaxy)**
Comp	Not given
Adm.	Oral
@	40-50 g od
Pres.	1 kg, 2 kg, 20 kg

Livex Pow	**Rakesh Pharma**			
Comp	100 g contains			
	Piehari	35 g	Virya	25 g
	Kirat	100 mg	Aspatra	3 g
	Kasni	200 mg	Rasayni	20 mg
	Arimarel	100 mg	Utkantak	100 mg
	Veervriksha	200 mg	Musahbar	100 mg
	Pbihaghna	100 mg	Birajasif	100 mg
	Pita	100 mg	Shaileyak	100 mg
	Shilatika	100 mg	Tikta	100 mg
	Gauri	100 mg	Faltric	100 mg
	Tiktak	15 mg	Jhau	200 mg
	Tandul	100 mg	Bhoonimbia	100 mg
Adm.	Oral			
@	30 g od			
Pres.	100 g, 1 kg			

Livomex Pow	**Rajshree**
Comp	Not given
Adm.	Oral
@	10 g od
Pres.	100 g

Livol Pow	**Indian Herbs**
Comp	Not given
Adm.	Oral
@	40-60 g bid
Pres.	100 g

Livron Pow	**Vets Farma**			
Comp	Tephrosia purpurea	40%	Terminalia chebula	10%
	Eclipta alba	20%	Ocimum sanctum	10%
	Andrographis paniculata	10%	Base	9.8 %
Adm.	Oral			
@	10 g od for 10 days			
Pres.	100 g, 500 g, 1kg			

Tefroli veg granules/ Syp	**TTK**	
Comp	1g or 5ml contains	
	Tephrosia purpurea	400 mg
	Andrographis paniculata	100mg
	Phyllanthus niruri	200 mg
	Ocimum sanctum	100 mg
	Eclipta alba	200 mg
	Terminalia chebula	100 mg
Adm.	Oral	
@	8 g tid 20 ml bid	
Pres.	100 g, 500 mg, 500 ml, 4.5L, 120 ml	

Linto Pow	**Cadila Pharma**
Comp	Not given
Adm.	Oral
@	5-10 g bid
Pres.	50 g, 1 kg

Livoguard Pow	**Carevet Pharma**
Comp	Not given
Adm.	Oral
@	50 g od 50 ml bid
Pres.	100 g, 1 kg, IL, 5L

Rumizyme Pow	**Arosol**
Comp	Not given
Adm.	Oral
@	25 g bid
Pres.	100 g, 500 g

Zigbir Pow	**Natural Remedies**	
Comp	Not given	
Adm.	Oral/ Feed	
@	250 g /Ton of feed	
Pres.	1 kg, 10 kg	

Yakritamrit Liq	**Patanjali**	
Comp	Not given	
Adm.	Oral	
@	8-100ml bid	
Pres.	IL	

Liv 52 Liq/Pow/Bol	**Himalya**	
Comp	Terminalia arjuna	Tinospora cardifolia
	Eclipta alba	Terminalia chebula
	Cassia occidentalis	Mandura bhasma
	Phyllanthus niruri	Cichorium intybus
	Capparis spinosa	Solanum nigrum
	Boerhavi diffusa	Raphanus sativus
	Fumaria officinalis	Plumbago zeylanica
	Berberis aristata	Tamarix gallica
	Achillea millefolium	Embellia ribes
Adm.	Oral	
@	2 Bol bid or 50 ml bid or 10 g bid	
Pres.	Strip of 4, 220 ml, 500 ml, IL, 5L, 100 g	

Kepoliv	**Kepler**	
Comp	Not given	
Adm.	Oral	
@	50 ml od	
Pres.	350 ml, IL	

Hepawell Forte Liq	**Venkys**	
Comp	Andographis paniculata	Sodium feredetate
	Silymarin	Zince and Copper
Adm.	Oral	
@	100 ml od x 3 - 5 days	
Pres.	IL, 5L	

Picliv	**Penetrant**
Comp	Not given
Adm.	Oral
@	100 ml od x 3-5 days
Pres.	500 ml

Hepagist	**Alembic**	
Comp	5 ml contains	
	Tephrosia purpurea	800 mg
	Andographis paniculata	200 mg
	Eclipta alba	400 mg
	Terminalis chebula	200 mg
	Phyllanthus niruri	400 mg
	Ocimum sanctum	200 mg
Adm.	Oral	
@	20 ml bid	
Pres.	IL, 5L	

Hepaking	**Herstel**
Comp	Not given
Adm.	Oral
@	100 ml od
Pres.	IL

Livol	**Natural Remedies**
Comp	Not given
Adm.	Oral
@	LA 30-40 ml od SA 7-10 ml od
Pres.	500 ml, IL

Livotas Tab/Susp	**Intas**
Comp	Not given
Adm.	Oral
@	Tab. LA 10 bid SA 3-7 bid Susp LA 30-40 ml bid SA 7-10 ml bid
Pres.	100 Tab, 500 ml, IL

Liv up Pow/Liq	**Century**
Comp	Not given
Adm.	Oral
@	LA 50 g bid SA 30 bid Liq. LA 50 ml SA 30 ml bid
Pres.	10 k g Pow. ,5L

Zigbo Bol/Liq	**Natural Remedies**
Comp	Not given
Adm.	Oral
@	LA 2 Bol or 30 ml od SA 1 Bol or 10 ml od
Pres.	Strip of 10, 30 ml, IL, 5L

Livol Classic Pow	**Indian Herbs**
Comp	Not given
Adm.	Oral
@	LA 40-60 g bid SA 15 g bid
Pres.	100 g, 1 kg

Appetaliv	**Argano**
Comp	Not given
Adm.	Oral
@	LA 60 ml Sa 25ml
Pres.	500 ml, IL, 5L

Vetliv Pow/ Liquid		**Carevet Pharma**	
Comp	10g	10 ml contains	
		Terminalia arjuna	400 mg
		Andrographis paniculata	200 mg
		Withania somnifera	300 mg
		Fumaria officinalis	100 mg
		Solanum nigrum	200 mg
		Ocimum sanctum	100 mg
		Embellia ribes	200 mg
		Phyllanthus niruri	400 mg
		Bombusa arundinacea	100 mg
		Asparagus racemosus	100 mg
		Calcium sulphate	100 mg
		Mytilus margratiferus shell	
		Sodium bicarbonate	300 mg
Adm.		Oral	
@		10 g od 50 ml od	
Pres.		100 g, 1 kg, 100 ml, 500 ml, IL, 5 L	

Hepacef Liquid			**Concept Pharma**
Indications: Generaltonic, Liverdisorder			
Composition: 10 ml Contains			
Kutaki	12.5 mg	Pippali	125.0 mg
Bhumyamalaki	375.0 mg	Shurithi	125.0 mg
Rohitak	375.0 mg	Maricha	125.0 mg
Punarnava	375.0 mg	Vacha	125.0 mg
Trifla	750.0 mg	Yashthimadhu	750.0 mg
Chitraka	125.0 mg	Sarapunkha	750.0 mg
Shatavari	187. mg	Sariva	437.5 mg
Ashwagandha	187.5 mg	Bhringraj	375.0 mg
Adm.: Oral			
@ : 20 ml twice daily			
Pres.: 100 ml, 460 ml, 5L			

Livex Pow.					**Alembic**
Indications: Hepatoprotective					
Composition: 100 g contains					
Plihari	35 g	Kasni	200 mg	Biranjasil	100 mg
Virya	25 g	Veervriksha	200 mg	Bhoonimb	100 mg
Rasayani	20 g	Jhag	200 mg	Musabbar	100 mg
Tiktak	15 g	Arimard	100 mg	Shilatika	100 mg
Asipatra	3 g	Utkantak	100 mg	Gauri	100 mg
Kirat	100 mg	Tandul	100 mg	Pita	100 mg
Shaileyak	100 mg	Faltrik	100 mg	Tikta	100 mg
Adm.: Oral					
@ : 30 g daily					
Pres.: 100 g, 1 kg					

VentrilivLiq./Pow. FS	**Venkys**
Indications: Hepatoprotective	
Composition: Not given	
Adm.: Oral	
@ : 50 ml daily, 500 g/ Ton of feed	
Pres.: 5 L,1 kg	

Meboliv Liq.	**Indian Herbs**
Indications: Hepatoprotective, Prevent Ketosis	
Composition: Not given	
Adm.: Oral	
@ : 30 ml twice daily for 10 days	
Pres.: 240 ml, 500 ml, 1L	

Macliv DS			**Macwell**
Indications: Hepatoprotective, Liver disorders, stress, sluggish liver			
Composition: 10 ml			
Silybum marianum	400 mg	Androphis paniculata	200 mg
Embelia ribes	200 mg	Piper longum	200 mg
Picrorrhiza kurroa	300 mg	Rheum offcinale	400 mg
Swertia chirata	200 mg	Rauwolfia serpentina	200 mg
Eclipta alba	300 mg	Terminalia arjuna	200 mg
Boerhaavia diffusa	300 mg	Terminalia chebula	150 mg
Ocimum sanctum	200 mg	Kuttutandal wak	200 mg
Adm.: Oral			
@ : 100 ml daily for 3 days.			
Pres.: 250 ml, 500 ml, 1 L, 5 L			

Liv62 Powder	**Pranav**
Indications: Hepatoprotective	
Composition: Not given	
Adm.: Oral	
@ : 50 g daily	
Pres.: 1kg	

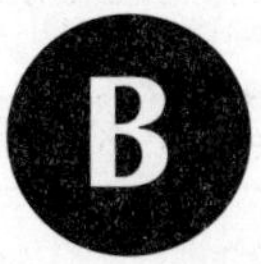

Anti-Infectives

Also known as antimicrobials, anti-infective agents. These are compounds that kill or control multiplication of micro-organisms. These are:

- **Antibacterial- kill bacterias**
- **Antiviral- kill viruses**
- **Antifungal- kill fungi**
- **Antiprotozoan- kill protozoa**

Bacterial Diseases

Actinobacillosis: (Wooden Tongue) caused by Actinobacillus lignierasi characterised by inflammation of tongue sometimes pharyngeal nodes.

Actinomycosis: (Lumpy Jaw) caused by Actinomyces bovis and is characterised by osteomyelitis of bones of head particularly mandible and maxilla

Anthrax: Caused by Bacillus anthracis and characterised by septicaemia and sudden death with exudation of tarry blood from all the orifices of body

Bacteriaemia: Presence of bacteria in the blood stream of animal

Black Disease: Caused by Clostridium novyi also called as infectious necrotic hepatitis. It is characterised by hyperaesthesia, rapid and shallow respiration recumbency and often dies within a few minutes. Associated symptoms are sudden depression, coldness of skin, absence of ruminal sounds, pain when palpated around liver

Black Leg: (Black Quarter) caused by Clostridium chauvi and characterised by inflammation of muscles, severe toxaemia and high mortality. It happens mostly in cattle. Lameness in leg is observed

Botulism: Caused by Clostridium bitulinum and characterised by muscle weakness, paralysis and death

Braxy: Caused by Clostridium septicum characterised by inflammation of abomasal wall, toxaemia and high mortality rate. Disease mostly in sheep only

Brucellosis: Caused by Brucella abortus characterised by abortion in last trimester of pregnancy followed by retained placenta, pyometra with higher rate of infertility. Opaque discharge from vagina is common.

Calf diphtheria: Caused by Fusiformis necroforus and characterised by fever, pain in mouth, cough, laboured breathing, necrotic patches in mouth, palate, gums, tongue and phanynx

Colibacillosis: Cause by E. coli manifested by bacteriemia, diarrhea and sudden death

Contagious bovine Pyelonephritis: Caused by Corynebactericum renale and is infectious urinary tract. It is characterised by chronic purulent inflammation of Kidney, Ureter and Urinary blandder

Contagious disease: Disease which is caused by pathogens and is transmitted from one animal to other by direct or indirect contact. All contagious diseases are infections

Contagious pustular dermatitis: Caused by Corynebacterium pseudotuberculosis in horses. It is characterised by development of pustules particularly where skin comes in contact with harness

Convalescence: Recovery phase

Enterotoxaemia: Caused by Clostridium perfingens Type B. it is highly Fatal disease. Animal dies within 12 hours. Symptoms are severe depression, haemoglobinurea, dyspnoea, collapse, rise in temperature, swollen Kidneys, dark brown and pulmonary oedema. In other form there can by dysentry

Eryisipelas: Caused by Erysipelas insidosa in sheep and swines. It is characterised by arthritis, laminitis and lameness

Foot rot: Caused by Spherophorus necrophorus and characterised by lameness, fever, depression in milk yield with swelling in coronet spreading to claws.

Glander: Caused by Actinobacillosis mallei. It is characterised by nodules or ulcers in respiratory tract and on the skin. It is highly fatel disease of horses.

Haemorrhagic septicaemia: (Pasteurellosis) caused by Pasteurella multocida and characterised by broncho pneumonia, swelling under jaw profuse salivation. Sudden onset of fever; submucosal petichiation, severe depression and death. In other form there can be fever and severe diarrhea.

Incubation period: It is the time of initial infection until symptoms of disease are observed

Incubation: Multiplication of micro-organisms without sign and symptoms

Infection: The invasion and proliferation of micro-organisms in the body tissue leading to some disease or disorder

Infectious bovine meningoencephelitis: Caused by Moraxella bovis and characterised by watery lachrymation, photophobia and fever

Infectious disease: Disease which is caused by micro-organisms

Inoculation: Multiplication of micro-organisms in the tissue

Johne's disease: (Paratuberculosis) caused by Mycobacterium paratuberculosis characterised by progressive emaciation, chronic diarrhea, thickening and corrugation of wall of intestine

Leptospirosis: Caused by Leptospira icterhaemorrhagiae characterised by high fever, anorexia, depression and acute haemolytic anaemia Dyspnoea is prominent

Listeriosis: Caused by Listeria monocytogenes characterised by meningo encephalitis, abortion or septicaemia

Malignant oedma: Caused by Clostridium perfingens and Clostridium sordellie characterised by inflammation at the site of infection and profound systemic toxaemia

Necrotic ulcers: Caused by Borrelia suilla and characterised by the development of chronic ulcers of skin and subcutaneous tissue

Non contagious disease: Disease which can not be transmitted from one to other animal by direct or indirect contact

Non infectious disease: Disease which is caused by injury, heat, cold or faulty nutrition

Salmonellosis: (Paratyphoid or Salmonellosis) caused by Salmonella typhimurium characterised by peracute septicaemia, acute enteritis or chronic enteritis, rise in temperature and discolouration of skin.

Septicaemia: Presence of bacteria and its multiplication in blood stream

Shigellosis: Caused by Shigella equirelis and characterised by sudden onset of fever, prostration, diarrhea and rapid respiration.

Strangles: (Distemper) It is disease of horses caused by Streptococcus equi and characterised by inflammation of upper respiratory tract and abscessation on the adjacent lymph nodes

Swine dysentry: Caused by Vibrio coli characterised by contagious enteritis

Tetanus: Caused by Clostridium tetani and characterised by convulsions and hyperaesthesia or wooden horse

Tuberculosis: Caused by Mycobacterium bovis characterised by progressive development of tubercles in any organ

Vibriotic abortion: Caused by Vibrio foetus but less severe effect after abortion

Viraemia: Presence of virus in blood

Virulence: Degree of pathogenicity of micro-organisms

Winter dysentry: Caused by Vibrio jejuni manifested by severe diarrhea associated with dysentery at the same time

Antibiotics / Antibacterial

Terms associated with Antibiotics

Aerobic: Which can live only in air

Anaerobic: Which do not need air for living or can live without air

Bacillus: Bacteria with rod shape

Bacteria: Single cellular organisms with a rigid cell wall. Nucleus is not well defined. These reproduce by binary fission. Animal body serves and host large number of biacteria.

Capnophillic: Micro-organisms which grow in Carbon Dioxide rich environment

Chalmydiae: These have filaments like branching structure and reproduce by means of spores.

Coccus: Bacteria which are spherical in shape

Colony: Collection or group of micro-organisms growing within a culture

Culture: Mass of micro-organisms in one or same kind of media

Endotoxins: Toxins liberated by bacterial disintegration

Exotoxins: Toxins exerted by pathogens in media in which they are grown

Facultative: Bacteria having anaerobes but can live with or without oxygen

Filamentous: Bacteria with filaments also called Tricho bacteria

Flora: Harmless micro-organisms are called flora or commensal

Gram +ve: Bacteria which can be stained

Gram –ve: Bacteria which can not be stained

Helical: Bacteria which are coiled in shape

Invitro: When bacteria placed on slide or patry dish not in living tissue.

Invivo: When micro-organism is within living tissue.

Micro-organisms: minute living beings which can not be seen with naked eye. Also known as microbes.

Mycoplasma: These assume various forms as do not have rigid cell wall. These can grow aerobically and anaerobically can be cultivated in liquid or solid media.

Obligate: Bacteria though anaerobes grow only in absence of oxygen

Pathogens: Micro-organisms which invade body, proliferate and cause disease. These can be internal or external pathogens.

Rickettsia: These are intermediate micro-organisms between virus and bacteria. These can grow inside living cells.

Spirillium: Bacteria with spiral shape

Spirochetes: Micro-organisms which are slender, motile and spiral in shape but multiply by transverse fission

Viruses: These are the smallest living organisms contains either DNA or RNA. These can grow only inside living cells. These grow by multiplication.

Aminoglycosides

These are group of natural semisynthetic antibiotics. These are products of research effective against Gram-ve bacteria. Streptomycin was first salt (1944) followed by Neomycin 1949. These diffuse through the outer coat of bacteria and inhibit bacterial protein synthesis via binding ribosomes. These are bactericidal Anaerobes are not sensitive. Aminoglycoside acquire resistance.

Injectables

Amikacin

It is semisynthetic aminoglycoside identical to the parent compound Kanamycin. This is effective against a variety of aerobic Gram+ve bacilli including those resistant to Gentamycin and other aminoglycosides. It is effective against penicillin and nonpenicillin producing Staphylococcus aureus. This has excellent activity against Mycobacteria. This is indicated in septicaemia, respiratory tract infection meningitis, skin and intra abdominal infections, lesions and burns and post operative infections.

Amikin	**Vets Pharma**
Comp	250 mg/ml Amikacin sulphate
Adm.	IM, IV, SC, IU
@	5-12 mg/kg B.wt
Pres.	2 ml, 10 ml, 30 ml

Akayci	**Brihans**
Comp	250 mg/ml Amikacin sulphate
Adm.	IM, IV, SC, IU
@	5-12 mg/kg B.wt
Pres.	2 ml, 10 ml, 30 ml

Amikacip	**Cipla**
Comp	250 mg/ml Amikacin sulphate
Adm.	IM, IV, SC, IU
@	5-12 mg/kg B.wt
Pres.	10 ml, 30 ml

Gentamicin

This is derived from Micromonospore purpurea. It is a broad spectrum (except Anaerobe Streptococcus) It is effective even in low concentration. It is indicated in female genital tract, urinary tract, Gastro-intestinal, skin, soft tissue infections, mastitis and Repeat Breeders.

Aminocin	**Neospark**
Comp	40 mg/ml of Gentamycin sulphate
Adm.	IM, IV, IU
@	2-5 mg/kg B.wt or Iml per 25-50 kg B.wt. first dose twice in a day followed by once daily. For IU 10-15 ml in Distt Water
Pres.	30 ml
Pro.	• Do not mix with other antibiotic in a vial or syringe. It can induce ototoxicity or nephrotoxicity. • For repent breeders insert 24 hours pre-insemination

G cin	**Indian Immunology**
Comp	40 mg/ml of Gentamycin sulphate
Adm.	IM, IV, IU
@	2-5 mg/kg B.wt or Iml per 25-50 kg B.wt. first dose twice in a day followed by once daily. For IU 10-15 ml in Distt Water
Pres.	10 ml

Genster inj	**Sterling**
Comp	40 mg/ml of Gentamycin sulphate
Adm.	IM, IV, IU
@	2-5 mg/kg B.wt or Iml per 25-50 kg B.wt. first dose twice in a day followed by once daily. For IU 10-15ml in Distt Water
Pres.	10 ml, 30 ml

Gentabiotic	**KAPL**
Comp	40 mg/ml of Gentamycin sulphate
Adm.	IM, IV, IU
@	2-5mg/kg B.wt or Iml per 25-50 kg B.wt. first dose twice in a day followed by once daily. For IU 10-15 ml in Distt Water
Pres.	10 ml, 30 ml

Gentabio	Cargill (Vetcare)
Comp	40 mg/ml of Gentamycin sulphate
Adm.	IM, IV, IU
@	2-5 mg/kg B.wt or Iml per 25-50 kg B.wt. first dose twice in a day followed by once daily. For IU 10-15 ml in Distt Water
Pres.	10 ml, 30 ml

Gentamicin	Alembic, TTK, Merial, Cadila Pharma
Comp	40 mg/ml of Gentamycin sulphate
Adm.	IM, IV, IU
@	2-5 mg/kg B.wt or Iml per 25-50 kg B.wt. first dose twice in a day followed by once daily. For IU 10-15ml in Distt Water
Pres.	30 ml, 100 ml

G Mycin	Carevet Pharma
Comp	40 mg/ml of Gentamycin sulphate
Adm.	IM, IV, IU
@	2-5 mg/kg B.wt or Iml per 25-50 kg B.wt. first dose twice in a day followed by once daily. For IU 10-15 ml in Distt Water
Pres.	30 ml

Lisarine	Zydus
Comp	40 mg/ml of Gentamycin sulphate
Adm.	IM, IV, IU
@	2-5 mg/kg B.wt or Iml per 25-50 kg B.wt. first dose twice in a day followed by once daily. For IU 10-15ml in Distt Water
Pres.	2 ml, 30 ml,

Lyramicin	Lyka
Comp	40 mg/ml of Gentamycin sulphate
Adm.	IM, IV, IU
@	2-5 mg/kg B.wt or Iml per 25-50 kg B.wt. first dose twice in a day followed by once daily. For IU 10-15ml in Distt Water
Pres.	30ml

Progenta	**Vets Farma**
Comp	40 mg/ml of Gentamycin sulphate
Adm.	IM, IV, IU
@	2-5 mg/kg B.wt or Iml per 25-50 kg B.wt. first dose twice in a day followed by once daily. For IU 10-15 ml in Distt Water
Pres.	10 ml, 30 ml, 90 ml

Vgenta	**Century**
Comp	40 mg/ml of Gentamycin sulphate
Adm.	IM, IV, IU
@	2-5 mg/kg B.wt or Iml per 25-50 kg B.wt. first dose twice in a day followed by once daily. For IU 10-15ml in Distt Water
Pres.	30 ml

Marcogenta	**Marc**
Comp	40 mg/ml of Gentamycin sulphate
Adm.	IM, IV, IU
@	2-5 mg/kg B.wt or Iml per 25-50 kg B.wt. first dose twice in a day followed by once daily. For IU 10-15 ml in Distt Water
Pres.	2 ml, 5 ml, 10 ml, 30 ml

Catlogenta	**Cattle Remedies**
Comp	40 mg/ml of Gentamycin sulphate
Adm.	IM, IV, IU
@	2-5 mg/kg B.wt or Iml per 25-50 kg B.wt. first dose twice in a day followed by once daily. For IU 10-15 ml in Distt Water
Pres.	10 ml, 30 ml

Primicin Vet	**HAL**
Comp	40 mg/ml of Gentamycin sulphate
Adm.	IM, IV, IU
@	2-5 mg/kg B.wt or Iml per 25-50 kg B.wt. first dose twice in a day followed by once daily. For IU 10-15 ml in Distt Water
Pres.	10 ml, 30 ml

Cipmycin	**Cipla**
Comp	40 mg/ml of Gentamycin sulphate
Adm.	IM, IV, IU
@	2-5 mg/kg B.wt or Iml per 25-50 kg B.wt. first dose twice in a day followed by once daily. For IU 10-15 ml in Distt Water
Pres.	10 ml, 30 ml

Kanamycin

A potent aminoglycoside which is bactericidal. It acts by inhibiting protein synthesis obtained form Streptomyces kanamyceticus (1957) It is effective against Streptomycin resistant Gram-ve organisms. It is broad spectrum and effective in Mastitis, Genital tract and respiratory tract infections and Calf Scours with chronic therapy it can be nephorotoxic.

Kancin	**Alembic**
Comp	Kanamycin acid sulphate powder
Adm.	IM, IV, IU after mixing with 10ml of distt water
@	LA 5-10 mg/kg B.wt SA 10-20mg/kg B.wt Repeat 12 hourly in severe infection
Pres.	I G, 500 mg
Sp. Pr.	Avoid using in cows with Hypocalcaemia

Neomycin

An aminoglycoside acts by inhibiting bacterial protein synthesis with bactericidal action. It is active against Gram-ve some Gram+ve cocci Ecoli, Staphylococcus, Streptococci, Klebiesela, Enterobacter, Shigella, Salmonella, Corynebacterium chronic usage can be nephrotoxic

Unimycin	**Cargill (Unichem)**
Comp	Neomycin sulphate 140 mg/ml
Adm.	IV, IM
@	2-5 mg/kg B.wt bid. In sever cases 10 mg/kg B.wt
Pres.	10 ml, 30 ml

N Mycin	Carevet Pharma
Comp	Neomycin sulphate 140 mg/ml
Adm.	IV, IM
@	2-5 mg/kg B.wt bid. In sever cases 10 mg/kg B.wt
Pres.	10 ml, 30 ml

Aminoglycosides Combinations

Neomycin + Doxycycline

Megadox N Pow	Neospark
Comp	Doxycycline 100 mg Neomycin sulphate 100 mg
Adm.	Oral
@	10-20 mg/kg B.wt for 3-5 days
Pres.	50 g, 100 g, 500 g

Neodox Bol	Cargill (Vetcare)
Comp	Doxycycline 100 mg Neomycin 40 mg
Adm.	Oral
@	4-5 Bolus/ day
Pres.	60 Bol. Pack

Sterdox N Pow	Sterling
Comp	Doxycycline 100 mg Neomycin sulphate 100 mg
Adm.	Oral
@	10-20 mg/kg B.wt for 3-5 days
Pres.	50 g,

Tenodoc	Vets Farma
Comp	Doxycycline 100 mg Neomycin sulphate 100 mg
Adm.	Oral
@	10-20 mg/kg B.wt for 3-5 days
Pres.	50 g,

Binodox Pow	Stallen
Comp	Doxycycline 100 mg Neomycin sulphate 100 mg
Adm.	Oral
@	10-20 mg/kg B.wt for 3-5 days
Pres.	50 g, 100 g, 500 g

Streptomycin

A potent bactericidal aminoglycoside and act by inhibiting bacterial protein synthesis. It is effective against Gram-ve organisms mainly Pasteurella, Brucella, Salmonella, Klebsiella, Shigella, Vibrio, Mycobacterium, Actinomyces, Erysipelothrix. It is indicated in Pasteurellosis, actinomycosis, actinobacillosis, brucellosis, tuberculosis, pink eye etc.

Ambistrin	Zydus (Sarabhai)
Comp	Streptomycin sulphate
Adm.	IM or SC
@	10 mg/kg B.wt dissolved in 10 ml water
Pres.	1 g vial
Sp. Pr.	Anaphylactic shock, ototoxicity, skin rash etc.

Streptomycin + Penicillin

Bistrepen V	Alembic	
Comp	Procaine penicillin	15 lac
	Benzyl penicillin	5 lac
	Streptomycin sulphate	2.5 g
Adm.	IM by adding 7.5 ml Distt water to make 10 ml	
@	LA 2 ml/50 kg B.wt SA 1 ml/5 kg B.wt	
Pres.	2.5 g, vial	

Vetopen 2.5	HAL	
Comp	Procaine penicillin	15 lac
	Benzyl penicillin	5 lac
	Streptomycin sulphate	2.5 g
Adm.	IM by adding 7.5 ml Distt water to make 10ml	
@	LA 2 ml/50 kg B.wt SA 1 ml/5 kg B.wt	
Pres.	2.5 g, vial	

Dicrysticin S	**Zydus (Sarabhai)**	
Comp	Procaine penicillin	15 lac
	Benzyl penicillin	5 lac
	Streptomycin sulphate	2.5 g
Adm.	IM by adding 7.5 ml Distt water to make 10 ml	
@	LA 2 ml/50 kg B.wt SA 1 ml/5 kg B.wt	
Pres.	2.5 g, vial	

Munomycin Forte	**Virbac**	
Comp	Procaine penicillin	15 lac
	Benzyl penicillin	5 lac
	Streptomycin sulphate	2.5 g
Adm.	IM by adding 7.5ml Distt water to make 10ml	
@	LA 2 ml/50 kg B.wt SA 1 ml/5 kg B.wt	
Pres.	2.5 g, vial	

Penstrep	**Cipla**	
Comp	Procaine penicillin	15 lac
	Benzyl penicillin	5 lac
	Streptomycin sulphate	2.5 g
Adm.	IM by adding 7.5ml Distt water to make 10ml	
@	LA 2 ml/50 kg B.wt SA 1 ml/5 kg B.wt	
Pres.	2.5 g, vial	

Dicristy	**Wesfa Pharma**
Comp	Streptomycin 2.5 g, Procaine penicillin 1500000 IU, Pen G sod. 500000 IU
Adm.	IM
@	Add 7.5 ml Diluent to make 10 ml LA 2 ml/50 kg B.wt SA 1 ml/5 kg B.wt
Pres.	Vial of 2.5 g

Aminoglycosides Powder/ Tablets or Bolus

Neomycin Bol.

Unimycin Bol	**Cargill (Uncihem)**
Comp	500 mg Neomycin sulphate equivalent to 350 mg of Neomycin
Adm.	Oral
@	I Bol per 25-50 kg B.wt
Pres.	500 mg Bol- Strip of 4

Neocare Pow	Cargill (Vetcare)
Comp	25% Neomycin sulplate
Adm.	Oral
@	50 mg/kg B.wt
Pres.	50 g, 250 g

Nubiotic SP	Neospark
Comp	20% Neomycin sulphate
Adm.	Oral
@	50-75/kg B.wt
Pres.	50 g, 100 g, 250 g, 500 g

Aminoglycosides Miscelaneous Dosage Form

Gentamycin cream

Gentamycin Cream	Lyka
Comp	Gentamycin sulphate 0.1%
Adm.	Apply localy after cleaning the wound. Apply a thin layer on hands during obstetrical manipulations
@	As per need
Pres.	50 g, 120 g tube

Cephalosporin

These are group of semisynthetic compound derived from a fungus cephalosporum. These are chemically related to penicillins. All cepharospornis are bactericidal. They have same mechanism of action as Penicillin. These inhibit bacterial cell wall synthesis but bind different proteins than those which Penicillins bind. These have potency against specific organisms. These are bactericidal. These are classified as per their period of research.

First Generation cephalosporins- (developed in 1960) e.g. Cephalexin, Cephaprin, Cefazoline, Cephaloridine, Cefadroxil, Cephradine

Second Generation- cephalosporins- (developed after 1970) e.g. Cefoxitin, Cefprozil, Cefaclor, Cefametazole, Cefuroxime, Cefamandole, Cefonicid, Cefotetan

Third Generation cephalosprins (developed in 1980-90) e.g. Cefataxime, Cefatoperizone, Ceftriaxone, Ceftiofur, Ceftizoxime, Cefoperazone, Cefexime, Cefotaxime, Maxalactain, Cefpodoxime

Some are not absorbed orally.IM use is very painful and in some cases it is used IV only. Sometimes these cause irritation and urticarias has been seen. Now these have been classified in 5 *i.e.* 4th generation and 5th generation.

4th Generation- cefquinone

Cephalexin

It belongs to 1st generation of cephalosporin. It is bactericidal and interferes with bacterial cell wall synthesis. It is effective against Staphylococcus, Streptococcus, Corynebacterium, E.coli, Proteus and Klebsiella. It is indicated in Respiratory infection, urinary tract infection, soft tissue and mixed bacterial infection. Avoid use in Penicillin hypersensitive animals.

Lixen Bolus	**Virbac (Glaxo)**
Comp	Each Bol 1.5g cephalexin
Adm.	Oral or IU
@	5-10 mg/kg B.wt 1 Bol/150 kg B.wt
Pres.	1.5 g Bolus x 2

Tricef Inj	**Cattle Remedies**
Comp	Cephalexin
Adm.	IM
@	2-5 mg/kg B.wt
Pres.	2 g vial

Safevet Inj	**Merial (Dosch)**
Comp	Cephalexin
Adm.	IM
@	2-5 mg/kg B.wt
Pres.	3 g vial

Cephaloridine

1st generation It's semisynthetic derivative of cephalosporine. It is bactericidal and effective in soft tissue and heavy infections. It's active against Penicillinase resistant bacteria

Kefelong Inj	**Virbac (Glaxo)**
Comp	Cephaloridine
Adm.	IM, IV
@	SA 15-30 mg/kg B.wt
Pres.	500 g, 1 g

Cephotoxamin

It belongs to 3rd generation of cephalosporin It is semisynthetic derivative and highly effective against Penicillinase producing bacteria. It is very rapid acting and safe bactericidial. It is indicated in Mastitis, Haemorrhagic septicaemia, Black quarter, Genital and Respiratory tract infections, severe enteritis and otitis.

Lyforan Inj	**(Lyka)**
Comp	Cephotoxamin sodium
Adm.	IM, IV
@	LA 10-20mg/kg B.wt SA 20-40mg/kg B.wt
Pres.	2 g vial

Vetaxime Inj	**Cattle Remedies**
Comp	Cephotoxamin sodium
Adm.	IM, IV
@	LA 10-20 mg/kg B.wt SA 20-40 mg/kg B.wt
Pres.	2 g vial

Britax Inj	**Brihans**
Comp	Cephotoxamin sodium
Adm.	IM, IV
@	LA 10-20 mg/kg B.wt SA 20-40 mg/kg B.wt
Pres.	2 g vial

Haltax Inj	**HAL**
Comp	Cephotoxamin sodium
Adm.	IM, IV
@	LA 10-20 mg/kg B.wt SA 20-40 mg/kg B.wt
Pres.	1 g

Cefotoxime

It belongs to 3rd generation. It's bactericidal and broad spectrum antibiotic

Bitax Inj	**Brihans**
Comp	Cefotaxime sod
Adm.	IM, IV
@	10-20 mg/kg B.wt or LA 2-3 g
Pres.	500 mg, 1 g, 2 g, 3 g

Mas X 3g inj	**Animax Healthcare** **19**
Comp	Ceftizoxime
Adm.	IM/ IV
@	5 mg/kg B.wt repeat after 72 hours if IV, 12 hourly if given IM
Pres.	3 g

Cefquinone

It belongs to 4th generation It has very short half life of 2.5 hour. It is active against Gram-ve species and some Gram+ve. Effective in all infection

Derilan Inj	**Wellcone**
Comp	Cefquinome (25mg/ml if liquid)
Adm.	IM, IV
@	5-10 mg/kg B.wt
Pres.	500 mg, 1500 mg vial

Ceftizoxime

It belongs to 3rd generation

Bovizox Inj	**Cargill**
Comp	Ceftizoxime sodium
Adm.	IV
@	5 mg/kg B.wt. Repeat within 96 hrs in mastitis
Pres.	2.5 g vial

Voxim Inj.	**Vetoquinol**
Comp	Ceftizoxime sodium
Adm.	IV
@	5 mg/kg B.wt. Repeat within 96 hrs in mastitis
Pres.	2.5 g vial

Ceftriaxone

It belongs to 3rd generation. It is semisynthetic derivative of cephalosporin. There are some side effects like diarrhea and colitis by its usage. It is bactericidal and active even against multi resistant bacteria. It is indicated in systemic bacterial infections like Mastitis, metritis, surgical wound infections.

Vetaceft Inj	**Cargill (Unichem)**
Comp	Ceftriaxone sodium
Adm.	IM, IV
@	LA 5-10 mg/kg B.wt SA 10-30 mg/kg B.wt bid
Pres.	1 g, 2 g

Intacef Inj	**Intas**
Comp	Ceftriaxone sodium
Adm.	IM, IV
@	LA 5-10 mg/kg B.wt SA 10-30 mg/kg B.wt bid
Pres.	2 g, 3 g, 4 g

Zydacef Inj	**Zydus**
Comp	Ceftriaxone sodium
Adm.	IM, IV
@	LA 5-10 mg/kg B.wt SA 10-30 mg/kg B.wt bid
Pres.	3 g

TT Cef Inj	**TTK**
Comp	Ceftriaxone sodium
Adm.	IM, IV
@	LA 5-10 mg/kg B.wt SA 10-30 mg/kg B.wt bid
Pres.	3 g

Bactogon Inj	**Bovian**
Comp	Ceftriaxone sodium
Adm.	IM, IV
@	LA 5-10 mg/kg B.wt SA 10-30 mg/kg B.wt bid
Pres.	3 g, 4 g

Aviceft Inj	**Avivet**
Comp	Ceftriaxone sodium
Adm.	IM, IV
@	LA 5-10 mg/kg B.wt SA 10-30 mg/kg B.wt bid
Pres.	3 g. 4 g

Cefnix Inj	**Phoenix**
Comp	Ceftriaxone sodium
Adm.	IM, IV
@	LA 5-10 mg/kg B.wt SA 10-30mg/kg B.wt bid
Pres.	3 g, 4 g

Ceftiforce Inj	**Vetkind**
Comp	Ceftriaxone sodium
Adm.	IM, IV
@	LA 5-10 mg/kg B.wt SA 10-30mg/kg B.wt bid
Pres.	3 g, 4 g

Sefwell Inj	**Macwell**
Comp	Ceftriaxone sodium
Adm.	IM, IV
@	LA 5-10 mg/kg B.wt SA 10-30 mg/kg B.wt bid
Pres.	3 g, 4 g

Saflar Inj	**Kepler**
Comp	Ceftriaxone sodium
Adm.	IM, IV
@	LA 5-10 mg/kg B.wt SA 10-30 mg/kg B.wt bid
Pres.	3 g

Safevet Inj	**Merial (Dosch)**
Comp	Ceftriaxone sodium
Adm.	IM, IV
@	LA 5-10 mg/kg B.wt SA 10-30 mg/kg B.wt bid
Pres.	3 g

Check B Inj	**Haster**
Comp	Ceftriaxone sodium
Adm.	IM, IV
@	LA 5-10 mg/kg B.wt SA 10-30 mg/kg B.wt bid
Pres.	3 g

Anicef S Inj	**PAIL**
Comp	Ceftriaxone sodium
Adm.	IM, IV
@	LA 5-10 mg/kg B.wt SA 10-30 mg/kg B.wt bid
Pres.	3 g

Wesceft Ceff inj 3 g, 4 g	Wesfa pharma 5
Comp Inj	Ceftriaxone
Adm.	IM/ IV
@	5-10 mg/ kg B.wt
Pres.	3 g, 4 g vial

Cifex 3/4 inj	Libra 96
Comp	Ceftriaxone
Adm.	IM/ IV
@	10-12 mg/kg B.wt
Pres.	3 g, 4 g, vial with Distt water

Axone inj	Cadila Pharma 208
Comp	Ceftriaxone
Adm.	IM/ IV/SC
@	5-10 mg/kg B.wt
Pres.	500 mg/3 g vial

Cefstan inj	Zydus 217
Comp	Ceftriaxone
Adm.	IM/IV/SC
@	10 mg/kg B.wt
Pres.	3 g vial

Bovizone inj	Herstel 295
Comp	Ceftriaxone
Adm.	IM/ IV
@	5-10mg/kg B.wt
Pres.	3 g vial

Ceftiofur

It belongs to 3rd generation. It gives longer action if mixed with a diluent of Methyl Pyrrolidone for 24 hour action. It is effective in Respiratory infections, post parturient disorders, Foot rot, surgical management. It should not be used in cats.

Saftifur Inj	Merial
Comp	Ceftiofur sodium
Adm.	IM
@	LA 2-2.4 mg/kg B.wt once daily for 3 days, SA 1.1-2.2 mg/kg B.wt
Pres.	500 mg, 1g

Ceft 1000 inj	**Hester**
Comp	Ceftiofur sodium
Adm.	IM
@	LA 2-2.4 mg/kg B.wt once daily for 3 days, SA 1.1-2.2 mg/kg B.wt
Pres.	1g + 20 ml distt water

Venceft inj	**Venky**
Comp	Ceftiofur sodium
Adm.	IM
@	LA 2-2.4 mg/kg B.wt once daily for 3 days, SA 1.1-2.2 mg/kg B.wt
Pres.	1 g + 20 ml distt water

Xceft inj	**Alembic**
Comp	Ceftiofur sodium
Adm.	IM
@	LA 2-2.4 mg/kg B.wt once daily for 3 days, SA 1.1-2.2 mg/kg B.wt
Pres.	4 g, 50 ml FFSWFI, 1g + 20 ml, 500 mg + 10 ml distt water

Weket LA inj	**Macwell**
Comp	Ceftiofur sodium
Adm.	IM
@	LA 2-2.4 mg/kg B.wt once daily for 3 days, SA 1.1-2.2 mg/kg B.wt
Pres.	1.25 g 20 ml distt water

Cefticure inj	**Cipla**
Comp	Ceftiofur sodium
Adm.	IM
@	LA 2-2.4mg/kg B.wt once daily for 3 days, SA 1.1-2.2 mg/kg B.wt
Pres.	4g

Wesceft Tazo inj 1.124g	**Wesfa pharma**
Comp	Ceftiofur sodium 1000 mg Tazobactam 125 mg
Adm.	IM
@	1-2 mg/kg B.wt
Pres.	1.124 g vial

Wesceft inj 1g	**Wesfa pharma**
Comp	Ceftiofur 1g
Adm.	IM
@	1-2 mg/kg B.wt
Pres.	1 g vial

Furticef LA inj	**Libra**
Comp	Ceftiofur
Adm.	IM/ SC
@.	1ml/25 kg B.wt
Pres.	1g vial with 20 ml Distt water

X-shot LA inj	**Nicosia**
Comp	Ceftiofur
Adm.	IM/ IV
@	1-2 mg/kg B.wt
Pres.	1.25 g vial

Eutifur inj	**Agilis**
Comp	Ceftiofur
Adm.	IM/ SC
@	1.1-2.2 mg/kg B.wt
Pres.	1 g with syringe and needle

Opticef inj	**Boehringer Ingelheim**
Comp	Ceftiofer
Adm.	IM/SC
@	1-1-2.2 mg/kg B.wt
Pres.	1 g

Cephalosporins and Combination

Ceftriaxone is 3rd generation cephalosporin and Sulbactam is a bacteriacidal antibiotic which kills Beta lactamase producing organisms. With their synergistic action it becomes broad spectrum for all systemic infections including Mastitis and resistant bacterias.

Ceftriaxone + Sulbactam

Cefwell Forte inj	**Macwell**
Comp	Ceftriaxone 3 g + Sulbactam 1.5 g
Adm.	IM or IV
@	5-10 mg/kg B.wt
Pres.	4.5 g vail with 20 ml Distt Water and Disposable syringe and needle

Vetceft XL inj	**Carrus**
Comp	Ceftriaxone 3g + Sulbactam 1.5g
Adm.	IM or IV
@	5-10 mg/kg B.wt
Pres.	4.5 g vail with 20 ml Distt Water and Disposable syringe and needle

Vetaceph plus inj	**Cargill**
Comp	Ceftriaxone 3g + Sulbactam 1.5 g
Adm.	IM or IV
@	5-10 mg/kg B.wt
Pres.	4.5 g vail with 20 ml Distt Water and Disposable syringe and needle

Ceftiforte SB3 inj	**Vetkind**
Comp	Ceftriaxone 3 g + Sulbactam 1.5 g
Adm.	IM or IV
@	5-10 mg/kg B.wt
Pres.	4.5 g vail with 20 ml Distt Water and Disposable syringe and needle

Sulbian inj	**Bovian**
Comp	Ceftriaxone 3 g + Sulbactam 1.5 g
Adm.	IM or IV
@	5-10 mg/kg B.wt
Pres.	4.5 g vail with 20 ml Distt Water and Disposable syringe and needle

Dimsy S inj	Macnor
Comp	Ceftriaxone 3 g + Sulbactam 1.5 g
Adm.	IM or IV
@	5-10 mg/ kg B.wt
Pres.	4.5 g vail with 20 ml Distt Water and Disposable syringe and needle

Cefsel inj	Carevet Pharma
Comp	Ceftriaxone 3g + Sulbactam 1.5g
Adm.	IM or IV
@	5-10 mg/kg B.wt
Pres.	4.5 g vail with 20 ml Distt Water and Disposable syringe and needle

Cefnix Forte inj	Phoenix
Comp	Ceftriaxone 3 g + Sulbactam 1.5 g
Adm.	IM or IV
@	5-10 mg/kg B.wt
Pres.	4.5 g vail with 20 ml Distt Water and Disposable syringe and needle

Safevet Forte inj	Merial
Comp	Ceftriaxone 3 g + Sulbactam 1.5 g
Adm.	IM or IV
@	5-10 mg/kg B.wt
Pres.	4.5 g vail with 20ml Distt Water and Disposable syringe and needle

Cifex S 3 or S 4.5 inj	Libra
Comp	Ceftriaxone 3 g + sulbactam 15 g or 2 gm and 1 g
Adm.	IM/ IV
@	5-10 mg/kg B.wt
Pres.	3 gm, 4.5 g vials

A4C SB inj	Agilis
Comp	Ceftriaxone 3 g + sulbactam 1.5 g
Adm.	IM/IV
@	5-10 mg/kg B.wt
Pres.	4.5 g vial

Axone Forte inj	Cadila Pharma
Comp	Ceftriaxone 3 g + sulbactam 1.5
Adm.	IM/ IV
@	5-10 mg/kg B.wt
Pres.	4.5 g vial with disposable syringe with water

Zydacef/ Zydaceft Forte inj	Zydus	
Comp	Ceftriaxone 3 g Ceftriaxone 5 g	Sulbactam 1.5 g Sulbactam 2.5 g
Adm.	IM/ IV	
@	10 mg/kg B.wt	
Pres.	Zydacef 3 g, 4 g, Zydacef Forte 4.5 g, 7.5 g	

Safevet inj	Boehringer Ingelheim
Comp	Ceftriaxone + sulbactam 1:5 ratio
Adm.	IM/ IV
@	10 mg/kg B.wt
Pres.	4.5 g and 7.5 g

Ceftriaxone + Tazobactam

It's same combinations as ceftriaxone with Sulbactam Tazobactam is bit superior to Sulbactam as far as stability is concerned. Action and activity is same.

Vetacef Tazo inj	Cargill
Comp	Cefotriaxione 4 g and Tazobactam 500 mg
Adm.	IM/IV
@	5-10 mg/kg B.wt for 3-5 days
Pres.	4.5 g

Cefnix Tazo inj	Phoenix
Comp	Ceftriaxione 4 g and Tazobactam 500 mg
Adm.	IM/IV
@	5-10 mg/kg B.wt for 3-5 days
Pres.	4.5 g with Distt water

Baceft TZ inj	Venky
Comp	Ceftriaxione 4g and Tazobactam 500mg
Adm.	IM/IV
@	5-10 mg/kg B.wt for 3-5 days
Pres.	4.5 g with Distt water

Ciptacef inj	**Cipla**
Comp	Ceftriaxione 3 g and Tazobactam 375 mg
Adm.	IM/IV
@	5-10 mg/kg B.wt for 3-5 days
Pres.	3.375 g

Cefnix Tazo 4.5 inj	**Phoenix**
Comp	Ceftriaxone 500 mg Tazobactam 62.5 mg Ceftriaxone 4 g Tazobactam 500 mg
Adm.	IM or IV
@	5-10 mg/kg B.wt
Pres.	4.5 g, 62.5 mg

A4C Tazo inj	**Agilis**
Comp	Ceftriaxone 4 g + 500 mg Tazobactam
Adm.	IM/ IV
@	5-10 mg/kg B.wt
Pres.	4.5 g vial with syringe and needle

Vetazo inj	**Zydus**
Comp	Ceftriaxone 3 g or 2 g Tazobactam 375 mg or 250 mg
Adm.	IM/ IV
@	5-10 mg/kg B.wt
Pres.	Vial of 2250 mg, 3375 mg

Cefoperazone + Sulbactam

Cefaject inj	**Cipla**
Comp	Cefoperazone 3 g + Sulbactam 1.5 g
Adm.	IM/IV
@	5-10 mg/kg B.wt
Pres.	4.5 g

Pathocef inj	**Zydus**
Comp	Cefoperazone 3 g + Sulbactam 1.5 g
Adm.	IM/IV
@	5-10 mg/kg B.wt
Pres.	4.5 g

Wesceft- Forte inj 4.5 g	**Wesfa pharma**
Comp	Cefoperazone 3g Sulbactam 1.5g
Adm.	IM/ IV
@	10-15 mg/kg B.wt
Pres.	4.5 g vial with water

Cefazone Plus inj	**Animax Healthcare**
Comp	Cefoperazone + Sulbactam 1.5 g
Adm.	IM/ IV
@	10-15 mg/kg B.wt
Pres.	4.5 g vial

Cefnix forte 4.5 inj	**Phoenix**
Comp	Cefoperazone 3 g Sulbactain 1.5 g
Adm.	IM/ IV
@	5-10 mg/kg B.wt
Pres.	4.5 g

Cefwell Forte inj	**Macwell**
Comp	Cefoperazone sod 3 g + sulbactam 1.5 g
Adm.	IM/ IV
@	10-15 mg/kg B.wt
Pres.	4.5 g via with 20 ml Distt water, Syringe and needle

Mastixome inj	**Boehringer Ingelheim** **268**
Comp	Cefoperazone with sulbactam
Adm.	IM/ IV
@	10 mg/kg B.wt
Pres.	4.5 g with water for injection

Cefixime

Best Bolus	**PAIL**
Comp	Cefixime trihydrate 1000mg
Adm.	Oral
@	1 bolus bid
Pres.	4's strip

Cifex Bolus	Libra
Comp	Cefixime 1g
Adm.	Oral
@	2 Bolus tid
Pres.	Strip of 2

Macrolids

Macrolid Injectables

These antibiotics have macrolytic 'lactone' ring with attached sugar. These are bacteriostatic at low but bactericidal at high concentration. Their cidal action depends on the organisms and its multiplication. Their action is by inhibiting bacterial protein synthesis. It is mostly safe group of antibiotics but painful when injected. It causes diarrhea when given orally. These are effective against Penicillin resistant organisms like Otitis, Pharygitis, Bronchitis, Dysentry and brucellosis etc. There are more than fifteen variants available. Commonly used macrolids are Azithromycin, Erythromycin, Vancomycin, Lincomycin, Tylosin, Spectinomycin, Spiramycin, Roxithromycin, Polymyxin B and Colilistin. In veterinary practice these are not much used injectable.

Spectinomycin

It is a macrolid and bacteriostatic in action. It acts by inhibiting Protein synthesis of bacterial cell. It is structurally different from other members of the group. It is rapidly absorbed after injection and lasts for 8 hrs. It's effective against Mycoplasama and other bacterial infection. There is pain during injection.

Spectin inj	Cipla
Comp	Spectinomycin 2 g
Adm.	IM
@	20-30 mg/kg B.wt
Pres.	2 g vial

Tylosin

It is a macrolid and similar in structure and chemistry as Erythromycin but different in activity. It has good absorption from G I. tract. There is no need of enteric coating for its stability. It is bacteriostatic in action. It is indicated in Pink Eye (Morexella bovis), Pneumonia, Foot not, metritis etc.

Trox pow	Virbac
Comp	50% Tylosin tartrate
Adm.	Oral
@	10-20 mg/kg B.wt
Pres.	20 g, 60 g, 120 g

Tylan pow	**Venky**
Comp	50% Tylosin tartrate
Adm.	Oral
@	10-20 mg/kg B.wt
Pres.	30 g

Tylogyl pow	**G. Loucatos**
Comp	50% Tylosin tartrate
Adm.	Oral
@	10-20 mg/kg B.wt
Pres.	75 g

Tylosip LA Inj.	**Cipla**
Comp	Tylosin 150 mg/ml
Adm.	IM
@	10-20 mg/kg B.wt
Pres.	30 ml, 100 ml

Lincomycin

It is a macrolid having some toxic properties and less potent. It causes higher incidence of diarrhea and colitis. It is effective in Respiratory infection, mastitis, metritis and infections caused by Gram+ve bacteria.

Lincomycin Powder	**Alembic**
Comp	4.4% Lincomycin
Adm.	Oral (can be given IM, IV or intramammary)
@	LA 10 mg/kg B.wt bid SA 15-25 mg/kg B.wt bid
Pres.	500 g, 10 kg

Lincospectin inj	**Generic**
Comp	Lincomycin hydrochloride 50 mg and Spectinomycin sulphate 100 mg each ml
Adm.	IM
@	1ml/20 kg B.wt
Pres.	20 ml

Erythromycin

A macrolid and derived from Streptomyces erythreus, slightly soluble but remains stable at cool temperature. It is normal spectrum antibiotic like Penicillin. It is indicated in Actinomycosis, Mastitis, Black quarter, urinary tract infection and pyomotra. Vomitting and diarrhea are its side effect.

Althrocin Sol Pow	Alembic
Comp	Erythromycin 50 mg/g
Adm.	Oral
@	LA 2.2-4.4 mg/kg B.wt SA 2.2-6 mg/kg B.wt
Pres.	100 g

Nitrobenzene Derivatives

It is also known as Nitrobenzol, Benzen-nitro. It is an organic compound. It is used in dye, pesticides. Only one member of this group chloramphenicol is used as antibiotic.

Chloramphenicol

It is isolated from Streptomyces venezuelac in 1947 and now manufactured synthetically. It is considered to be the first Broad Spectrum antibiotic affecting Gram +, Gram-ve organism, aerobic and many intracellular organisms. It acts by inhibiting protein. It is bacteriostatic but bactericidal when in high concentration. Its acts on E.coli, Ricketsia Mycoplasma, Chlamydia. It is indicated in Neonatal septicaemia, Pasteurellosis, Pink eye, calf diphtheria, Mastitis, acute pneumonia, calf scocrs and meningitis. It can be used orally as well as by parental route, Hypersensitivity, bone marrow depression and resistance is developed.

Chloretec inj	Neospark
Comp	100 mg of Chloramphenicol Sod succinate/ml
Adm.	IM, slow IV
@	LA 20-30 mg/kg B.wt IM or 2-4 mg/kg B.wt IV SA 10 mg/kg B.wt IM or 2 mg/kg B.wt IV
Pres.	30 ml

Neochlor inj	Cargill (Vetcare)
Comp	100 mg of Chloramphenicol Sod succinate/ml
Adm.	IM, slow IV
@	LA 20-30 mg/kg B.wt IM or 2-4 mg/kg B.wt IV SA 10 mg/kg B.wt IM or 2 mg/kg B.wt IV
Pres.	10 ml, 30 ml

Chlorvet inj	**G. Loucatos**
Comp	100 mg of Chloramphenicol Sod succinate/ml
Adm.	IM, slow IV
@	LA 20-30 mg/kg B.wt IM or 2-4 mg/kg B.wt IV SA 10 mg/kg B.wt IM or 2 mg/kg B.wt IV
Pres.	30 ml

Chloramphenicol inj	**KAPL**
Comp	1g of Chloramphenicol
Adm.	IM
@	LA 20-30 mg/kg B.wt SA 10 mg/kg B.wt
Pres.	1g

Ranphenicol inj	**Zydus (Ranbaxy)**
Comp	1 g Chloramphenicol succinate
Adm.	IM
@	LA 20-30 mg/kg B.wt SA 10 mg/kg B.wt
Pres.	1 g

Chlorectin inj	**Merial (Dosch)**
Comp	2.5 g Chloramphenicol succinate
Adm.	IM
@	LA 20-30 mg/kg B.wt SA 10 mg/kg B.wt
Pres.	2.5 g

Agichlor inj	**Agilis**
Comp	Chloramphenicol
Adm.	IM
@	2-4 mg/kg B.wt
Pres.	3 g vial

Nitrofurazone Derivatives

Nitrofurans comprise several synthetic compounds derived from 5 Nitrofurans and possess antimicrobial activity. Over 3500 Nitrofurans have been synthesized. Only a few are useful in animal chemotherapy. Nitrofurans and Furazolidones are used very less in food producing animals. These are bacteriostatic in activity. They deprive the organisms of vital energy producing pathway. They are active against

Gram +ve, Gram-ve and protozoa. These can be administered orally or topically. Their oral absorptions is enhanced by administering wet food. Some of these have carcinogenic effect and also produce systemic toxicity.

Furaltadone

It is a Nitrofuran and indicated in Salmonella infections, Coccidiosis, Pneumonia and synovitis.

Altasol pow	**Vets Pharma**
Comp	20% Furaltadone
Adm.	Oral
@	100-125 mg/kg B.wt for LA 5-7 days
Pres.	50 g

Fucox Pow	**Virbac**
Comp	20% Furaltadone
Adm.	Oral
@	100-125 mg/kg B.wt for LA 5-7 days
Pres.	50 g

Furazolidone

A Nitrofuran active against Gram-ve bacilli including Salmonella, Shigella, Giardia and protozoa like Trichomonas. It is effective in Bacterial enteritis and Bacillary diarrhea. Side effect can be colouration of urine and dizziness.

Furazolidon Tab	**KAPL**
Comp	200 mg Furazolidone
Adm.	Oral
@	10-12 mg/kg B.wt
Pres.	200 mg Tab

Scorid Tab	**Vet Farma**
Comp	200 mg Furazolidone
Adm.	Oral
@	10-12 mg/kg B.wt
Pres.	200 mg Tab

Neftin Tab	**Zydus (Pfizer)**
Comp	200 mg Furazolidone
Adm.	Oral
@	10-12 mg/kg B.wt
Pres.	200 mg Tab

Nitrofurazone

It is a powerful broad spectrum Nitrofuran. It is bactericidal. There is no cross resistance. Mostly it is used topically as it is active in the presence of blood, pus or serum and does not effect healing. No side effect has been seen.

Furacin Powder/ Ointment	**Zydus (Pfizer)**
Comp	Nitrofuazone 0.2%
Adm.	Topically to be applied. Powder to be used IU
@	As per need
Pres.	28 g Tube, 10 g sachet

Furazone Liq	**Vets Farma**
Comp	Nitrofurazone 0.2%
Adm.	IU
@	30-50 ml
Pres.	30 ml, 90 ml

Nitromidazole

There are antiprozoan group of antibiotics. These are active especially against anaerobic bacteria as well as protozoas. Their mechanism of action is not well understood. These are completely absorbed from the small intestine. These are indicated in protozoan infections like amaebiasis, Trichomoniasis, Giardiasis, Balantidium and other anaerobic infections. Their higher dosage can lead to adverse reaction. These have synergistic action with various antibiotics.

Metronidazole

It is indicated in Protozoan infection. It is very potent against anaerobic bacteria. It is used in Genital tract infection, intestinal amebiasis etc. brown discolouration of urine is often observed after its usage which is due to pigmented active metabolite of Metronidazole. Its side effect may be anorexia, dryness of mouth and higher doses may cause neurological disturbances.

Anarobin inj	Cargill (Unichem)
Comp	Metronidazole 5 mg/ml
Adm.	Oral, IV, IU
@	20 mg/kg B.wt/day
Pres.	50 ml

Metron	Vets Farma
Comp	Metronidazole 5 mg/ml
Adm.	Oral, IV, IU
@	20 mg/kg B.wt/day
Pres.	90 ml

Tinidazole

A nitromidazole equally efficacious congener Metronidazole similar to every way except its metabolism is slower so action is for longer period. Hence it suits for once daily therapy. Some reports on antiamaebiasis have reported its higher use rate with comparatively low side effect. It is indicated in Amaebiasis, Giardiasis, Trichomoniasis and anaerobic infection. Avoid its use in pregnants.

Zil Tab	Zydus (Sarabhai)
Comp	Tinidazole 1 g, 300 mg, 600 mg
Adm.	Oral or IU
@	20 mg/kg B.wt
Pres.	Tablet of 300 mg, 600 mg, 1G

Tinilica Tab	Cadila
Comp	Tinidazole
Adm.	Oral or IU
@	20 mg/kg B.wt
Pres.	300 mg Tab

Nitromidazole Combination

Furazolidone and Metronidazole

Both are combined for better synergistic action. Furazolidone is poorly absorbed whereas Metrinidazole is rapidly absorbed leading to drug presence in lumen and cell. Both are effective against Protozoa and anaerobic bacterial infection. It is indicated in diarrhea with foul smell, dysentery, bovine coccidiosis, protozoan infection and uterine infections.

Fazole Bol	Cargill (Unichem)
Comp	Metronidazole 1 G Furazolidone 200 mg
Adm.	Oral
@	Oral 1 Bolus/50 kg B.wt IU- 3-4 boli
Pres.	Strip of 4

Furazolidone and Nitrofurazone

Their combination is effective against Gram + ve, Gram- ve bacteria. Nitrofuran is quickly eliminated from the system. Danger of residues in the milk (when treated against mastitis) is considerably reduced. Thus this milk can be consumed by humans 24 hrs after last treatment. This is indicated in Mastitis and coccidiosis

Nefrun Bol	Zydus (Pfizr)
Comp	Nitrofurazone 150 mg and Furazolidone 150 mg
Adm.	Oral
@	One Bol / OD for 3 days
Pres.	Pack of 12

Penicillin

Penicillin was first clinically used antibiotic. It was originally obtained from Penicillin notatum, a fungus but presently from Penicillium chrysogenum. Its also known as Beta lactam antibiotic. These are narrow spectrum antibiotic and their action is limited to Gram + ve bacteria. Due to production of penicillinase the resistance develops. It acts by inhibiting cell wall synthesis. It is active in presence of blood, pus and tissue fluids. It is bactericidal. These are active against penicillin sensitive organisms- Actinomyces, Bacillus anthracis, Streptococus, Clostridia and Corynebacterium.

Injectables

Ampicillin

It is synthetic is Penicillin broad spectrum antibiotic. It inhibits bacterial cell wall synthesis and bactericidal in action. Its bio-availability is high. It is sensitive to Gram + ve, Gram – ve bacteria. It is well absorbed from G I tract. It is inactivated by Penicillanse producing organisms.

Bacipen	Alembic
Comp	Ampicillin sodium B. P
Adm.	IM, IV
@	LA 2-7 mg/kg B.wt IM IV for 3-5 days in SA 7mg/ kg B.wt
Pres.	2 g, 2.5 g

Albercillin	Novartis (Hoechst)
Comp	Ampicillin sodium B. P
Adm.	IM, IV
@	LA 2-7 mg/kg B.wt IM IV for 3-5 days in SA 7 mg/ kg B.wt
Pres.	1 g

Campicillin	Cadila Healthcare
Comp	Ampicillin sodium B. P
Adm.	IM, IV
@	LA 2-7mg/kg B.wt IM IV for 3-5 days in SA 7mg/kg B.wt
Pres.	1 g, 2 g

Catcillin	Cattle Remedies
Comp	Ampicillin sodium B. P
Adm.	IM, IV
@	LA 2-7 mg/kg B.wt IM IV for 3-5 days in SA 7 mg/ kg B.wt
Pres.	2.5g

Dynacil	HAL
Comp	Ampicillin sodium B. P
Adm.	IM, IV
@	LA 2-7 mg/kg B.wt IM IV for 3-5 days in SA 7 mg/ kg B.wt
Pres.	1 g

Kampibiotic	KAPL
Comp	Ampicillin sodium B. P
Adm.	IM, IV
@	LA 2-7 mg/kg B.wt IM IV for 3-5 days in SA 7 mg/ kg B.wt
Pres.	1 g, 2 g, 2.5 g

Marcollin	**Marc**
Comp	Ampicillin sodium B. P
Adm.	IM, IV
@	LA 2-7 mg/kg B.wt IM IV for 3-5 days in SA 7 mg/kg B.wt
Pres.	2 g, 2.5 g

Conampi	**Concept**
Comp	Ampicillin sodium B. P
Adm.	IM, IV
@	LA 2-7 mg/kg B.wt IM IV for 3-5 days in SA 7 mg/kg B.wt
Pres.	1 g, 2 g,

Ampish	**Merial (Dosch)**
Comp	Ampicillin sodium B. P
Adm.	IM, IV
@	LA 2-7 mg/kg B.wt IM IV for 3-5 days in SA 7 mg/kg B.wt
Pres.	2 g, 2.5 g

Animycin G	**Cipla**
Comp	Ampicillin sodium B. P
Adm.	IM, IV
@	LA 2-7 mg/kg B.wt IM IV for 3-5 days in SA 7 mg/kg B.wt
Pres.	2 g, 2.5 g

Brandocillin	**Intas**
Comp	Ampicillin sodium B. P
Adm.	IM, IV
@	LA 2-7 mg/kg B.wt IM IV for 3-5 days in SA 7 mg/kg B.wt
Pres.	2 g, 2.5 g

L Cin	**Phoenix**
Comp	Ampicillin sodium B. P
Adm.	IM, IV
@	LA 2-7 mg/kg B.wt IM IV for 3-5 days in SA 7 mg/kg B.wt
Pres.	2 g, 2.5 g

Solampi	Brihans
Comp	Ampicillin sodium B. P
Adm.	IM, IV
@	LA 2-7 mg/kg B.wt IM IV for 3-5 days in SA 7 mg/kg B.wt
Pres.	2 g, 2.5 g

Tinampi	Tineta
Comp	Ampicillin sodium B. P
Adm.	IM, IV
@	LA 2-7 mg/kg B.wt IM IV for 3-5 days in SA 7 mg/kg B.wt
Pres.	2 g, 2.5 g

Vetampin	Wockhardt
Comp	Ampicillin sodium B. P
Adm.	IM, IV
@	LA 2-7 mg/kg B.wt IM IV for 3-5 days in SA 7 mg/kg B.wt
Pres.	2 g, 2.5 g

Ampicillin	Cadila Pharma
Comp	Ampicillin sodium B. P
Adm.	IM, IV
@	LA 2-7 mg/kg B.wt IM IV for 3-5 days in SA 7 mg/kg B.wt
Pres.	1 g, 2 g, 2.5 g

Stancillin	Zydus (Sarabhi)
Comp	Ampicillin sodium B. P
Adm.	IM, IV
@	LA 2-7 mg/kg B.wt IM IV for 3-5 days in SA 7 mg/kg B.wt
Pres.	2 g,

Ampicillin cloxacillin

These have synergistic bactericidal action. It covers Gram +ve, Gram –ve and act against Penicillinase producing organisms. Their action is also prolonged. Thus it becomes a broad spectrum in all types of infection.

AC Vet	**Intas**
Comp	Ampicillin 50% + cloxacillin 50%
Adm.	IM, IV
@	5-10 mg/kg B.wt for 3 to 5 days
Pres.	2 g, 3 g, 4 g

Baxivet	**Lyka**
Comp	Ampicillin 50% + cloxacillin 50%
Adm.	IM, IV
@	5-10 mg/kg B.wt for 3 to 5 days
Pres.	2 g

Betalactin	**Cargill (Unichem)**
Comp	Ampicillin 50% + cloxacillin 50%
Adm.	IM, IV
@	5-10 mg/kg B.wt for 3 to 5 days
Pres.	1 g, 2 g

Binocin	**Concept**
Comp	Ampicillin 50% + cloxacillin 50%
Adm.	IM, IV
@	5-10 mg/kg B.wt for 3 to 5 days
Pres.	1 g, 2 g

Catlox	**Cattle Remedies**
Comp	Ampicillin 50% + cloxacillin 50%
Adm.	IM, IV
@	5-10 mg/kg B.wt for 3 to 5 days
Pres.	2 g

Cenclox	**Century**
Comp	Ampicillin 50% + cloxacillin 50%
Adm.	IM, IV
@	5-10 mg/kg B.wt for 3 to 5 days
Pres.	2 g

Clampivet	**Merial (Dosch)**
Comp	Ampicillin 50% + cloxacillin 50%
Adm.	IM, IV
@	5-10 mg/kg B.wt for 3 to 5 days
Pres.	2 g

Cloxam	**Marc**
Comp	Ampicillin 50% + cloxacillin 50%
Adm.	IM, IV
@	5-10 mg/kg B.wt for 3 to 5 days
Pres.	2 g

Vetclox	**Zydus**
Comp	Ampicillin 50% + cloxacillin 50%
Adm.	IM, IV
@	5-10mg/kg B.wt for 3 to 5 days
Pres.	2 g

Inclox	**Brihans**
Comp	Ampicillin 50% + cloxacillin 50%
Adm.	IM, IV
@	5-10 mg/kg B.wt for 3 to 5 days
Pres.	1 g, 2 g, 2.5 g

Glycin	**Tineta**
Comp	Ampicillin 50% + cloxacillin 50%
Adm.	IM, IV
@	5-10 mg/kg B.wt for 3 to 5 days
Pres.	2.5 g

Tablet/ Liquid/ Powder

Ampicillin

Nepocil	**TTK**
Comp	Ampicillin 500 mg/g
Adm.	Oral
@	1-2 g/10 kg B.wt
Pres.	50 g

Campisol Pow	**Cadila**
Comp	Ampicillin 500 mg/g
Adm.	Oral
@	1-2 g/10 kg B.wt
Pres.	50 g

Roscillin	**Zydus (Ranbaxy)**
Comp	Ampicillin 500 mg/g
Adm.	Oral
@	1-2 g/10 kg B.wt
Pres.	50 g

Amoxicillin

It is synthetic penicillin, Betalactam antibiotic with broad spectrum activity via inhibiting bacterial cell wall synthesis. It is close congeneous to Ampicillin and resistance is common. In respect to oral absorption it is similar to Ampicillin. It provides higher and sustained blood level. With cloxacillin it has synergistic action. It's superior to Ampicillin pharmacokinetically. It is indicated in bacterial diarrhea pyrexia of unknown orgin, Respiratory and urinary infections, otits. In small dose also gives effective plasma concentration.

Amoxirum Bol	**Virbac**
Comp	Amoxycillin 1500 mg
Adm.	Oral
@	1 Bol/ 200 kg B.wt
Pres.	1.5 g x 2 Bol

Symoxyl Bol	**Zydus**
Comp	Amoxicillin 750 mg
Adm.	Oral
@	750 mg/kg 100 kg B.wt
Pres.	750 mg Bol x 4

Combination

Amoxycillin + Cloxacillin

Their combination has synergistic action and becomes broad spectrum with Beta lactamase resistance antibiotic.

Conmox	**Concept**
Comp	Amoxicillin 50% + cloxacillin 50%
Adm.	IM, IV
@	LA 5-10 mg/kg B.wt SA 15-25 mg/kg B.wt
Pres.	2 g

Megamycin Forte	**Zydus (Pfizer)**
Comp	Amoxicillin 50% + cloxacillin 50%
Adm.	IM, IV
@	LA 5-10 mg/kg B.wt SA 15-25 mg/kg B.wt
Pres.	2 g, 3 g

Intamox	**Intas**
Comp	Amoxicillin 50% + cloxacillin 50%
Adm.	IM, IV
@	LA 5-10 mg/kg B.wt SA 15-25 mg/kg B.wt
Pres.	2 g, 2.5 g, 3.5 g, 4.5 g

Nepoclox	**TTK**
Comp	Amoxycillin 50% + cloxacillin 50%
Adm.	IM, IV
@	5-10 mg/kg B.wt for 3 to 5 days
Pres.	2 g

Kloxamp	**KAPL**
Comp	Amoxycillin 50% + cloxacillin 50%
Adm.	IM, IV
@	5-10 mg/kg B.wt for 3 to 5 days
Pres.	1 g, 2 g

Amcox	**PAIL**
Comp	Amoxycillin 50% + cloxacillin 50%
Adm.	IM, IV
@	LA 5-10 mg/kg B.wt SA 15-25 mg/kg B.wt
Pres.	3 g

Clomox	**Tineta**
Comp	Amoxycillin 50% + cloxacillin 50%
Adm.	IM, IV
@	LA 5-10 mg/kg B.wt SA 15-25 mg/kg B.wt
Pres.	2.5 g

Clomoxy	**Brihans**
Comp	Amoxycillin 50% + cloxacillin 50%
Adm.	IM, IV
@	LA 5-10 mg/kg B.wt SA 15-25 mg/kg B.wt
Pres.	2 g, 3 g, 4 g

CMox	**Carevet Pharma**
Comp	Amoxycillin 50% + cloxacillin 50%
Adm.	IM, IV
@	LA 5-10 mg/kg B.wt SA 15-25 mg/kg B.wt
Pres.	3 g, 4.5 g

Crilmox	**Cattle Remedies**
Comp	Amoxycillin 50% + cloxacillin 50%
Adm.	IM, IV
@	LA 5-10 mg/kg B.wt SA 15-25 mg/kg B.wt
Pres.	2.5 g

Dosmox	**Merial (Dosch)**
Comp	Amoxycillin 50% + cloxacillin 50%
Adm.	IM, IV
@	LA 5-10 mg/kg B.wt SA 15-25 mg/kg B.wt
Pres.	3 g

Hipenox	**Cadila Health**
Comp	Amoxycillin 50% + cloxacillin 50%
Adm.	IM, IV
@	LA 5-10 mg/kg B.wt SA 15-25 mg/kg B.wt
Pres.	1 g, 2 g

Inimox	**Indian Immunology**
Comp	Amoxycillin 50% + cloxacillin 50%
Adm.	IM, IV
@	LA 5-10 mg/kg B.wt SA 15-25 mg/kg B.wt
Pres.	2 g, 4 g

Mamox	**Sushima**
Comp	Amoxycillin 50% + cloxacillin 50%
Adm.	IM, IV
@	LA 5-10 mg/kg B.wt SA 15-25 mg/kg B.wt
Pres.	3 g

Moxel	**Alembic**
Comp	Amoxycillin 50% + cloxacillin 50%
Adm.	IM, IV
@	LA 5-10 mg/kg B.wt SA 15-25 mg/kg B.wt
Pres.	2.5 g, 3 g, 4 g

Moxyclox	**Wockhardt**
Comp	Amoxycillin 50% + cloxacillin 50%
Adm.	IM, IV
@	LA 5-10 mg/kg B.wt SA 15-25 mg/kg B.wt
Pres.	3 g

Novaclox	**Cipla**
Comp	Amoxycillin 50% + cloxacillin 50%
Adm.	IM, IV
@	LA 5-10 mg/kg B.wt SA 15-25 mg/kg B.wt
Pres.	2 g, 3 g

Synkron	**Cadila Pharma**
Comp	Amoxycillin 50% + cloxacillin 50%
Adm.	IM, IV
@	LA 5-10 mg/kg B.wt SA 15-25 mg/kg B.wt
Pres.	0.5 g, 2 g, 2.5 g

Amclox	**Novartis**
Comp	Amoxycillin 50% + cloxacillin 50%
Adm.	IM, IV
@	LA 5-10 mg/kg B.wt SA 15-25 mg/kg B.wt
Pres.	2 g

Amoxirum Forte	Virbac
Comp	Amoxycillin 50% + cloxacillin 50%
Adm.	IM, IV
@	LA 5-10 mg/kg B.wt SA 15-25 mg/kg B.wt
Pres.	3 g

Centamox	Century
Comp	Amoxycillin 50% + cloxacillin 50%
Adm.	IM, IV
@	LA 5-10 mg/kg B.wt SA 15-25 mg/kg B.wt
Pres.	2 g, 3 g

Bovimox 4 inj	Herstal	
Comp	Amoxycillin 2 g	Cloxacillin 2 g
Adm.	IM	
@	5-7 mg/kg B.wt	
Pres.	4 g vial	

Amoxycyllin + Clavulanate Potassium

Potassium clavulanate or clavulanic acid is betalactamase resistance. It inhibits beta lactamase produced by some micro-organisms and make them susceptible to Amoxycillin which is hydrolysed by betalactamase. Action is bactericidal. It is indicated in Mastitis, Respiratory infection, metritis and soft tissue infections. It should not be given by IV route.

Synulox	Zydus (Pfizer)	
Comp	Amoxycillin trihydrate Potassium clavulanate	140 mg/ml 35 mg/ml
Adm.	IM	
@	1ml/20 kg B.wt once daily 3-5 days	
Pres.	40 ml vial	

Temobax	(Ranbaxy)	
Comp	Amoxycillin Cl. Pott	140 mg/5ml 28.5 mg/5ml
Adm.	IM	
@	1 ml/20 kg B.wt	
Pres.	6.6 g vial	

Amoxycyllin Sulbactam

Wesceft S Forte	Wesfa pharma	
Comp	Amoxycillin 3 g	Sulbactam 1.5 g
Adm.	IM/ IV	
@	1-10 mg/kg B.wt	
Pres.	4.5 g vial	

Wellmox Forte inj	Macwell	
Comp	Amoxicillin 3 g	Sulbactam 1.5 g
Adm.	IM/ IV	
@	10-15 mg/kg B.wt	
Pres.	4.5 g via with 20 ml Water	

NMox Forte inj	Macnor	
Comp	Amoxycyline 3 g	Sulbactam 1.5 g
Adm.	IM/ IV	
@.	10-15 mg/kg B.wt	
Pres.	4.5 g via with 20 ml Water	

Synkrone Forte inj	Cadila Pharma	
Comp	Amoxicillin 3 g	Sulbactam 1.5 g
Adm.	IM/ IV	
@	7-10 mg/kg B.wt	
Pres.	4.5 g with water and disposable syringe	

Sodamox inj	Boehringer Ingelheim
Comp	Amoxycillin + sulbactam 1:0.5 ratio
Adm.	IM/ IV
@	10 mg/kg B.wt
Pres.	4.5 g and 7.5 g

Benzathin Penicillin

It is narrow spectrum Penicillin act via interfering wall synthesis of bacteria. It's long acting bactericidal. Activity is from 74-120 hours. It can be given in Actinobacillosis, Actinomycosis, Black leg, Tetanus, Mastitis, Haemorrhagic septicaemina, Pyelonephritis. It should be given deep IM. Avoid in animals with hypersensitive to Penicillin.

Benthipen LA	**Carevet Pharma**
Comp	Benzathin sod
Adm.	IM
@	12000 IU/kg B.wt
Pres.	24 Lacs, 48 Lacs

Benzapen	**KAPL**
Comp	Benzathin sod
Adm.	IM
@	12000 IU/kg B.wt
Pres.	24 L, 48 L

Longacillin	**HAL**
Comp	Benzathin sod
Adm.	IM
@	12000 IU/kg B.wt
Pres.	6 L, 12 L, 24 L, 48 L

Pencom	**Alembic**
Comp	Benzathin sod
Adm.	IM
@	12000 IU/kg B.wt
Pres.	6 L, 12 L, 24 L

Benpen	**Cipla**
Comp	Benzathin sod
Adm.	IM
@	12000 IU/kg B.wt
Pres.	6 L, 12 L, 24 L, 48 L

Benzyl Penicillin

This penicillin is limited to Gram +ve bacteria and few others. It is bactericidal and acts by inhibiting cell wall synthesis. Resistance develops due to Penicillinase production by Staphylococcus and coli. It is indicated in wounds. Tetanus, B. Q, Anthrax, Infection. Leptospirosis, Actinomycosis, Mastitis, Respiratory infection and foot rot.

Bepen 20	**KAPL**
Comp	Sodium benzyl pencillin
Adm.	IM
@	5-10 mg/kg B.wt or 8000-12000 IU/kg B.wt
Pres.	20 L

Sodicillin	**HAL**
Comp	Sodium benzyl pencillin
Adm.	IM
@	5-10 mg/kg B.wt or 8000-12000 IU/kg B.wt
Pres.	5 L

Procain Penicillin or Fortified procaine Peniclin

Activity and indication as Benzyl Peniclin but the Plasma concentration obtained by it is lower but sustained for 1-3 days. It is the most nontoxic antibiotic.

Procain Penicillin	**Alembic**
Comp	Procaine penicillin G 30 L + Penicillin G sod 10 L PPG 15 L + PG 5 L
Adm.	IM
@.	4000 IU/kg B.wt
Pres.	15 L+ 5 L, 30 L+10 L

Crys 4	**Zydus**
Comp	Procaine penicillin G 30L + Penicillin G sod 10L PPG 15L + PG 5L
Adm.	IM
@	4000 IU/kg B.wt
Pres.	20L, 40L Vial

Kalpen Forte	**KAPL**
Comp	Procaine penicillin G 30 L + Penicillin G sod 10 L PPG 15 L + PG 5 L
Adm.	IM
@	4000 IU/kg B.wt
Pres.	20L, 40L

Omnacillin	**Novartis**
Comp	Procaine penicillin G 30 L + Penicillin G sod 10 L PPG 15 L + PG 5 L
Adm.	IM
@.	4000 IU/kg B.wt
Pres.	20 L, 40 L

Procillin 20	**HAL**
Comp	Procaine pnicillin G 30 L + Penicillin G sod 10 L PPG 15 L + PG 5 L
Adm.	IM
@	4000 IU/kg B.wt
Pres.	20 L, 40 L

Procain Penicillin in oil

To sustain the activity PP is used

PAM	**Zydus**
Comp	Procaine Pencillin G 30 L+2%. Aluminium monosteorate in oil base
Adm.	IM for LA
@	8000 IU/kg B.wt
Pres.	30 L

Quinolones or Floraquinolones

The members of this group have unique mechanism of action. These inhibit bacterial enzyme DNA gyrase responsible for multiplication of bacteria. These are bactericidal and active against Gram+ve, Gram-ve bacteria. These are absorbed rapidly when given orally and excreted through urine. These are used in various infections as systemic drug. There can be side effect of restlessness or abdominal pain.

Ciprofloxacin

It is one of quinolones. It is very potent and broad spectrum. Normally it does not disturb normal anaerobic ruminal and intestinal microflora. Their spectrum is wider than aminoglycosides and cephalosporins. It is not recommended in young ones. It is indicated Respiratory, urinary, Genital, Gastro-intestinal tract, bone and joint infections, systemic infections. Mastitis, Anthrax and severe dysentery.

Injectable

Ciprobid	**Cadila Healthcare**
Comp	Ciprofloxacin 100 mg/ml
Adm.	IM IV
@	4-5 mg/kg B.wt
Pres.	50 ml, 100 ml

C Flox	Intas
Comp	Ciprofloxacin 100 mg/ml
Adm.	IM IV
@	4-5 mg/kg B.wt
Pres.	50 ml

Ciplox IV	Cipla
Comp	Ciprofloxacin 100mg/ml
Adm.	IM IV
@	4-5 mg/kg B.wt
Pres.	50 ml, 100 ml

Enrofloxacin

It is Fluroquinolone member with very wide bactericidal spectrum. It is active against Gram+ve, Gram-ve bacteria, mycoplasma. It acts by inhibiting enzyme. DA gyrase to inhibit DNA synthesis. It acts within 20 minutes of its exposure in optimal concentration in the bacterial cell. It is indicated in Broncho pneumonia, Contagious Bovine Caprine pleuro pneumonia, Dermatitis, Mastitis, Metritis, Pyometra, Woodentongue, Brucellosis and in mixed infection. It's half life is 15 hours and has low MIC. It is non allergic and safe for pregnants. It is not to be used in horses. It has weak activity against streptococci and anaerobic bacteria.

Injectables

Conflox	Concept
Comp	Enrofloxacin 50mg/ml
Adm.	IM, IV
@	2.5-5 mg/ kg B.wt
Pres.	30 ml

Enrocin	Zydus (Ranbaxy)
Comp	Enrofloxacin 50 mg/ml
Adm.	IM, IV
@	2.5-5 mg/ kg B.wt
Pres.	15 ml, 50 ml

Enrogil	G. Lucatos
Comp	Enrofloxacin 50 mg/ml
Adm.	IM, IV
@	2.5-5 mg/ kg B.wt
Pres.	15 ml, 50 ml

Roflox	**Novartis**
Comp	100 mg/ml of Enrofloxacin
Adm.	IM, IV
@	2.5-5 mg/ kg B.wt
Pres.	15 ml, 30 ml, 50 ml, 100 ml

Quinintas	Intas
Comp	100 mg/ml of Enrofloxacin
Adm.	IM, IV
@	2.5-5 mg/ kg B.wt
Pres.	15 ml, 30 ml, 50 ml, 100 ml

Meriquin	**Merial (Wokhardt)**
Comp	100 mg/ml of Enrofloxacin
Adm.	IM, IV
@	2.5-5 mg/ kg B.wt
Pres.	15 ml, 50 ml, 100 ml

K flox	**KAPL**
Comp	100mg/ml of Enrofloxacin
Adm.	IM, IV
@	2.5-5 mg/ kg B.wt
Pres.	15 ml, 50 ml

Gyroflox	**Indian Immunology**
Comp	Enrofloxacin 50mg/ml
Adm.	IM, IV
@	2.5-5 mg/ kg B.wt
Pres.	2 ml, 15 ml, 50 ml

Floxidin	**Hoechst**
Comp	Enrofloxacin 50mg/ml
Adm.	IM, IV
@	2.5-5 mg/ kg B.wt
Pres.	15 ml, 50 ml

Enrox	**Alembic**
Comp	100 mg/ml of Enrofloxacin
Adm.	IM, IV
@	2.5-5 mg/ kg B.wt
Pres.	15 ml, 50 ml

Enrotreat	**Cadila Pharma**
Comp	100 mg/ml of Enrofloxacin
Adm.	IM, IV
@	2.5-5 mg/ kg B.wt
Pres.	30 ml, 100 ml

Enrocare	**Cargill (vetcare)**
Comp	Enrofloxacin 50 mg/ml
Adm.	IM, IV
@	2.5-5 mg/ kg B.wt
Pres.	20 ml

Enrobest	**TTK**
Comp	100 mg/ml of Enrofloxacin
Adm.	IM, IV
@	2.5-5 mg/ kg B.wt
Pres.	15 ml, 30 ml, 50 ml

Enrovet	**Vets Farma**
Comp	100 mg/ml of Enrofloxacin
Adm.	IM, IV
@	2.5-5 mg/ kg B.wt
Pres.	15 ml, 30 ml, 50 ml

Zona	**Century**
Comp	100 mg/ml of Enrofloxacin
Adm.	IM, IV
@	2.5-5 mg/ kg B.wt
Pres.	15 ml, 50 ml

Enrodac	**Cadila Health**
Comp	100 mg/ml of Enrofloxacin
Adm.	IM, IV
@	2.5-5 mg/ kg B.wt
Pres.	15 ml, 50 ml

Enrovet	**Cipla**
Comp	100 mg/ml of Enrofloxacin
Adm.	IM, IV
@	2.5-5 mg/ kg B.wt
Pres.	15 ml, 50 ml

Quroflox	**PAIL**
Comp	100 mg/ml of Enrofloxacin
Adm.	IM, IV
@	2.5-5 mg/ kg B.wt
Pres.	15 ml, 30 ml, 50 ml, 100 ml

Kenrol	**Kepler**
Comp	100 mg/ml of Enrofloxacin
Adm.	IM, IV
@	2.5-5 mg/ kg B.wt
Pres.	15 ml, 30 ml, 50 ml, 100 ml

Vetrocin Forte	**Boehringer**
Comp	100 mg/ml of Enrofloxacin
Adm.	IM, IV
@	2.5-5 mg/ kg B.wt
Pres.	15 ml, 30 ml, 50 ml, 100 ml

Wesfloxin inj	**Wesfa pharma**
Comp	Enrofloxacin 100 mg/ml
Adm.	IM/ SC
@	5 mg/kg B.wt or 1 ml per 20 kg B.wt
Pres.	30 ml, 100 ml

Enroplasm inj	**Libra**
Comp	Enrofloxacin 10%
Adm.	IM
@	2.5-5 mg/kg B.wt or 1 ml/20-40 kg B.wt
Pres.	30 ml, 100 ml

Enrofloxacin combination

Penrocin Z inj	**Carevet Pharma**
Comp	Zinc 50 mg Enrofloxacin 500 mg Pefloxacin 1500 mg
Adm.	IM
@	1 vial for 400 kg B.wt by adding 15 ml od Distt water in vial 1 ml/24 kg B.wt
Pres.	Vial having 0.25% Zinc, 2.5% Enrofloxacin, 7.5% Pefloxacin

Fluxishot inj	Nicosia	
Comp	Each ml contains Enrofloacin Flunixin meglumine	 100 mg 50 mg
Adm.	IM	
@	1 ml/25/kg B.wt bid	
	30 ml, 100 ml	

Quinolone Tablet/Pow/Liq

Ciprofloxacin

C Flox Pow	Intas
Comp	Ciprofloxacin 10%
Adm.	Oral
@	LA 30 gm bid
Pres.	100 g, 500 g

Ciprost pow	Sterling
Comp	Ciprofloxacin 10%
Adm.	Oral
@	LA 30 gm bid
Pres.	100 g, 500 g

Ciprofloxacin Combination

Ciprofloxacin and Tinidazole

These have synergistic action.

C Flox TZ Bol.	Intas
Comp	Ciprofloxacin 1500 mg, Tinidazole 1800 mg
Adm.	Oral
@	LA 2 Bol. Bid, SA ½ Bol bid
Pres.	Strip of 2

Floxanil TZ	Marc
Comp	Ciprofloxacin 1500 mg, Tinidazole 1800 mg
Adm.	Oral
@	LA 2 Bol. Bid, SA ½ Bol bid
Pres.	Strip of 2

Enrofloxacin Liquid

Conflox Liquid	**Concept**
Comp	Enrofloxacin 100 mg/ml
Adm.	Oral
@	10 mg/ kg B.wt
Pres.	100 ml, 500 ml

Bayrocin Liq	**Bayer**
Comp	Enrofloxacin 100 mg/ml
Adm.	Oral
@	10 mg/ kg B.wt
Pres.	100 ml

Enrodac Liq	**Zydus**
Comp	Enrofloxacin 100 mg/ml
Adm.	Oral
@	10 mg/ kg B.wt
Pres.	100 ml

Enrovet Liq/ Tab	**Cipla**
Comp	Enrofloxacin 100 mg/ml Tab 50 mg, 150 mg
Adm.	Oral
@	10 mg/ kg B.wt
Pres.	100 ml/50 mg × 10 150 mg × 10

Enrox Liq.	**Alembic**
Comp	Enrofloxacin 100 mg/ml
Adm.	Oral
@	10 mg/ kg B.wt
Pres.	100 ml, 500 ml

Quinrocin Liq.	**Neospark**
Comp	Enrofloxacin 100 mg/ml
Adm.	Oral
@	10 mg/ kg B.wt
Pres.	500 ml, IL

Quinintas Liq.	**Intas**
Comp	Enrofloxacin 100 mg/ml
Adm.	Oral
@	10 mg/ kg B.wt
Pres.	IL

Fortius Liq.	**Virbac**
Comp	Enrofloxacin 100 mg/ml
Adm.	Oral
@	10 mg/ kg B.wt
Pres.	IL

Zona Liq.	**Century**
Comp	Enrofloxacin 100mg/ml
Adm.	Oral
@	10 mg/ kg B.wt
Pres.	500 ml, IL

Meriquin Tab	**Merial (Wockhardt)**
Comp	Enrofloxacin 50mg
Adm.	Oral
@	5 mg/kg B.wt
Pres.	Strip of 10

Gyroflox Tab	**IIL**
Comp	Enrofloxacin 50mg
Adm.	Oral
@	5 mg/kg B.wt
Pres.	Strip of 10

Ofloxacin

One of the latest quinolone of second generation having acting against, Gram+ve, Gram-ve and not on anaerobic one. Risk of resistance is low. It is very good in urinary tract infection, skin and soft tissue, skeletal and surgical infections. It is capable of overcoming Brucellosis. It is not recommended in young. There can be hypersensitive action.

Ofloxacin Bol

Oflokind	**Vetmankind**
Comp	Ofloxacin 1000 mg
Adm.	Oral
@	One bolus bid x 5-7 days
Pres.	2's strip

Maclone	**Macwell**
Comp	Ofloxacin 1200 mg
Adm.	Oral
@	2 Bol bid
Pres.	Strip of 2

Oflaxcin Cominaiton

Oflokind OZ Bol	**Vetkind**
Comp	Ofloxacin 100o mg + Ornidazole 2500 mg
Adm.	Oral
@	One Bol od
Pres.	Strip of 2

Pefloxacin

It is quinolone with broad spectrum activity. It is very effective in Gram+ve, Gram-ve infections including mixed infections caused by one or more type of organisms and multidrug resistance bacteria. It can be combined with metronidazole.

Pelwin inj	**Merial (Wockhardt)**
Comp	400 mg Pefloxacin with 5G Dextrose in water
Adm.	IV
@	5-10 mg/kg B.wt for 3 days
Pres.	100 ml

Peflocin Bol	**Neospark**
Comp	Pefloxacin 1000 mg
Adm.	Oral
@	5-10 mg/kg B.wt
Pres.	Strip of 2

Pelwin Tab	**Merial (Wockhardt)**
Comp	Pefloxacin 400 mg
Adm.	Oral
@	5-10 mg/kg B.wt
Pres.	Strip of 4

Pelorid Pow	**Sterling**
Comp	Each gm contain 200 mg of Pefloxacin
Adm.	Oral
@	5-10 mg/kg B.wt
Pres.	50 g, 100 g

Anflox Pow	**Anmark**
Comp	Each gm contain 50 mg of Pefloxacin
Adm.	Oral
@	5-10 mg/kg B.wt
Pres.	50 g, 100 g

L Cin inj	**Phoenix**
Comp	Levofloxacin 100mg/ml
Adm.	IM/ IV
@	LA 0.5-1 ml/kg B.wt SA 1-1.5 ml/ 100 kg B.wt
Pres.	30 ml

Flumiquine

It is a synthetic fluoroquinolone antibiotic of 1st generation. It is used in treatment of enteric and all intestinal infections given only orally.

Fluquin Powd.	**Cadila Pharma**
Comp	Flumequin
Adm.	Oral
@	6 g/100 kg B.wt
Pres.	25 g Sache

Zydaquin Pow	**Cadila Healthcare**
Comp	Flumequin
Adm.	Oral
@	6 g/100 kg B.wt
Pres.	25 g Sache

Sulphonamides

These were first antimicrobial agents effective against Pyrogenic infections. All Sulphonamides are considered to be derivative of Sulphonamide. These are bacteriostatic against Gram+ve and Gram-ve bacteria. Depending upon their usage sensitivity has been changing. Resistance is developing. These are mostly known as chemotherapeutic agents. Basically all have same spectrum. These have been classified according to their absorption.

Short acting (4-8 hrs)	Sulpha acetamide Sulphadiazine Suplhadimidine Sulphamethazine
Medium acting (8-16 hrs)	Sulphamethazole Sulphamethoxazole Sulphamoxale
Long acting (1-7 days)	Sulphamethoxine Sulphadoxine Sulphamethoxy pyridazine
Poorly absorbed	Sulphathiazole succinyl Sulphathiazole Pasualyl Sulphaguandine

Sulpha Injectables

Sulphadimidine

It is a short acting Sulphonamide. It's a broad spectrum and bacteriostatic. It acts by inhibiting bacterial folate synrhetase. Folic acid is not formed and a number of essential metabolic reactions suffer. It is indicated in Respiratory, Gastrointestinal, urinogenital tract infections, skin and joint infection, wounds and foot rot.

Sulfan	**Pranav**
Comp	33.3% Sulphadimidine
Adm.	IM
@	200 mg/kg B.wt on 1st day followed by 100 mg/kg B.wt
Pres.	100 ml

Sulfamin	Indian Immunology
Comp	33.3% Sulphadimidine
Adm.	IM
@	200 mg/kg B.wt on 1st day followed by 100 mg/kg B.wt
Pres.	100 ml, 450 ml

Brimidine	Brihans
Comp	33.3% Sulphadimidine
Adm.	IM
@	200 mg/kg B.wt on 1st day followed by 100 mg/kg B.wt
Pres.	100 ml

Sulfacip	Cipla
Comp	33.3% Sulphadimidine
Adm.	IM
@	200 mg/kg B.wt on 1st day followed by 100 mg/kg B.wt
Pres.	100 ml

Sulphadimethyl Pyrimidine

It's long acting and its status is similar to Sulphamethoxy pyridiazine. Not in Injectable form.

Sulphamethoxy Pyridizine

It is long acting Sulphonamide and excreted very slowly. Duration of action is 1-2 days. It is very good in acute infection. It is indicated in Surgical intervention, urinary tract infection.

Aldazine LA	(Alved)
Comp	250 mg of Sulphomethoxy pyridizine
Adm.	IM
@	1 ml/10 kg B.wt
Pres.	30 ml

Sulpha Liquid- Bolus Dosage form

Sulpha dimidine

Aldin Bolus	Alembic
Comp	5 gm Sulphadimidine in 1 Bol.
Adm.	Oral
@	200 mg/kg B.wt followed by 100 mg/kg B.wt od
Pres.	Pack of 50

Entradin	**Neospark**
Comp	5 gm Sulphadimidine in 1 Bol.
Adm.	Oral
@	200 mg/kg B.wt followed by 100 mg/kg B.wt od
Pres.	Pack of 50

Diadin	**Zydus (Pfizer)**
Comp	5 gm Sulphadimidine in 1 Bol.
Adm.	Oral
@	200 mg/kg B.wt followed by 100 mg/kg B.wt
Pres.	Pack of 50

Hamidin	**HAL**
Comp	5 gm Sulphadimidine in 1 Bol.
Adm.	Oral
@	200 mg/kg B.wt followed by 100 mg/kg B.wt
Pres.	Pack of 50

Pabadin	**Intas**
Comp	5 gm Sulphadimidine in 1 Bol.
Adm.	Oral
@	200 mg/kg B.wt followed by 100 mg/kg B.wt
Pres.	Pack of 50

Sulphadimidine	**Carevet Pharma/ sterling**
Comp	5 gm Sulphadimidine in 1 Bol.
Adm.	Oral
@	200 mg/kg B.wt followed by 100 mg/kg B.wt
Pres.	Pack of 50

Sulpha Bolus	**Zydus**
Comp	5 gm Sulphadimidine in 1 Bol.
Adm.	Oral
@	200 mg/kg B.wt followed by 100mg/kg B.wt
Pres.	Strip of 4

Sulfamin	**Indian Immunology**
Comp	5 gm Sulphadimidine in 1 Bol.
Adm.	Oral
@	200 mg/kg B.wt followed by 100mg/kg B.wt
Pres.	Pack of 50

Sulphadin	Vets Farma
Comp	5 gm Sulphadimidine in 1 Bol.
Adm.	Oral
@	200 mg/kg B.wt followed by 100 mg/kg B.wt
Pres.	Pack of 50

Sulfasys	KAPL
Comp	5gm Sulphadimidine in 1 Bol.
Adm.	Oral
@	200mg/kg B.wt followed by 100mg/kg B.wt
Pres.	Pack of 50

Cipadine Bol	Cipla
Comp	5gm Sulphadimidine in 1 Bol.
Adm.	Oral
@	200mg/kg B.wt followed by 100mg/kg B.wt
Pres.	Pack of 50

Dimidos	Merial (Dosch)
Comp	5gm Sulphadimidine in 1 Bol.
Adm.	Oral
@	200mg/kg B.wt followed by 100mg/kg B.wt
Pres.	Pack of 50

Sulfam	Parnav
Comp	5 gm Sulphadimidine in 1 Bol.
Adm.	Oral
@	200 mg/kg B.wt followed by 100 mg/kg B.wt
Pres.	Pack of 50

Sulphadimidine Solution

Sulphadimidine sol.	Generic
Comp	16% Sulphadimidine
Adm.	Oral
@	200mg/kg B.wt followed by 100mg/kg B.wt
Pres.	450ml

Sulphaguanidine

Due to slow absorsption it acts on gut and is antidiarrheal to treat specific and non-specific diarrhea including Calf Scours, Salmonellosis, E.Coli and Bacillary infection.

Suplhagut Bol	**KAPL**
Comp	5 g Sulphagunidine
Adm.	Oral
@	200 mg/kg B.wt followed by 100 mg/kg B.wt
Pres.	Pack 50 mg

Sulphaguanidine bol	**Carevet Pharma**
Comp	5g Sulphaguanidine
Adm.	Oral
@	200 mg/kg B.wt followed by 100 mg/kg B.wt
Pres.	Pack of 50

Sulphaquinoxaline

It specifically acts against coccidosis. It is highly effective when used with diamino pyrimidine in coccidiosis.

Coxter Pow	**Sterling**
Comp	Sulphaquinoxaline 18.7% + Diaveridine 3.3%
Adm.	Oral
@	13mg/kg B.wt
Pres.	100g

Sulphadiazine + Trimethoprim/ Sulphamethoxazole + Trimethoprim

Sulphadiazine is widely used in live stock in combination with Trimethoprim and can be combined with Sulphamethazine, Sulphamerazine and Tylosin for use. Combination is rapidly absorbed and excreted in urine. It is soluble and can be used only IU and not SC route by injection. Sulphamethazole has slower absorption.

Trimethoprim is a derivative related to antimicrobial drug Pyremethazone. This combination or with Sulphadiazine or Sulpamethoxazole is called Cotrimazine. Many additional micro-organisms are killed including some Sulpha resistants. Combination is of Sulpha + Trimethoprim. Indicated in Mixed bacterial infection and other systemic infections.

Injectable

Trisul inj	**Pranav**
Comp	Sulphadiazine 200 mg + Trimethoprim 40 mg
Adm.	IM IV
@	1ml/10 kg B.wt
Pres.	30 ml

Biotrim	**Zydus (Ranbaxy)**
Comp	Sulphadiazine 200 mg + Trimethoprim 40 mg
Adm.	IM IV
@	1 ml/10 kg B.wt
Pres.	30 ml

Bovisulf	**Bovina**
Comp	Sulphadiazine 200 mg + Trimethoprim 40mg
Adm.	IM IV
@	1 ml/10 kg B.wt
Pres.	30ml

Duaprim	**Brihans**
Comp	Sulphadiazine 200 mg + Trimethoprim 40 mg
Adm.	IM IV
@	1 ml/10kg B.wt
Pres.	30 ml

Sulprim	**Cargill (Unichem)**
Comp	Sulphadiazine 200 mg + Trimethoprim 40 mg
Adm.	IM IV
@	1 ml/10 kg B.wt
Pres.	30 ml

Trepin Inj	**Cadila Pharma**
Comp	Sulphamethoxazole 400 mg Trimethoprim 80 mg/ml
Adm.	IV
@	1 ml/10 kg B.wt
Pres.	30 ml

Oriprim	**Cadila Health**
Comp	Sulphamethoxazole 400 mg Trimethoprim 80 mg/ml
Adm.	IV
@	1 ml/10 kg B.wt
Pres.	30 ml

Cobact DS	Cipla
Comp	Sulphamethoxazole 400 mg + Trimethoprim 80 mg/ml
Adm.	IV
@	1 ml/10 kg B.wt
Pres.	30 ml

Trimasol	Novartis
Comp	Sulphamethoxazole 400 mg + Trimethoprim 80 mg/ml
Adm.	IM, IV
@	1 ml/10 kg B.wt
Pres.	10 ml, 30 ml, 50 ml

Sulphatrim	Vets Farma
Comp	Sulphadiazine 400 mg Trimethoprim 80 mg/ml
Adm.	IV
@	1 ml/10 kg B.wt
Pres.	30 ml

Sparktrim	Neospark
Comp	Sulphadiazine 200 mg Trimethoprim 40 mg/ml
Adm.	IV
@	1 ml/10 kg B.wt
Pres.	30 ml

Other Dosage Form Sulpha + Trimethoprim

Cobact Bol	Cipla
Comp	Sulphamethoxazole 2 g Trimethoprim 400 mg.
Adm.	Oral
@	4-6 Bol od
Pres.	Strip of 4

Duaprim Bol.	Brihans
Comp	Sulphamethoxazole 2 g + Trimethoprim 400 mg
Adm.	Oral
@	3-4 Bol od
Pres.	Strip or 4

Duxprim Pow.	Neospark
Comp	Sulphamethoxazole 10% Trimethoprim 2%
Adm.	Oral
@	10-20 g od
Pres.	100 g, 500 g, 1 kg

Metaprim Pow	**Vets Farma**
Comp	Sulphamethoxazole 10% Trimethoprim 2%
Adm.	Oral
@	10-20 g od
Pres.	100 g, 500 g

Oriprim Bol.	**Cadila Health**
Comp	Sulphamethoxazole 2 g + Trimethoprim 400 mg
Adm.	Oral
@	3-4 Bol
Pres.	2 Bol strip

Sterbac Pow/Bol	**Sterling**
Comp	Sulphamethoxazole 10% Trimethoprim 2%
Adm.	Oral
@	10-20 g od
Pres.	Strip of 4, 100 g, 500 g

Trepin Pow	**Cadila Pharma**
Comp	Sulphamethoxazole 10% Trimethoprim 2%
Adm.	Oral
@	10-20 g od
Pres.	100 g, 500 g, 1 kg

Uptran Bol.	**UnJha**
Comp	Sulphamethoxazole 1 g Trimethoprim 200 mg
Adm.	Oral
@	4-6 Bol od
Pres.	Strip of 4

Woktrin Bol.	**Merial (Wocknardt)**
Comp	Sulphamethoxazole 2 g + 400 mg Trimethoprim
Adm.	Oral
@	4-6 Bol od
Pres.	Strip of 4

Zintrid Bol.	**Zydus (Sarabhai)**
Comp	Sulphamethoxazole 2 g + Trimethoprim 400 mg
Adm.	Oral
@	3-4 Bol od
Pres.	Strip or 4

Cotrimal Bol	**Alembic**
Comp	Sulphamethoxazol 2.5 g Trimethoprim 500 mg
Adm.	Oral
@	3-4 Bol od
Pres.	10 x 4

Sulcoprim Bol/Pow	**Concept**
Comp	Sulphadiazine 2 g + Trimethoprim 400 mg Same for Powd
Adm.	Oral
@	3-4 Bol od
Pres.	10 Bol strip, 100 g, 500g

Vetran Bol	**Vets Farma**
Comp	Sulphadiazine 100 mg Trimethoprim 20 mg
Adm.	Oral
@	8-10 Tab od
Pres.	10 Tab strip

Vetran LA Bol	**Vets Farma**
Comp	Sulphadiazine 1000 mg Trimethoprim 200 mg
Adm.	Oral
@	4-6 Bol od
Pres.	Strip or 4

Trizine Pow	**KAPL**
Comp	Sulphadiazine 10% Trimethoprim 2%
Adm.	Oral
@	25-50 g/od
Pres.	100 g, 500 g

Trisul Bol	**Pranav**
Comp	Sulphadiazine 1 g Trimethoprim 200 mg
Adm.	Oral
@	4-6 Bol od
Pres.	Strip or 4

Sparktrim DS Bol	**Neospark**
Comp	Sulphadiazine 2 g + Trimethoprim 400 mg Same for Powd
Adm.	Oral
@	3-4 Bol od
Pres.	10 Bol strip, 100 g, 500 g

Robatrim bol	**TTK**
Comp	Sulphadiazine 1g Trimethoprim 200 mg
Adm.	Oral
@	4-6 Bol od
Pres.	Strip or 4

Macroprim	**Marc**
Comp	Sulphamethoxazole 2 g + Trimethoprim 400 mg
Adm.	Oral
@	3-4 Bol
Pres.	2 Bol strip

Initrim bol	**Indian Immunology**
Comp	Sulphamethoxazole 2 g + Trimethoprim 400 mg
Adm.	Oral
@	3-4 Bol od
Pres.	Strip or 4

Hatrix Bol	**HAL**
Comp	Sulphamethoxazole 2 g + Trimethoprim 400 mg
Adm.	Oral
@	3-4 Bol
Pres.	2 Bol strip

Duocidal bol	**KAPL**
Comp	Sulphamethoxazole 2 g + Trimethoprim 400 mg
Adm.	Oral
@	3-4 Bol
Pres.	2 Bol strip

Solbac SP Sol/ Pow	**Cargill (Vetcare)**
Comp	Sulphamethoxazole 2 g + Trimethoprim 400 mg
Adm.	Oral
@	10-20 g od
Pres.	100 g, 500 g

Tetracyclin

These are class of antibiotic derived from soil Actinomyces. First introduced member was chlortetracycline in 1984. Tetracycline is group of broad spectrum antibiotic. Primarily these are bacteriostatic. These inhibit protein synthesis. These are active against Gram+ve, Gram-ve, spirochets, Rickettsia, Mycplasma and a few protozoan organisms. These can be given orally and parentally. Sometimes these have side effect of vomiting and diarrhea when given orally.

Chlortetracyclin

It was first Tetracyclin discovered and introduced in 1948. Their absorption, distribution, metabolism and excrction is as for all Tetracyclins. Action is bacteriostatic. It is ued orally in mixed infection or as feed additive for promotion of growth as well as for treating Salmonellosis.

Aureomycin Tab	**Cynamid**
Comp	Chloretracyclin 500 mg
Adm.	Oral or IU
@	LA 10-15 mg/kg B.wt SA 20-25 mg/kg B.wt 4 Tab IU
Pres.	4's Strip

Doxycyclin

It is a broad spectrum antibiotic of Tetracyclin group. It is active against Ricketssia, Eschirichia and some protozoa. It is also a bacteriostatic acts by inhibiting protein synthesis. Potency is very high. It can be given in mixed bacterial infection of Respiratory, urinal, genital tract, Mastitis usually given orally alone or with other antibiotic.

Doxyterin	**Zydus**
Comp	2.5% Doxycyclin
Adm.	Oral or IU
@	2-4 g/50 kg B.wt
Pres.	50 g, 100 g

Xidox	**Sarabhai**
Comp	12.5 mg/g Doxycyclin
Adm.	Oral
@	2-4 g/50 kg B.wt
Pres.	100 g, 500 g

Bidox granule	**Merial (Wockhardt)**
Comp	100 mg/gm
Adm.	Oral
@	1-2 g/100 kg B.wt
Pres.	10 g, 50 g, 250 g

Oxytetracyclin

It is broad spectrum antibiotic of Tetracyclin group derived from Streptomyces rimosus. It is active aginst Gram+ve, Gram-ve bacteria, astercocci, chlamydae, Rickettsia, some protozoa and large viruses. It inhibits protein synthesis particularly the formation of peptide linkage. In low concentration it is bacteriostatic and in higher doses its bacteriocidal. It is indicated in mixed infection of Respiratory, urinary, genital, Gastro intestinal tract, post operative infections and mastitis. It can be given IM, IV, SC, orally and can be used topically. When given orally in young ones it effects teeth and bone formation and temporarily interferes with digestion in ruminants when given orally.

Injectables

Terrramycin	**Pfizer**
Comp	50 mg/ml of oxytetracycline hydrochloride
Adm.	IM, IV, SC
@	5-10 mg/kg B.wt bid or 1-2 ml/25 kg B.wt 20 mg/kg B.wt for Anaplasmosis and Theileriasis
Pres.	10 ml, 30 ml, 100 ml

Alcyclin	**Alembic**
Comp	50mg/ml of oxytetracycline hydrochloride
Adm.	IM, IV, SC
@	5-10 mg/kg B.wt bid or 1-2 ml/25 kg B.wt 20 mg/kg B.wt for Anaplasmosis and Theileriasis
Pres.	30 ml, 50 ml, 100 ml

Amoly	**Pranav**
Comp	50 mg/ml of oxytetracycline hydrochloride
Adm.	IM, IV, SC
@	5-10 mg/kg B.wt bid or 1-2 ml/25 kg B.wt 20 mg/kg B.wt for Anaplasmosis and Theileriasis
Pres.	100 ml

Brioxy	**Brihans**
Comp	50mg/ml of oxytetracycline hydrochloride
Adm.	IM, IV, SC
@	5-10 mg/kg B.wt bid or 1-2 ml/25kg B.wt 20 mg/kg B.wt for Anaplasmosis and Theileriasis
Pres.	10 ml, 30 ml, 50 ml, 100 ml

Intamycin	**Intas**
Comp	50 mg/ml of oxytetracycline hydrochloride
Adm.	IM, IV, SC
@	5-10 mg/kg B.wt bid or 1-2ml/25 kg B.wt 20 mg/kg B.wt for Anaplasmosis and Theileriasis
Pres.	30 ml, 100 ml

Oxysure	**Sterling**
Comp	50 mg/ml of oxytetracycline hydrochloride
Adm.	IM, IV, SC
@	5-10 mg/kg B.wt bid or 1-2 ml/25 kg B.wt 20 mg/kg B.wt for Anaplasmosis and Theileriasis
Pres.	30 ml, 100 ml

Oxysteclin	**Sarabhai**
Comp	Oxytetracyclin dihydrate 50 mg/ml
Adm.	IM, IV, SC
@	5-10 mg/kg B.wt bid or 1-2 ml/25 kg B.wt 20 mg/kg B.wt for Anaplasmosis and Theileriasis
Pres.	10 ml, 30 ml, 50 ml

Oxtetracyclin	**Concept , G.Loucatos, TTK**
Comp	50 mg/ml of oxytetracyclin hydrochloride
Adm.	IM, IV, SC
@	5-10 mg/kg B.wt bid or 1-2 ml/25 kg B.wt 20 mg/kg B.wt for Anaplasmosis and Theileriasis
Pres.	30 ml, 100 ml

Wolicyclin	**Merial (Wockhardt)**
Comp	50 mg/ml of oxytetracyclin hydrochloride
Adm.	IM, IV, SC
@	5-10 mg/kg B.wt bid or 1-2 ml/25 kg B.wt 20 mg/kg B.wt for Anaplasmosis and Theileriasis
Pres.	30 ml, 50 ml, 100 ml

Tetroxin	**Indian Immunology**
Comp	50mg/ml of oxytetracyclin hydrochloride
Adm.	IM, IV, SC
@	5-10mg/kg B.wt bid or 1-2ml/25kg B.wt 20mg/kg B.wt for Anaplasmosis and Theileriasis
Pres.	30ml, 100ml

Vetoxy	Vets Farma
Comp	50mg/ml of oxytetracyclin hydrochloride
Adm.	IM, IV, SC
@	5-10mg/kg B.wt bid or 1-2ml/25kg B.wt 20mg/kg B.wt for Anaplasmosis and Theileriasis
Pres.	30ml, 90ml

Ultrox	Neospark
Comp	50 mg/ml of oxytetrauycli oxytetracyclin hydrochloride
Adm.	IM, IV, SC
@	5-10 mg/kg B.wt bid or 1-2 ml/25kg B.wt 20 mg/kg B.wt for Anaplasmosis and Theileriasis
Pres.	30 ml, 50 ml

Double Strength Oxytetracyclin Injections

Wolicyclin DS	Merial (Wockhardt)
Comp	Oxytetracyclin hydrochloride 100 mg/ml
Adm.	IM, IV, SC
@	5-10 mg/kg B.wt
Pres.	30 ml, 100 ml

Amoly Ds	Pranav
Comp	Oxytetracyclin hydrochloride 100 mg/ml
Adm.	IM, IV, SC
@	5-10 mg/kg B.wt
Pres.	30 ml, 100 ml

Oxy DS	Carevet Pharma
Comp	Oxytetracyclin hydrochloride 100 mg/ml
Adm.	IM, IV, SC
@	5-10 mg/kg B.wt
Pres.	30 ml, 100 ml

Ultrox DS	Neospark
Comp	Oxytetracyclin hydrochloride 100 mg/ml
Adm.	IM, IV, SC
@	5-10 mg/kg B.wt
Pres.	30 ml, 100 ml

Long acting oxytetracyclin

It forms depot in muscle and released slowly so that blood level is maintained for more than 72 hour.

Centrocyclin LA	**Century**
Comp	Oxytetracyclin hydrochloride 200 mg/ml + Aqueous 2 Pyrrolidone
(vehicle)	Oral
Adm.	Im
@	20 mg/kg B.wt or 1 ml/10 kg B.wt
Pres.	30 ml, 50 ml

Intamycin LA	**Intas**
Comp	Oxytetracyclin hydrochloride 200 mg/ml + Aqueous 2 Pyrrolidone
Adm.	IM, IV, SC
@	5-10 mg/kg B.wt
Pres.	30 ml, 100 ml

Oxy Vet LA	**Zydus**
Comp	Oxytetracyclin hydrochloride 200 mg/ml + Aqueous 2 Pyrrolidone
Adm.	IM, IV, SC
@	5-10 mg/kg B.wt
Pres.	30 ml, 100 ml

Telon LA	**Zydus**
Comp	Oxytetracyclin hydrochloride 200 mg/ml + Aqueous 2 Pyrrolidone
Adm.	IM, IV, SC
@	5-10 mg/kg B.wt
Pres.	30 ml, 100 ml

Ultrox LA	**Merial**
Comp	Oxytetracyclin hydrochloride 200 mg/ml + Aqueous 2 Pyrrolidone
Adm.	IM, IV, SC
@	5-10 mg/kg B.wt
Pres.	30 ml, 100 ml

Vetran LA	Neospark
Comp	Oxytetracyclin hydrochloride 200 mg/ml + Aqueous 2 Pyrrolidone
Adm.	IM, IV, SC
@	5-10 mg/kg B.wt
Pres.	30 ml, 100 ml

Wolicyclin LA	Wockhardt
Comp	Oxytetracyclin hydrochloride 200 mg/ml + Aqueous 2 Pyrrolidone
Adm.	IM, IV, SC
@	5-10 mg/kg B.wt
Pres.	30 ml, 100 ml

Tetracyclin

It is broad spectrum antibiotic of group Tetracyclin and derived from Streptomyces. It is active against Gram+ve, Gram-ve Rickettsia, Streptomyces, large virus and certain blood protozoan affecting livestock. Acion is usually bacteriostatic by inhibiting Protein synthesis. It is indicated in all infections as oxytetracyclin.

Injectable

Streclin inj IM	Zydus Sarabhai
Comp	Tetracyclin 500 mg + Xylocain 200 mg, vit C 1500 mg Magnesium Chloride 35 mg
Adm.	IM
@	2-4 mg/kg b.wt for 2-3 days bid
Pres.	Vial

Other Dosage form of Tetracyclin/Oxytetracyclin

Alcyclin Bol	Alembic
Comp	Tetracyclin 500mg
Adm.	Oral, IU
@	4 Bol bid, 2-3 Bol IU
Pres.	Strip of 4 Bol
Pres.	Strip of 4 Bol.

Neocyclin Bol	**Intas**
Comp	Tetracyclin 500mg
Adm.	Oral, IU
@	4 Bol bid, 2-3 Bol IU
Pres.	Strip of 4 Bol

Steclin bol	**Zydus**
Comp	Tetracyclin 500mg
Adm.	Oral, IU
@	4 Bol bid, 2-3 Bol IU
Pres.	Strip of 4 Bol

Terramycin Liq	**Zydus (Pfizer)**
Comp	Oxytetracyclin hydrochloride 50 mg/ml
Adm.	Oral, IU topical
@	5-10 mg/kg B.wt 30 ml IU
Pres.	100 ml

Oxy Liquid	**Carevet Pharma**
Comp	Oxytetracyclin hydrochloride 50 mg/ml
Adm.	Oral, IU topical
@	5-10 mg/kg B.wt 30ml IU
Pres.	100 ml

Hostacyclin Powder	**Novartis (Hoechst)**
Comp	56 mg/g of Tetracyclin Pow
Adm.	Oral
@	1 g/3 kg B.wt
Pres.	30 g, 1 kg

Vetcillin Pow	**Zydus (Sarabhai)**
Comp	Tetracyclin hydrochloride 112 mg/g
Adm.	Oral
@	2.5 g/30 kg Preventive, 5 g/30 kg Treatment
Pres.	100 g

Amoly Bol	**Pranav**
Comp	Oxytetracycline hydrochloride 500 mg
Adm.	Oral, IU
@	10 mg/kg B.wt 4 Bol IU
Pres.	Strip of 4

Oxysure Tab	**Sterling**
Comp	Oxytetracycline hydrochloride 500 mg
Adm.	Oral, IU
@	10 mg/kg B.wt 4 Bol IU
Pres.	Strip of 4

Oxytra Tab	**HAL**
Comp	Oxytetracycline hydrochloride 500 mg
Adm.	Oral, IU
@	10 mg/kg B.wt 4 Bol IU
Pres.	Strip of 4

Tetrakal Bol	**KAPL**
Comp	Oxytetracycline hydrochloride 500 mg
Adm.	Oral, IU
@	10 mg/kg B.wt 4 Bol IU
Pres.	Strip of 4

Ultrox Tab	**Neospark**
Comp	Oxytetracycline hydrochloride 500 mg
Adm.	Oral, IU
@	10 mg/kg B.wt 4 Bol IU
Pres.	Strip of 4

Vetoxy	**Vets Farma**
Comp	Oxytetracycline hydrochloride 500 mg
Adm.	Oral, IU
@	10 mg/kg B.wt 4 Bol IU
Pres.	Strip of 4

Wolicyclin Tab	**Merial (Wockhardt)**
Comp	Oxytetracycline hydrochloride 500 mg
Adm.	Oral, IU
@	10 mg/kg B.wt 4 Bol IU
Pres.	Strip of 4

Terramycin Tab	**Zydus (Pfizer)**
Comp	Oxytetracycline hydrochloride 500 mg
Adm.	Oral, IU
@	10 mg/kg B.wt 4 Bol IU
Pres.	Strip of 4

Tetrakal Forte Bol	**KAPL**
Comp	Oxytetracycline hydrochloride 1000 mg
Adm.	Oral, IU
@	10 mg/kg B.wt 4 Bol IU
Pres.	Strip of 4

Tettra Bol	**Marc**
Comp	Oxytetracycline hydrochloride 1000 mg
Adm.	Oral, IU
@	10 mg/kg B.wt 4 Bol IU
Pres.	Strip of 4

Marbofloxacin

Marbodac/ Marbodac 16	**Zydus**
Adm.	IM
@	8-10 mg/kg B.wt
Pres.	30 ml

Antifungal Drugs

Fungal Infections/ Diseases

- Nuclear Directed Antifungal
- Cell membrance Directed Antifungal
  - Imidazoles
  - Clotrimazole
  - Fluconazole
  - Ketoconazole
  - Miconazole
- Cell wall Directed Antifungal
  - Amphotericin
  - Combination antifungals

Fungal Diseases

Aspergillosis: Caused by Aspergillosis species, a comman cause of abortion in cattle and mares, specially during 6th to 8th month of pregnancy. Infection occurs by inhaling spores from mouldy hay or straw.

Coccidomycosis: Found in all species but common in dogs and caused by Coccidiodes immitis.Infection occurs by inhalation of spores of fungus growing in soil and ingestion or through cutaneous abrasions Severe emaciation, fluctuating temperature odema of legs and anaemia, may be death due to rupture of liver.

Epizootic lymphangitis: Chronic Contagious disease of horses characterized by suppurative lymphangitis and ulcers of skin with or without Pneumonia. It is caused by Histoplasma farciminosum. Infection spreads through objects and cutaneous abrasions. In most cases lesions develop on limbs. Disease persist for 3-12 months Spontaneous recovery occurs and immunity after an attack is permanant.

Histoplasmosis: Caused by Histoplasma capsulatumEffected animals show chronic emaciation diarrhea, dyspnea, enlarged oedematous liver and thickening of large intestine can cause death.

Ring worm: Also called dermatomycosis Fungi grow on hair and skin with Trichophyton spp. in different animals. Lesions are heavy, grey white crust above skin roughly circular surface below crust. Lesions are mostly on neck, head or perineum region. These may be deep or superficial. There is no itching.

Rhinosporidiosis: Caused by Rhinosporidia secheriLesions Consist of small nodules to nasal Cavity mucosa. Dyspnea with mucoprulent nasal discharge, sometime blood stained from both nostrils. Abnormal respiratory sounds.

Sporotrichosis: Contagious disease of horses characterized by cutaneous nodules and ulcer on limbs may or may not be accompanied by lymphangitis. It is caused by Sporotrichum schencki Nodules are generally on lower part of legs and are painless, discharge a small amount of pus and heal in 3-4 weaks.

Nuclear directed Antifungal agent

These are fungistatic antibiotics. These disrupt mitotic spindle and interferes with polymerization of microtubular protein into microtubuler of dermatophytes. Therapy must be continued till shedding of infected area. It is terratoginic, so should be avoided in pregnants.

Griseofulvin

Grisovin FD	**Virbac**
Comp	Griseofulvin 250 mg, 500 mg
Adm.	Oral
@	LA 7.5-10 mg/kg B.wt for 30 days. SA 20 mg/kg B.wt for 3 days
Pres.	250 mg x 10 500 mg x10

Cell membrane directed Antifungal

These have multiple action on fungal cells. These are highly fungicidal at low concentration by inhibiting crgosterol synthesis of fungal cell membrance and changes its flucidity and barrier functions. At high concentration it can cause oxidation and damage the fungal cell. It is indicated in coccidoodomycosis, Blastomycosis.

Imidazoles

Cotrimazole

It is imidazole derivatine. It acts by inhibition of ergosterol synthesis. It is applied locally.

Myconil Pow	**Ranbaxy**
Comp	Clotrimazole 1%
Adm.	Apply locally
@	As per need
Pres.	100 g

Canesten Sol/ Cream	**Bayer**
Comp	Clotrimazole Sol 1% Cream 10 ml/g
Adm.	Local
@	As per need
Pres.	Sol 15 ml Cream 15 g tube

Imidil Pow/ Cream/ Sol	**Lyka**
Comp	Sol 1% Powder 1% Cream 1% of clotrimazole
Adm.	Local application
@	As per need
Pres.	Pow 30 g, Cream 15 g tube, Sol 15 ml

Fluconazole

It is imidazole derivative. It is fungistatic in action. It is indicated in Aspergillosis, Sporotrichasis. It is applied local for dermatophytosis and can be given orally.

Alfucoz Tab	**Sarabhai**
Comp	Fluconazole 200 mg
Adm.	Oral
@	5-10 mg/kg B.wt
Pres.	150 mg x 10, 100 mg x 10

Ketoconazole

It is imidiazole derivative. It inhibits ergosterol synthesis. It is indicated in coccidiomycosis, dermatomycosis, histoplasmosis etc. it is given orally. It is terratogenic so must be avoided in pregnants. It is hepatatoxic. It can be applied directly.

Sheen N Clean Lotion	**Venky's**
Comp	2% Ketoconazole
Adm.	Apply locally
@	As per need
Pres.	100 ml

Miconazole

It is imidazole derivative. Its action is to inhibit ergosterol synthesis. It is indicated in dermatomycosis or ringworm. It is applied locally.

Micogel Cream	**Cipla**
Comp	Miconazole 2%
Adm.	Local application
@	As per need
Pres.	15 g tube

Cell Wall directed antifungal agents

These are narrow spectrum in action and cause severe damage to the cell wall of fungal cell. These are under clinical evaluation and in development process.

Amphotericin B

These are Plyene antibiotics. These act on cell wall by inhibiting ergosterol synthesis. It is indicated in Histoplasmosis, Coccidiomycosis, blastomycosis and candidiasis. It should be diluted in dextrose 5% solution and infused IV. It is ineffective against ringworm if diluted. Side effect involve renal toxicity.

Fungizone IV inj	**Sarabhai**
Comp	Vial of 50 mg
Adm.	IV in dilution with 500 ml or of 5% Dextrose
@	1.8 mg/kg B.wt
Pres.	50 mg vial

Combination of Antifungal

Two antifungal compound were found to be very effective than used alone. So various combination of antifungal are used to treat fungal infection. Antifungals are also combined with other antimicrobial agents to enhance their action.

Conesten 3 cream	**Bayer**
Comp	Clotrimazol 10 mg/g Beclomethasone 0.25 mg/g
Adm.	Local application
@	As per need
Pres.	10 g tube

Spectrazole	**Ranbaxy**	
Comp	Miconazole nitrate Gentamicin Clobetasole	2% 0.1% 0.025%
Adm.	Local application	
@	As per need	
Pres.	20 g tube	

Tenovate M cream	**Virbac**
Comp	Miconazole 2% Clobetasole 0.05%
Adm.	Local application
@	As per need
Pres.	15 g tube

Indigenous

Anbioflam Pow	**Indian Herbs**
Comp	Not given
Adm.	Oral as supportive in skin diseases
@	LA 2 g/100 kg B.wt
Pres.	500 g

Charmaid Cap	Ayurvet
Comp	Not given
Adm.	Oral
@	Upto 10kg body weight 1 Cap od above 10kg B.wt 2 Cap od
Pres.	30's

Teeburb Cap	Natural Remedies
Comp	Not given
Adm.	Oral
@	LA 2 Cap bid SA 1 Cap bid
Pres.	24's

Antiviral

Viral Diseases

African Horse Sickness: Signs are intermittent fever 105-106 0 F in pulmonary or cardic form. Laboured breathing, coughing mucus with bluish oral mucosa and oedema in head region are prominent signs. Death is there within 4-5 days

African Swine Fever: High fever persists with other signs marked cyanotic clotching of skin, anorexia, depression, weakness and incoordination.

Blue Tongue: It appears with Catarrhal stomatitis, rhinitis, enteritis and lameness due to inflammation of coronary band and sensitive laminae of feet

Cow pox: (Pox disease) Appearance of typical lesions of pox on teats, udder. Fever, pinpoint red spots, papules of mustard size are signs.

Enzootic Pneumonia: Dry cough, transient diarrhea, sneezing and retardation of growth. There can be pneumonia

Ephemeral fever: Inflammation of mesodermal tissues evidenced by muscular severity, stiffness and lameness with enlargement of lymph nodes

Foot and Mouth disease: Acute disease of clone feeted animals and is characterised by fever and vesicular eruption in mouth and feet. Vesicles may be seen on teats, tongue and dental pad. Abortion and infertility may be sequalae

Infectious Bovine Rhinotracheitis: There is fever, nasal and ocular discharge, abortion and a relatively short course and high recovery rate

Malignant catarrhal fever: Highly fatal characterised by development of catarrhal inflammation of upper respiratory tract and alimentry epithelium and enlargement of lymph nodes

Papillomatosis: Warts or solid outgrowth of epidermis may be sessible or pedunculated

Rabies: Highly fatal infection of central Nervous System characterised by motor irritation with signs of mania, central ascending paralysis

Rinderpest: It is characterised by high fever, local erosive lesions confined largely by to the mucosa of alimentary tract. Disease is very fatal

Vesicular stomatitis: There is development of vesicles in mouth and feet there is salivation. Recovery is rapid.

Miscellaneous Diseases

Contagious agalactia: It's fungal disease caused by Mycoplasma agalactia characterised by mastitis ophthalamitis, arthritis with painful swelling of affected joints

Contagious Bovine Pleuro preumonia: It's fungal disease caused by Mycoplasma spp. Characterised by focalisation of lungs and pleura. In goats it is called contagious caprine pleuro pneumonia.

Dengue or three days sickness: It is caused by moderate infections

Enzootic abortion: A chlamydial disease in which there is abortion in sheep and goats caused by Chlamydia psittaci

Kerato conjunctivitis: Caused by Mycoplasma conjunctiva and Chlamydia ovis. It is characterised by loss of body condition and blindness. Lot of tear spills over face. Pink eye or redness of cornea followed by thick mucopurulant discharge with sticky eyes

Mycotoxicosis: (Aflatoxicosis) Caused by member of fungi produced mycotoxins, toxic metabolites. Their consumption can lead to deaths in zero grazing. It is characterised by hydropericardium local heamorrhages, necrosis of kidney, hyperplasia of mammany epithelium. Milk production and reproduction is affected. There can be acute nervous signs depending on the type of mycotoxins. It is also known as Degnala disease caused by specially exclusively feeding of paddy straw. Skin lesions alopecia, scales, cracking of skin and ulcerative wounds are also there

Peste des petits ruminitis: (PPR) It is found in sheep and goats. Dull animals with high rise of temperature, rhinitis, pharyngitis and entero-colitis, arched back, mucopurulant, nasal and eye discharge. There can be severe diarrhea, weakness, depression and death. It is misunderstood as Rinderpest. It is a viral and called Goat Plague.

Spirotrichosis: Caused by Spirotrichium schenkiand characterised by development of cutaneous nodules and ulcers on the limbs associated with or not lymphangitis

Tickborn fever: It is caused by Rickettsia bovina and characterised by high lethargy, polyponea. Animal may abort in last trimester of pregnancy.

Protozoan Diseases

Protozoa are single celled organisms found in blood, rumen, genital tract, intestine etc. These lead to specific infection and disease.

Anaplasmosis: It is also known as Gall sickness. It is caused by Anaplasma marginale in cattle, sheep and goats. It is transmitted by ticks. Acutely effected animals loose condition rapidly Breathlessness, fall in milk production and loss of co-ordination are main symptoms. Urine may become brown. Fever is very high about 106°F Mucous membrance becomes pale. Pregnants may abort. Death may occur due to anaemia and jaundice.

Babesiosis: It is caused by Babesia bigemina in domestic and wild animals. Ticks transmit the disease. First sign is fever 41°C or higher accompanied with inappetence, increased respiration, anemia, Jaundice, loss of weight and finally haemoglobinurea. There may be diarrhea or constipation Pregnants may abort. Babesia are also known as Piroplasma and infection is known as Piroplasmosis.

Coccidiosis: It is contagious enteritis caused by infection with Eimeria species. It occurs in all domestic animals. It is characterised by diarrhea, dysentery, anaemia and emaciation. Source of infection is ingestion of contaminated feces causative protozoa are:

Cattle: Eimeria bovis, E.elliapsaidalis, E.zurnii

Sheep: E.arloingi, E.absata

Pigl: E.debliecki, E.perminuta, E.scabra

Horses: E.lecikarti

Filariasis: Filaria cause intrammscular or subcutaneous or cutaneous lesions in domestic animals. There may be nodules which ulcerate, bleed, heal and disappear spontaneously usually in summer infected by flies Parafilaria bovicola or P.multipapillosa are cause of infection in cattle.

Schistosomiasis: Also known as Nasal granuloma of cattle caused by Schistosoma nasalis. Most common affected animals are between 6 months to 4 years of age. Granulomatous nodules of 1-4mm in diameter and height grow first from inside of nostrils. Sometime mucopurulent with blood discharges. Respiratory distress caused by obstruction of air flow leads to loss of body conditions and reduction in milk.

Theileriasis: It is caused by Theileria parva and T.annulata. It is transmitted by ticks. Temperature of animal goes very high upto 42°C or more through out the course of infection. Lymphnode swelling becomes pronounced and generialised. There is anorexia, loss of condition, nasal discharge and lacrimation. There is fall in temperature before death. Animals that recover are immune to subsequent challenge with same strain.

Toxoplasmosis: It is contagious disease of all species including man. Causal protozoan is Toxoplasma gondi and transmitted mainly by ingestion. It is characterised by encephalitis when infection is common. There is fever, dyspnea, coughing, sneezing and nasal discharge with grinding of teeth. There are tremors of head and neck.

Trichomoniasis: Trichomonas foetus is cansative organism. It's venereal disease that leads to infertility but also cause abortion in first half of gestation. Foetus does not show any special lesions.

Trypanosomiasis: There are various species of Trypanosome which affect all domestic animal. Major species are Trypanosoms congolense, T.vivax, T.brucei, T.simae. These are transmitted by tosetsefly. There is fever, anaemia, weight loss, mortality (if poor nutrition) Surra is another form of Trypansomiasis caused by T.evansi. It is mostly in camels and horses but other animals are also susceptible with all above symptoms.These is fever, circling of animal and even death if not treated.

Antiprotozoans

These are the agents to treat protozoan disease. To control protozoan disease specific antiprotozoans are used.

Antiamoebiasis/ Antiflagellate

Nitromidazole

A group of antibiotic like compound. It is antiprotozoal and antibacterial.

Tinidozole

It is active against intestinal amoebiasis giardiasis, trichomoniasis, gingivitis and anaerobic bacterial infection. It is used orally and IU. It affects DNA in the pathogen.

(Refer Antimicrobial)

Metronidazole

Its activity is as good as Tinidazole. It can be given orally and IV.

(Refer Antimicrobial)

Nitrofurans

Refer Antibiotics

Tetracyclins

Refer Antibiotics

Antihaemoprotozoan

Buparvaquone

It is active against both schizont and piroplasmal stages of Theileria spp.

Butalex inj	**Zydus**
Comp	Buparvaquone 50 mg/ml
Indi	Theileriasis
Adm.	IV or SC
@	2.5 mg/kg B.wt
Pres.	20 ml

Bupalet inj	**Alivira 305**
Comp	Buparvaquone 50 mg/ml
Adm.	IM
@	1ml/20 kg B.wt
Pres.	30 ml

Butazyd inj	**Zydus**
Ind	Theilariasis
Comp	Buparvaquone 50 mg/ml
Adm.	IM
@	2.5 mg/kg B.wt or 1 ml/20 kg B.wt
Pres.	20 ml

Diminazine aceturate

It is potent babesicidal and trypanocidal. Total dose should not be more than 9 g/ animal in a day. Contraindicated in Camels.

Berenil inj	**Novartis**
Comp	0.444 g/g Diminazine aceturate
Indi	Babesiasis, Trypanosomiasis
Adm.	IM
@	0.8-1.6/100 kg B.wt
Pres.	5g m, 22.5 g granules 20 ml (70 mg/ml)

Dimaze inj	**Merial**
Comp	0.444 g/g Diminazine aceturate
Indi	Babesiasis, Trypanosomiasis

Adm.	IM
@	0.8-1.6/100 kg B.wt
Pres.	5 gm

Pronil-4	**Wockhardt**
Comp	0.444 g/g Diminazine aceturate
Indi	Babesiasis, Trypanosomiasis
Adm.	IM
@	0.8-1.6/100 kg B.wt
Pres.	4.8 g

Diminagal inj	**G. Loucatos**
Comp	Diaceturate 70 mg with Phenazone 375 mg in 1ml
Indi	Babesiasis, Trypanosomiasis
Adm.	IM
@	5 ml/100 kg B.wt
Pres.	20 ml, 30 ml

Nilbery inj	**Intas**
Comp	Diaceturate 70 mg with Phenazone 375 mg in 1ml
Indi	Babesiasis, Trypanosomiasis
Adm.	IM
@	5 ml/100 kg B.wt
Pres.	30 ml, 90 ml

Prozomin inj	**Virbac**
Comp	Diacetruate 70 mg with Phenazone 375 mg in 1ml
Indi	Babesiasis, Trypanosomiasis
Adm.	IM
@	5 ml/100 kg B.wt
Pres.	30 ml

Trityl granule	**Lyka**
Comp	Diaceturate 70 mg with Phenazone 375 mg in 1ml
Indi	Babesiasis, Trypanosomiasis

Adm.	IM
@	5 ml/100 kg B.wt
Pres.	5 g, 23.6 g

Sequene RTO inj	**Alivira**	
Comp	Diminazene diaceturate	70 mg/ml
	Phenazone	375 mg/ml
Adm.	IM	
@	3.5 mg/kg B.wt	
Pres.	30 ml, 90 ml	

Other

Babimido inj	**Zydus**
Ind	Babesiosis
Comp	Imidocarb dipropionate 120 mg/ml
Adm.	IM/SC
@	1 ml/100 kg B.wt Bevention 2.5 ml/100 kg B.wt (Effect upto 2 months)
Pres.	5 gm, 22.5 g granules 20 ml (70 mg/ml)

Lithium Antimony Thiomalate

It is an organic compound which is effectives in the therapy of nasal granuloma, papilomatosis and haemoprotozoan conditions.

Anthiomoline	**M and B**
Comp	6% Lithium antimony
Indi	Nasal granuloma
Adm.	IM
@	LA 15-30 ml repeated on alternate days SA 10-15 ml in a week
Pres.	50 ml

Lithomany	**Indian Immunology**
Comp	6% Lithium antimony
Indi	Nasal granuloma
Adm.	IM
@	LA 15-30 ml repeated on alternate days SA 10-15 ml in a week
Pres.	50 ml

Quinapyramine

It is haemoprotozoal agent Quinapyramine salts (Sulphate and chloride), inhibit the growth and cell divison of haemoprotozoa. It is used against Trypanosomiasis and Surra. There can be salivation restlessness and muscular tremors overdose may cause trembling also.

Antrycide Prosalt	**Virbac**
Comp	Quinapyramine sulphate 1.5 g Quinapyramine chloride 1 g vial
Indi	Trypanasomiasis and Surra
Adm.	SC
@	2.5 ml/100 kg B.wt after adding 15 ml of sterile water
Pres.	2.5 g vial

Corridan	**HAL**
Comp	Quinapyramine sulphate 1.5 g Quinapyramine chloride 1 g vial
Indi	Trypanasomiasis and Surra
Adm.	SC
@	2.5 ml/100 kg B.wt after adding 15 ml of sterile water
Pres.	2.5 g vial

Dyequin	**Marc**
Comp	Quinapyramine sulphate 1.5 g Quinapyramine chloride 1 g vial
Indi	Trypanasomiasis and Surra
Adm.	SC
@	2.5 ml/100 kg B.wt after adding 15 ml of sterile water
Pres.	2.5 g vial

Triquin	**Merial (Wockhardt)**
Comp	Quinapyramine sulphate 1.5 g Quinapyramine chloride 1 g vial
Indi	Trypanasomiasis and Surra
Adm.	SC
@	2.5 ml/100 kg B.wt after adding 15 ml of sterile water
Pres.	2.5 g vial

Teevansi	Zydus (Ranbaxy)
Comp	Quinapyramine sulphate 1.5 g Quinapyramine chloride 1 g vial
Indi	Trypanasomiasis and Surra
Adm.	SC
@	2.5 ml/100 kg B.wt after adding 15 ml of sterile water
Pres.	2.5 g vial

Triquin S	Merial (Wockhardt)
Comp	Quinapyramine sulphate 2g/vial
Indi	Surra
Adm.	SC
@	2.5 ml/100 kg B.wt after adding 15 ml of sterile water
Pres.	2 g

Babesan inj	ICI-Virbac
Comp	Q. Sulphate 0.5% or 5%
Indi	Babesiasis
Adm.	SC
@	1 ml 5% sol /50 kg B.wt SA 2-4 ml 0.5%
Pres.	0.5%-10 ml 5% 6 ml

Suramin

It is antihaemoprotozoan. It has potent trypanocidal action. It is used for Surra and Trypanosomiasis. Subcutaneously, can be used for prevention therapy. Local reaction may occur with IM inj.

Gilpol inj	G. Loucotos
Comp	IG Suramin sod
Indi	Preventive surra
Adm.	SC or IM
@	0.5 g/45 kg B.wt for treatment IV
Pres.	25 g.

Nagnol inj	**Bayer**
Comp	IG Suramin Sod
Adm.	SC or IM
@	IG/100 kg B.wt Camels 5 g for adult
Pres.	2.5 g.

Coccidiostats/ Sulfonamides

Coccidiostats

(SULPHAS refer under Antibiotics)

Dihydrofolate Reluctass Agents.

Trimethoprim, Pyrimethamine, ormethoprim are several agents. Thse are diamino pyrimidine derivatives. It selectively inhibits bacterial dihydrofolate reductase are, in combination with Sulphamethaxazole (1969) as cotrimoxazole.

Refer Antibiotic

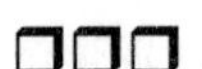

Cardio Vascular System

Disease/ Terms Related to Cardiovascular System

Adenitis: Inflammation of glands.

Anaemia: Deficiency of Haemoglobin concentration per unit volume of blood.

Angina Pectoris: A syndrome characterised by pain below sternum on exertion or excitement caused by ischaemia of heart muscles usually due to coronary artery disease.

Arrhythmia: Rhythmical variation in heart rate.

Arterial Thrombosis: Thrombosis formation due to arteritis.

Arteritis: Inflammation of arteries.

Bradycardia: Normal heart action at a reduced rate.

Endrocarditis: Inflammation of endocardium of heart.

Epistaxis: Bleeding form nose.

Hematoma: Swelling containing blood.

Haemorrhage: Bleeding or rapid loss of blood.

Leucopenia: Reduction in number of leucocytes and resistance is reduced.

Leukemia: Increased number of lymphocytes circulating in blood with enlargement of lymph-nodes and progressive loss of condition. It is a form of cancer.

Lymphangitis: Inflammation and enlargement of lymph vessels.

Myocardial Asthenia: Decreased power of contraction of heart.

Myocarditis: Inflammation of myocardium of heart.

Oedema: Excessive accumulation of fluid in tissue spaces characterised by swelling of area. It can be in subcutaneous tissue.

Pericarditis: Inflammation of pericardium of heart.

Pus: Thick often yellowish fluid found in abcesses and on surface of ulcers and inflamed area where skin is broken.

Septicaemia (or Viraemia): Condition compounded with pyrexia, toxaemia and presence of large number of infectious agents like bacteria, virus and blood protozoa.

Shock: Peripheral circulatory failure without evidence of blood loss after trauma, sub normal temperature cold body with weak pulse and heart rate.

Tachycardia: Increased heart rate.

Thrombosis: Clot formation in heart or blood vessels.

Toxaemia: Presence of toxins in the blood stream.

Venous Thrombosis: Formation of thrombosis due to development of Vein thrombin.

Hematinics / Antianaemic

Anaemia is regarded as an important clinical sign indicative of an underlying pathophysiological process. Agents used to treat or control anaemia are known as antianaemics or haematinics. Anaemia is inadequate red blood cell mass and is a secondary condition in diseases and not a primary disease. Haematinics should be used depending upon the identification of etiologic factors.

It can be:-

(a) Blood loss from intravascular space.

(b) Impaired RBC formation due to bone marrow depression (hypoplastic anaemia) deficiency of essential factors i.e. iron, vit B12, Folic acid and Copper.

(c) Increased destruction of RBC (hemolytic).

Iron Preparations

Therapeutic use of Iron is indicated in certain situations for prevention of iron deficiencies. For oral administration Ferrous salts are believed to be absorbed more efficiently in most species. Ferrous sulphate and other iron salts are commercially available under a variety of trade names. All contain iron and other haematinic drugs. These can be given during pregnancy or in heavy worm infestation showing PICA etc.

Ferrous Sulphate Pow	**Generic**
Comp	Ferrous sulphate
Adm.	Oral
@	LA 8-15 g od, SA 0.5-2 g od for 2 weeks
Pres.	100 g, 450 g

Haematic Powder	**Generic**	
Comp	5 g contains	
	Dried Ferrous sulphate	4.5 g
	Copper sulphate	300 mg
	Magnesium sulphate	100 mg
	Cobalt sulphate	100 mg
Adm.	Oral	
@	LA 8-15 g bid, SA ½ -1 g bid	
Pres.	20 g, 100 g	

Imferon inj	Intas
Comp	Iron dextran providing 50 mg/ml of elemental iron
Adm.	IM
@	LA 0.5-1 mg/kg B.wt or ½ -1 ml/50 kg B.wt
Pres.	10 ml

Macferon inj	Macwell
Comp	Iron dextran providing 50 mg/ml of elemental iron
Adm.	IM
@	LA 0.5-1 mg/kg B.wt or ½ -1 ml/50 kg B.wt
Pres.	10 ml

Copper Preprations

Microcytic anaemia similar to that seen with dietary deficiency can be due to copper deficiency. Sustained release methods of copper administration provide longer time protection against copper deficiency with greater margin of safety. It is indicated in haemoglobinuria and haemoprotozoan infections to prevent anaemia.

Curan inj	Carevet Pharma
Comp	Copper glycinate 75 mg/ml
Adm.	S/C
@	0.5 mg/kg B.wt (Sufficient for 60 days)
Pres.	2 ml, 20 ml

Curan BH	Carevet Pharma
Comp	Copper glycinate 500 mg
Adm.	IV with normal saline
@	LA single dose of 500 mg
Pres.	500 mg vial

Others

Feritas Bol / Inj	Intas
Comp	Bolus-Ferrous fumerate 1500 mg, Vit B_{12} 75 mcg, Folic acid 7500 mcg Inj-Iron sorbitol citric acid complex equal to Iron 50 mg, Folic acid 500 mcg, hydroxycobalamine acetale equal to 50 mcg of hydroxycobalamine per ml

Adm.	Inj IM, Bol orally
@	LA 1 ml/50 kg B.wt and 2 Bol bid
Pres.	10 ml inj, 5 Bol strip

Ferrocom	**Indian Herbs**
Comp	Not given
Adm.	Oral
@	LA 2 g/100 kg B.wt
Pres.	10 g

Anticoagulants

These are agents used to prevent clotting of blood for diagnostic use or transfusion in vitro and prevent development of thrombi in vitro. A variety of chemicals are used to prevent coagulation of shed blood in vitro Systemic anticoagulants are used therapeutically for the prevention of enlargement of thrombi.

Heparin

It is a powerful and instantaneously acting anticoagulant effective both invitro and in vivo. It acts indirectly by activating plasma antithrombin. It is indicated in thromboembolic conditions, prophylaxis of deep vein effects like transient and reversible alopecia.

Beparine inj	**Baif**
Comp	Heparin Sodium 500 IU/ml
Adm.	SC
@	25-100 IU/kg B.wt (IM use is contraindicated)
Pres.	5 ml

Antihaemorrhagic/ Haemostatics

These are used to prevent bleeding or control of haemorrhage.Several substances are used to provide help in control of bleeding. Some topical haemostatics are available for human use. It is indicated in Mastitis where blood is mixed with milk.

Adrenaline

It belongs to class catecholomine. It is potent Vasconstrictor of cutaneous and muscular blood vessels. It is indicated in animals in haemorrhage and epistaxis. It is potent alpha agonist with a presser action or smaller arterioles and precapillary sphincters.

Adrenaline inj	Generic
Comp	1.819 mg/ml of Adrenaline tartarate (1:1000 solution)
Adm.	IV or SC
@	LA 2-4 ml IV, 2-8 ml SC, SA 0.1-0.3 ml IV or 0.1-0.5 ml SC
Pres.	10 ml

Adrenuchrome Monosemi Carbazone

It is a systemic haemostatic. It is an epinephrine oxidation product which reduces capillary fragibity effecting haemostatic action. It is indicated in pre and post operative haemorrhages and haemorrhages of various origin. Hypersensitivity reaction may be seen.

Adchrome inj	G Loucatos
Comp	5 mg Adrenochrome per ml
Adm.	IV or IM
@	20-25 mg total
Pres.	10 ml

Stytichrome	Dr. Reddy
Comp	750 mcg/ Adrenochsome
Adm.	20-25 mg total
@	IV or IM
Pres.	2 ml

Etamsylate

It acts by stimulating thromhopoiesis and their release from bone marrow. It stabilizes capillaries and encourages vaso constriction.

Maclote inj	Macnor
Comp	125 mg/ ml of Etamsylate
Adm.	IM or IV
@	6-8 mg/kg B.wt or 20-30 ml for large animal.
Pres.	30 ml, 100 ml

Clotex inj	**PAIL**
Comp	125 mg/ ml of Etamsylate
Adm.	IM or IV
@	6-8 mg/kg B.wt or 20-30 ml for large animal.
Pres.	30 ml, 100 ml

Wesclote inj	**Wesfa pharma**
Comp	Etamsylate 125 mg/ml
Adm.	IM/ IV
@	5-10 mg/kg B.wt for 2.3 days
Pres.	30 ml

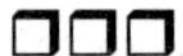

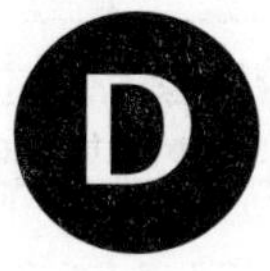

Central Nervous System

Disease/ Terms Related to Nervous System

Anxiety: Feeling of apprehension, uncertainity and fear without apparent stimulus.

Cerebral Anoxia: When the supply of oxygen to brain is reduced. Initially there are signs of irritation followed terminally by signs of loss of function.

Circling Disease of Sheep: It is a symptom of Gid, encephalitis or enterotoxaemia.

Coma: Sate of unconsciousness.

Convulsions: Widespread spasms involving whole body.

Diplegia: Extensive paralysis of both sides of body.

Distress: Physical or mental anguish or suffering.

Dummy Syndrome: Animals remain standing, able to move but does not respond all external stimuli.

Encephalitis: Inflammation of brain.

Encephalomalacia: Softening of brain with neurosis of grey matter.

Gid: Also called coenurosis caused by development of cyst in brain or spinal cord which are intermediate host of Taenia mulitceps a dog, parasite. Fever, blindness, ataxia, muscle tremors, excitement and collapse are the symptoms.

Grass Tetany: Tetany, convulsions, reduced milk and death caused due to disturbed calcium & magnesium ratio in blood.

Hydrocephalus: Increase in intracranial pressure. Irritation, signs of mania head pressing muscle and convulsions occur.

Meningitis: Inflammation of meninges of brain/spinal cord.

Myelitis: Inflammation of spinal cord

Neuralgia: Sharp pain alongwith the course of nerve.

Paralysis: Physiological and result in all cases of motor nerve injury with loss of voluntary movement.

Paraplegia: Paralysis of hind limbs characterised by staggering gait, incoordination of movements of hind legs. General prostration.

Paresis: Incomplete immobility of muscles.

Anaesthetics

Anaesthesia is a Greek word which means insensible or without feeling not loss of consciousness.

Anaesthesiology is defined as the art and science of administration of anaesthesia. The role of anaesthesia is to minimize or eliminate pain, relax muscles and facilitate patient restrain during surgical, obstetrical and other diagnostic & therapeutic procedures. It also helps to monitor and support life function during operative period or critically ill or injured.

Anaesthesia can be local or regional i.e., when desensitize a localized or regional area of body.

Local Anaesthesia

Lidocaine (Lignocaine)

It is versatile anaesthetic and good for both for surface application as well as injection. It blocks conditions within three minutes. Anaesthesia is more intense and long lasting. Side effect of blurred vision tremors, convulsions and respiratory arrest.

Gesicaine	**Zydus (Sarabhai)**
Comp	Lignocaine 2%
Indi	Epidural, Spinal, regional anaesthesia. Topically useful in pain and itching due to insect bite or fissures.
Adm.	Local or IM route, SC route Epidural
@	As per need and body weight for epidural
Pres.	30 ml

Novocaine	**Novartis (Hoechst)**
Comp	Lignocaine 2%
Indi	Epidural, Spinal, regional anaesthesia. Topically useful in pain and itching due to insect bite or fissures.
Adm.	Local or IM route, SC route Epidural
@	As per need and body weight for epidural
Pres.	30 ml, 100 ml

Xylocaine	**Astral IDL**
Comp	Lignocaine 2%
Indi	Epidural, Spinal, regional anaesthesia. Topically useful in pain and itching due to insect bite or fissures.

Adm.	Local or IM route, SC route Epidural
@	As per need and body weight for epidural
Pres.	30 ml

Plainocaine	**Primavet**
Comp	Lignocaine 2%
Indi	Epidural, Spinal, regional anaesthesia. Topically useful in pain and itching due to insect bite or fissures.
Adm.	Local or IM route, SC route Epidural
@	As per need and body weight for epidural
Pres.	20 ml

Xylocaine with Adrenaline	**Astral IDL**	
Comp	Lignocaine hydrochloride Adrenaline bitartrate Sodium chloride	21.3 mg 5 mcg 6 mg/ml
Indi	Anaesthesia	
Adm.	Local or IM route, SC route Epidural	
@	As per need and body weight for epidural	
Pres.	30 ml	

Bupivacaine

It is long acting and used for obstetric epidural block. It has slow onset of action app. 30 minutes to effect. There can be CNS depression, cardiac effect, allergy, rashes or oedema as side effects.

Marcain	**Sarabhai**
Comp	Bupivacaine hydrochloride 5 mg/ml
Indi	Epidural anaesthesia in prolapse or in surgical operation to block hind region
Adm.	Local infilteration & epidural
@	As per need
Pres.	20 ml

Sensorcaine	**Astral IDL**
Comp	Bupivacaine hydrochloride 5mg/ml
Indi	Epidural anaesthesia in prolapse or in surgical operation to block hind region

Adm.	Local infilteration & epidural
@	As per need
Pres.	20 ml

General Anaesthesia

General Anaesthesia: In which CNS depression is controlled and is reversible. It is induced by one or two methods. In this there is loss of all sensation, unconsciousness and muscle relaxation with abolition of reflexes.

There are various stages of General Anaesthesia:

(i) Stage of analgesia: Beginning of anaesthetic action and lasts upto loss of consciousness.

(ii) Delirium stage: From loss of consciousness to beginning of regular respiration, jaws are lightly closed, pupil dilates.

(iii) Surgical stage: Extends from onset of regular respiration to cessation of spontaneous breathing.

These are the derivatives of Barbituric acid (Malonyl urea) result from the compensation of malonic acid and urea. These are of 2 types:

(a) **Oxybarbiturates:** It is hygroscopic and decomposes on exposure to light white in colour.

(b) **Thiobarbiturates:** It is yellow in colour and contains Sulphur. These also effect transmission of automatic neuro effctor junction. These are short acting and long acting. Long acting are Phenobarbital sodium and Barbital sodium. Where as short acting are Thiopentone sodium

Thiopentone Sodium

It is ultra short barbiturate, highly soluble in water which should be prepared fresh before injection.

Intraval Sod inj	**Primavet**
Comp	Thiopentone sod 50 mg vial, 1 g vial
Adm.	IV
@	LA 10-5 mg/kg B.wt SA 10 mg/kg B.wt
Pres.	50 mg, 1g

Ketamine

It produces anaesthesia called dissociative anaesthesia profound analgesia, immobility and feeling of dissociation from one's own body and surroundings. Respiration is not depressed. Reflexes are not abolished and muscle tone increases due to sympathetic stimulation. Heart rate and cardiac output are elevated overdose may cause respiratory depression, Anorexia nausea and vomiting

Ketamine Inj.	Generic
Comp	Ketamine hydrochloride 10 mg/ml, 20 mg/ml
Indi	Surgical operation in head and neck, patients which had excessive bleeding and for short duration surgery.
Adm.	IM, IV, SC
@	LA 2.2 mg/kg B.wt SA 22-44 mg/kg B.wt
Pres.	10 ml, 30 ml

Anticonvulsants

Convulsions are periodic and un-predictable occurrence of seizures in epilepsy. seizure is transient alteration of behavior due to various reasons. Tetanic convulsions occur in tetanus or Strychrine poisoning. Some diseases also cause convulsions. Drugs used to control such convulsions and overcome excitement of CNS are known as anticonvulsants. These are used for treating epilepsy. It is suitable for use either alone or in combination with other anti convulsants since the origins of convulsion is in the brain. These have psychotropic action by producing CNS depression in the brain and blocking the reflexes.

Diazepam

It is a Benzodizepam derivative. It acts on CNS by blocking the spiral polysynaptic reflexes. It has sedative tranquilizing effects.

Calmpose inj / Tab	Ranbaxy
Comp	Diazepam 10 mg/ml/ 5 mg, 10 mg Tab
Indi	Sedative, Anticonsvulsant
Adm.	Inj. IV – Oral tablet
@	LA 0.1-0.2 mg/kg B.wt Horses 80 mg/ animal
Pres.	2 ml, 10 Tab Strip

Antihistamins /Autocoids

Substances classed as autocoids are histamines, serotonins. These are released by the cells initiated by variety of stressful stimuli including anaphylaxis, allergy, different drugs, chemicals or physical injury. With the release of histamine antigen antibody reactions are evoked in the body leading to physiological manifestations of such reactions e.g. itching, rashes, urticarial, muscle contraction, edema, bronchial constriction, laryngeal edema, nausea, vomiting etc allergic like symptoms. Anti allergic or antihistaminic drugs have property of antagonizing histamine by blocking histamine receptors.

Chlorpheniramine maleate

It is antihistamine and also provides soothing effect. It is generally called CPM.

Anistamin inj	**Intas**
Comp	Chlorpheniramine maleate 10 mg/ml
Adm.	IM
@	3-5 ml IM, 0.5-1 ml SA
Pres.	10 ml, 30 ml, 50 ml

Anthisan inj	**Primavet**
Comp	Chlorpheniramine maleate 10 mg/ml
Adm.	IM
@	3-5 ml I M, 0.5-1 ml SA
Pres.	30 ml

Baifonil inj	**Baif**
Comp	Chlorpheniramine maleate 10mg/ml
Adm.	IM
@	3-5 ml I M, 0.5-1 ml SA
Pres.	10 ml, 30 ml

Cadistin inj	**Zydus**
Comp	Chlorpheniramine maleate 10 mg/ml
Adm.	IM
@	3-5 ml IM, 0.5-1 ml SA
Pres.	10 ml, 30 ml

Catalon inj	**Cattle Remedies**
Comp	Chlorpheniramine maleate 10 mg/ml
Adm.	IM
@	3-5 ml IM, 0.5-1 ml SA
Pres.	10 ml, 30 ml

Chlorazin inj	**Ranbaxy**
Comp	Chlorpheniramine maleate 10 mg/ml
Adm.	IM
@	3-5 ml IM, 0.5-1 ml SA
Pres.	10 ml, 30 ml

Chloril inj	**TTK**
Comp	Chlorpheniramine maleate 10 mg/ml
Adm.	IM
@	3-5 ml IM, 0.5-1 ml SA
Pres.	10 ml, 30 ml,100 ml

Chlor pheniramine maleate inj	Sushima
Comp	Chlorpheniramine maleate 10 mg/ml
Adm.	IM
@	3-5 ml IM, 0.5-1 ml SA
Pres.	10 ml, 30 ml

Cural inj	Wockhardt
Comp	Chlorpheniramine maleate 10 mg/ml
Adm.	IM
@	3-5 ml IM, 0.5-1 ml SA
Pres.	10 ml, 30 ml

Histal inj	Cargill
Comp	Chlorpheniramine maleate 10 mg/ml
Adm.	IM
@	3-5 ml IM, 0.5-1 ml SA
Pres.	30 ml

Lorfen inj	Vets Farma
Comp	Chlorpheniramine maleate 10 mg/ml
Adm.	IM
@	3-5 ml IM, 0.5-1 ml SA
Pres.	30 ml

Vetistin DS	Carevet Pharma
Comp	Chloropheniramine maleate 20 mg/ml
Adm.	IM
@	LA 3-5 ml SA 0.3-0.5 ml 1 mg/kg B.wt
Pres.	30 ml

Zoet	Alembic
Comp	Chloropheniramine maleate 20 mg/ml
Adm.	IM
@	LA 3-5 ml SA 0.3-0.5 ml 1 mg/kg B.wt
Pres.	10 ml

Alervil	Marc
Comp	Chlorpheniramine maleate 10 mg/ml
Adm.	IM
@	3-5 ml IM, 0.5-1 ml SA
Pres.	10 ml, 30 ml

Avil	**Hoechst**
Comp	Chlorpheniramine maleate 10 mg/ml
Adm.	IM
@	3-5 ml IM, 0.5-1 ml SA
Pres.	10 ml, 30 ml

Cadistin	**Cadila Health**
Comp	Chlorpheniramine maleate 10 mg/ml
Adm.	IM
@	3-5 ml IM, 0.5-1 ml SA
Pres.	10 ml, 30 ml

Hisloc	**Cadila Pharma**
Comp	Chlorpheniramine maleate 10 mg/ml
Adm.	IM
@	3-5 ml IM, 0.5-1 ml SA
Pres.	10 ml, 30 ml

Neohista	**Wellcone**
Comp	Chlorpheniramine maleate 10 mg/ml
Adm.	IM
@	3-5 ml IM, 0.5-1ml SA
Pres.	10 ml, 30 ml

Weschlorm	**Wesfa pharma**
Comp	Chlorpheniramine maleate 10 mg/ml
Adm.	IM/ SC
@	1ml/50 kg B.wt
Pres.	100 ml

Chlorazin	**Zydus**
Comp	Chlorpheniramine inalcate 10 gm/ml
Adm.	IM
@	LA 3-5 ml SA 0.502 ml
Pres.	100 ml

Halopyramine Hydrochloride

Synistamin	**Sarabhai**
Comp	Halopyramine hydrochloride 10 mg/ml
Adm.	IM

@	LA 4-10 ml SA 0.5-1 ml
Pres.	2 ml

Mepyramine Maleate

It in given is conditions associated in acute nature. In conjunction with antibacterial treatment it has a place in the treatment of acute infections.

Anthisan	**M & B**
Comp	Mephyramine Maleate 2.5% sol, 5% sol
Adm.	IM
@	LA 10-30 ml SA 5-10 ml
Pres.	10 ml, 2.5%-2 ml

Pheniramine Maleate

This gives quick relief from allergic condition. It is used for its potent, rapid and prolonged antihistaminic action as well as for its excellent tolerance. It is indicated in seasonal allergic condition itching due to eczema, dermititis, rhinitis, drug rashes, anaphylactic shocks. It is also recommended in all inflammatory conditions where histamine is liberated due to tissue damage. It is symptomatic treatment and is helpful as a supportive treatment. This eliminates specific or contributing etiological factors.

Pheniramine Maleate	**Novartis**
Comp	Pheniramine Maleate 22.75 mg/ml
Adm.	IM or IV
@	LA 5-10 ml or more SA 0.5-1 ml or more
Pres.	30 ml

Pheniramine Maleate	**Primavet**
Comp	Pheniramine Maleate 22.75 mg/ml
Adm.	IM or IV
@	LA 5-10 ml or more SA 0.5-1 ml or more
Pres.	10 ml, 30 ml

Malprim inj	**National vet Farma**
Comp	Pheniramine Maleate 22.75 mg/ml
Adm.	IM or IV
@	LA 5-10 ml or more SA 0.5-1 ml or more
Pres.	30 ml

Cistamin	**Century**
Comp	Pheniramine Maleate 22.75 mg/ml
Adm.	IM or IV
@	LA 5-10 ml or more SA 0.5-1ml or more
Pres.	30 ml

Promethazine

Apart from antihistaminic it can be used as a sedative or hypnotic also. It also belongs to Phenothiazine derivative. CNS excitement, G.I disturbances Tretatogenic effect are the side effects. It may cause anorexia, nausea, vomiting, constipation or diarrhea.

Phenergan inj	**M & B**
Comp	Promethazine hydrochloride 5%
Adm.	IM
@	LA 15-20 ml SA 2.5-5 ml
Pres.	2 ml, 5 ml

Promethazine	**Primavet**
Comp	Promethazine hydrochloride 5%
Adm.	IM
@	LA 15-20 ml SA 2.5-5ml
Pres.	5 ml

CNS Stimulants

These are drugs having primary action of CNS stimulation. Many drugs are capable of CNS stimulation as side effect or at high doses. Thus mostly produce a generalized action which may at high dose result in convulsions. There are

(i) Analeptics- Nikethamide, Doxapram

(ii) Cerebro acting- Piracetam, Pento oxyphylline

(iii) Convulsants- Strychrime, Picrotoxin

(iv) Psychostimulants- Caffeine, Theophyllin, Cocaine, Amphetamine

Nikethamide

It is related to Nicotinic acid and Nicotinamide. It is a life saving drug mainly a respiratory stimulant. It results increase in respiratory rate and depth by stimulating medullary centre and acting on chemoreceptors of carotid artery. Orally not much effective.

Coramine inj	Intas
Comp	Nikethamide 25%
Adm.	IM/ IV
@	LA 10-25 ml SA 3-5 ml
Pres.	5 ml, 25 ml

Strychnine

It is an alkaloid from the seeds of Strydinos nuxvomica. It is potent convulsant. It has been labelled as spinal convulsant resulting in exaggerated muscular response following slight sensory stimulation. It has been used as nervine tonic and GI stimulant. Strychnine hydrochloride or sulphate or nitrate or phosphate salts are used. Presently it has been banned.

Strychnine inj	Generic
Comp	5 mg/ml of Strychnine hydrochloride
Adm.	IM/ SC
@	LA 15-60 mg SA 5-15 mg
Pres.	10 ml, 30 ml, 100 ml.

Aminophylline

It is also called Theophyline ethylene diammine which acts directly on bronchial smooth muscles. It is used in broken wind in horses and to relieve bronchial spasms in anaesthetic emergencies.

Aminophylline inj	Generic
Comp	Aminophylline 25 mg/ml, 50 mg/ml
Adm.	IV
@	LA 1 vial for
Pres.	10 ml

Hypnotics / Sedatives

A drug that induces or maintains sleep similar to normal drowsable sleep. This is more or less general CNS depressants with differing time actions and dose action relationship. Sedative is a drug that subdues excitement and calms without inducing sleep though drowsiness may be produced. Drug with quicker onset, shorter duration and steeper dose are preferred as hypnotics and slow acting drug with flatter dose are preferred as sedative. Sometimes a hypnotic except Benzodiazepines given in high dose produce general anaesthesia.

Barbiturates

(Refer General anaesthesia)

Long acting- Phenobarbitone

Short acting- Pentobarbitone

Ultra short acting- Thiopentone

Benzodiazepines

Hypnotics- Diazepam, Nitrazepam

Diazepam

This is Benzodiazepine derivative. Primarily it is hypnotic, sedative, anxiolytic, anticonvulsant and skeletal mucle relaxant. It should not be used in breeding animal.

Calmpose inj/Tab	**Ranbaxy**
Comp	Diazepam 5 mg/ml Tab 5 mg, 10 mg
Adm.	IM or IV / oral
@	LA 0.1-0.2 mg/kg B.wt Horses 80 mg/kg B.wt
Pres.	2 ml amp 5 mg x 10 10 mg x 10 Tab

Valeum Tab	**General**
Comp	Diazepam 2 mg, 5 mg, 10 mg
Adm.	Oral
@	LA 0.1-0.2 mg/kg B.wt Horses 80 mg/kg B.wt
Pres.	All from in 10's

Dizep Tab	**Intas**
Comp	Diazepam 5 mg/ml Tab 5 mg, 10 mg
Adm.	Oral
@	LA 0.1-0.2 mg/kg B.wt Horses 80 mg/kg B.wt
Pres.	5 mg x 10 10 mg x 10

Preanaesthetic Medication

These are used before administering anaesthesia to make it more safe and pleasant. It relieves anxiety, decreases secretion and vagal stimulation. It supplements analgesic action and has antiemetic effect. Different drugs achieve different purpose.

Chloral Derivatives

Chlorpromazine

It is phenothiazine derivative. It is also used as preanaesthetic. It has central sedative effect on sympathetic system. Mostly indicated for immobilization of animal. It is not recommended in equines as causes excitability, drowsiness, depression and ataxia. Avoid its use in debilitated animals. Solution should be protected from light.

Chlorpromazine inj, Tab	**General**
Comp	Chlorpromazine 25 mg/ml Tab of 10 mg, 25 mg, 50 mg, 100 mg, 200 mg
Adm.	IM or IV Tab orally
@	LA 1-2 mg/kg B.wt IM- 0.5-1mg/kg B.wt IV SA 2 mg/kg B.wt
Pres.	2 ml, Tablets in 10's

Megatil inj , Tab	**General**
Comp	Chlorpromazine 25 mg/ml Tab of 10 mg, 2 5 mg, 50 mg, 100 mg, 200 mg
Adm.	IM or IV Tab orally
@	LA 1-2 mg/kg B.wt IM- 0.5-1 mg/kg B.wt IV SA 2 mg/kg B.wt
Pres.	2 ml Tablets in 10's

Largactil	**Rhone Poulenc**
Comp	Chlorpromazine hydrochloride 25 mg/ml, 50 mg/ml
Adm.	IM or IV Tab orally
@	LA 1-2 mg/kg B.wt IM- 0.5-1 mg/kg B.wt IV SA 2 mg/kg B.wt
Pres.	25 mg/ml- 1 ml, 25 ml, 10 ml 50 mg/ml- 5 ml

Promethazine

Refer Antihistamincs

Triflupromazine

It is also phenothiazine derivative. It is neuraleptic agent having property of antagonism at central dopamide D receptors. It is used as preanaesthetic and in resistance for clinical examination or minor surgical procedures, vomiting etc.

Anicalm inj, Tab	**Intas**
Comp	Triflupromazine 20 mg/ml, 5 mg, 10 mg Tab
Adm.	IM or IV oral Tablet
@	LA 0.11-0.18 mg/kg B.wt IV SA 0.1 mg/kg B.wt IV LA 0.22-0.33 mg/kg B.wt IM SA 0.2 mg/kg B.wt IM
Pres.	5 ml, Tab 10's maximum dose 100 mg

Siquil inj	**Sarabhai Zydus**
Comp	Triflupromazine 20 mg/ml, 5 mg, 10 mg Tab
Adm.	IM or IV oral Tablet
@	LA 0.11-0.18 mg/kg B.wt IV SA 0.1 mg/kg B.wt IV LA 0.22-0.33 mg/kg B.wt IM SA 0.2 mg/kg B.wt IM
Pres.	5 ml, Tab 10's maximum dose 100 mg

Antiaxiety Drugs

Phenobarbitones

These depress the motor centres of the cerebral cortex by potentiation of synaptic inhibition on GABA receptors. This action inhibits eleptic seizures. These are used symptomatic or prophylactic control of convulsive seizures. Can be given oral or IM and IV route.

Gardenal inj Tab	**Rhona Poulnec**
Comp	Phenobarbitone sodium inj 200 mg/ml, Tab 30 mg, 60 mg
Adm.	Oral, IM and IV
@	SA 1.5-5mg/kg B.wt bid IV or 1-1.5mg/kg B.wt IM 2.2 to 6.6 mg/kg B.wt oral
Pres.	1 ml, 2 ml, 20 Tab

Luminal Tab	**Bayer**
Comp	Phenobarbitone sodium 30 mg
Adm.	Oral
@	2.2 to 6.6 mg/kg B.wt oral
Pres.	30 mg Tab x10

Diazepam

(Already covered)

Atropine Sulphate

It is anti cholinergic agent i.e. Parasympatholytic which antagonizes the action of ache at its muscarinic receptors. Relaxes smooth muscles of bronchi and gut and reduces glandular secretion hence render excellent preanaesthetic action. More dose may cause atropine poisoning. It is contraindicated in respiratory diseases and pyloric stenosis. It is used as antidote for many poisoning cases.

Atropine sulphate	**Generic**
Comp	Atropine sulphate 0.6 mg/ml or 100 mg/ml
Adm.	IV
@	LA 0.05 mg/kg B.wt same in SA
Pres.	1 ml, 5 ml, 10 ml

Xylazine

It is Alpha 2 adrenergic agonist used as sedative, analgesic and muscle relexant. Its action is sympathomimetic on CNS and controls superficially arising pain. It is contraindicated in obstruction of oesophagus, hernia and late stage of pregnancy. Its duration depends upon dose and route of administration. It is indicated in sedation, analgesic, muscle relexant, immobilization of excited animal or as pre anaesthetic.

Bomazine inj	**Sarabhai Zydus**
Comp	Xylazine hydrochloride 20 mg/ml
Adm.	IM or IV
@	LA 0.03-0.2 mg/kg B.wt IV 0.1-0.2 mg/kg B.wt IM SA 0.01-0.5 mg/kg B.wt IV 0.05-0.5 mg/kg B.wt
Pres.	10 ml

Izine	**Intas**
Comp	Xylazine hydrochloride 20 mg/ml
Adm.	IM or IV
@	LA 0.03-0.2 mg/kg B.wt IV 0.1-0.2 mg/kg B.wt IM SA 0.01-0.5 mg/kg B.wt IV 0.05-0.5 mg/kg B.wt
Pres.	10 ml

Xylazine inj	**Indian Immunology**
Comp	Xylazine hydrochloride 23.32 mg/ml
Adm.	IM or IV
@	LA 0.03-0.2 mg/kg B.wt IV 0.1-0.2 mg/kg B.wt IM SA 0.01-0.5 mg/kg B.wt IV 0.05-0.5 mg/kg B.wt
Pres.	2 ml, 10 ml, 30 ml

Xylocad inj	**Cadila Pharma**
Comp	Xylazine hydrochloride 20 mg/ml
Adm.	IM or IV
@	LA 0.03-0.2 mg/kg B.wt IV 0.1-0.2 mg/kg B.wt IM SA 0.01-0.5 mg/kg B.wt IV 0.05-0.5 mg/kg B.wt
Pres.	5 ml

Xylodac inj	**Sarabhai Zydus**
Comp	Xylazine hydrochloride 20 mg/ml
Adm.	IM or IV
@	LA 0.03-0.2 mg/kg B.wt IV 0.1-0.2 mg/kg B.wt IM SA 0.01-0.5 mg/kg B.wt IV 0.05-0.5 mg/kg B.wt
Pres.	2 ml, 10 ml

Tranquilizers

These are the drugs used to restrain the animals for various diagnostic and clinical procedures. These are useful in quieting and calming unfriendly and apprehensive animals. These provide relief from anxiety, supplement analgesic action of anaesthesia and potentiate them so that less anaesthesia is needed. It decrease secretions and vagal stimulation. It has antiemetic action. Different drugs used are:-

Chlorpromazine Hydrochloride

(Already covered)

Diazepam

(Already covered)

Promethazine Hydrochloride

(Already covered)

Triflupromazine

(Already covered)

Xylaziine Hydrochloride

(Already covered)

□□□

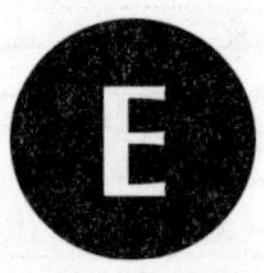

Musculoskeletal System

Disease of Musculoskeletal System

Ankylosis: A condition of joints in which movement is restricted by malformation by union of bones.

Arthritis: Inflammation of synovial membrane & articular surface.

Caries: Decay of teeth in which enamel is decalcified followed by softening and discolouration.

Incoordination: Irregularity in movement.

Myopathy: Non inflammatory degeneration of skeletal muscles seen by muscular weakness.

Myositis: Inflammation of muscles with swelling heat and pain.

Osteoarthritis: Non inflammatory lesion of joint cavities, lameness which increases with exercise.

Osteodystrophy: Diseases of bones where there is abnormal growth of bone and failure of normal bone development.

Osteoma: Small hard swelling with little or no pain in bone.

Osteomyelitis: Inflammation of bone marrow.

Osteoporosis: Loss of bone density caused by excessive absorption of calcium and Phosphorus from bone.

Rheumatism: A general term indicating diseases of muscles, tendons, joints, bones or nerves resulting in pain and disability.

Ringbone: Common in forefeet, lameness usually in all gaits and upon turning. Heat and swelling is present over involved area.

Spondylitis: Inflammation of vertebrae.

Sprains: Wrenching of joint often with simultaneous tearing of a ligament.

Tetany: Condition of muscular hyperexcitability in which mild stimuli produces cramps & spasms.

Analgesics / Antipyretics / Antiinflammatory

Algesia is unpleasant sensation usually evoked by internal or external noxious stimulus. It is generally known as pain.

Analgesic is a drug that selectively relieves pain by acting on CNS or peripheral pain mechanism without significantly altering consciousness. Pain is a signal & primarily protective in nature. Analgesics relieve pain symptom without affecting its cause.

Fever or hyperthermia is again a symptom or signal of problem in the body. The normal temperature of animal body rises. It can be during infection in which pyrogen a protein increases prostaglandin syntheses in hypothalamus thus raising its temperature.

Antipyretic drugs are used to reset the body temperature but not below the normal temperature of animal by different mode of action.

Inflammation can occur in any Vascularised tissue in the body. Symptoms after inflammation are redness, heat, swelling, pain or loss of function. Anti-inflammatory drugs are used to reduce the inflammation symptomatically by inhibiting mediators of inflammation.

Most of the drugs have all the three qualities but with different strength i.e. a drug can be primarily analgesic but with secondary function of antipyretic or anti-inflammatory. Similarly a drug can be antipyretic with secondary analgesic property and so. Collectively we called these analgesics.

Basically analgesics are-

(a) **Opoid analgesics:** Derived from poppy which contains alkaloids e.g. Morphine, Codiene, Narcotine etc.

(b) **Non Opoid analgesics:** These are weaker analgesics or called antipyretic analgesics. These can be Non-steroidal anti-inflammatory drugs and Steroidal anti-inflammatory drugs.

Rumalya Cream/tablets	**Himalya**
Indi: Sprain, Arthritis	
Comp: Not given	
Adm: Oral	
@ : 8-12 tablet thrice daily Applylocally	
Pres: 28 g tube 100 tab. pack	

Inflamin	**Himalya**
Indi: Mastitis for swelling	
Comp: Not given	
Adm: Topical	
@ : Apply on affected part	
Pres: 50 gm, 125 g tube	

Anbioflam 400 Cap.			**Indian Herbs**
Indi: Antiinflamatory, Skin diseases, Ringworm			
Comp:			
Alstonia scholaris	3%	Godanti bhasam	4%
Hermodactylus gol	1%	Ptychotis ajowan	4%
Cinchona officinale	3%	Yavkshar	10%
Tenospora cordifolia	4%	Madarkshar	10%
Swertia chirata	4%	Epsum salt	30%
		base	q.s.
Adm: Oral			
@ : 50-100 g bd for 2-3 days			
Pres: 150 g, 1 kg			

Feverdon Pow.	**Vets Farma**
Indi: HighTemperature due to infection, swelling	
Comp: Not given	
Adm: Oral	
@ : 50-100 g bd for 2-3 days	
Pres: 150 g, 1 kg	

Herbina Cap.	**Indian Herbs**
Indi: Antipyretic	
Comp: Not given	
Adm: Oral	
@ : 2 Cap .6 hourly	
Pres: 6 Cap. 12 Cap. vial	

R Compound tab	**Alarsin**
Indi: Rheumatism, Sprain, Arthritis	
Comp: Not given	
@ : 5-10 tab. twice daily for10-20 days	
Pres: Pack of 100 tablets	

Opoid Analgesics

Morphine

It is the principle opium alkaloid. It effects sensation through CNS. Apart from analgesic action it has sedative effect also. It is given for prolonged relief of severe and intractable pain. It is contraindicated in respiratory depression.

These control anxiety and apprehension of operation. These produce pre and post operative analgesia. These reduce the dose of anaesthetics. These depress respiration and interfere with pupillary signs of anaesthetics. These lead to urinary retention and constipation. In certain animals (Cattle, sheep, goat, horses) morphine produce thermia. These are also given in spasmodic colic.

Morphine inj	**Burroughs Wellcome**
Comp	1.1 ml contains 11 mg morphine 1.1 ml contains 22 mg morphine
Adm.	IM, IV
@	LA 0.12 mg/kg B.wt IV 0.22 mg/kg B.wt IM As preanaesthetic 0.1-2 mg/kg B.wt IM or SC LA 150-600 mg SC SA 30-60 mg SC
Pres.	1.1 ml ampoule for both

Morphine Sulphate inj Tab	**Generic**
Comp	30 mg, 60 mg Tab, Inj 15 mg/ml (Delayed release Tablet)
Adm.	IM/ IV Tablet oral
@	LA 0.5-1 mg/kg B.wt SA 0.1-0.2 mg/kg B.wt
Pres.	30 mg, 60 mg tab, 1ml inj

Pentazocine

It is opioid analgesic. This exerts against antagonist action on opioid receptors. Principle analgesic effect is exerted upon CNS and smooth muscle. Action is short as preanaesthetic etc. It is indicated in severe traumatic pain, surgery, colic, burns, fracture incoordination and muscular tremors can be side effects.

Fortwin inj	Ranbaxy
Comp	Pentazocine 30 mg/ml
Adm.	IM/ IV
@	LA 0.5-1 mg/kg B.wt SA 0.25-0.50 mg/kg B.wt 200-400 mg total dose
Pres.	2 ml, 5 ml

Pethidine

It is also known as Meperidine hydrochloride which is a synthetic drug. Its action resembles Morphine. It is analgesic and antispasmodic in action. It also produces sedation.

Pethidine inj	Generic
Comp	Pethidin 25 mg/ml, 5 mg Tab
Adm.	IV, IM
@	LA 500 mg/ml SA 1-2 mg/ml
Pres.	5 ml, Tab 10's maximum dose 100 mg

Non Opoid Analgesics

They do not depress CNS and act primarily on peripheral pain mechanism. These are grouped differently.

(a) Potent anti-inflammatory & Good Analgesic:

Aspirin, Sodium salicylate.

(b) Potent anti-inflammatory & Poor Analgesic:

Oxyphenylbutazone, Indomethacin.

(c) Moderate anti-inflammatory & Moderate Analgesic:

Ibuprofen, Naproxen, Diclofenac, Piroxicam, Mefenamic acid.

(d) Poor anti-inflammatory & good Analgesic:

Paracetamol, Phenacetin, Metamizol.

These are grouped as

NSAID- Non steroid anti-inflammatory drugs

SAID- Steroid anti-inflammatory drugs

NSAID

Non steroidal anti-inflammatory drugs is a group of analgesic with more than 200 compounds varying in dose, action, distribution, metabolism and excretion. This group has varying effect of killing pain, reducing inflammation and restoring animal normal body temperature. These are injected as well as given orally or applied topically but not all.

Analgin

It is a NSAID derivative and used for relieving pain, fever, swelling and spasmodic condition during parturition, rheumatic conditions, neuritis, neuralgia and other painful conditions. It also acts as antispasmodic and helps in relaxation of intestinal spasm. It has good analgesic and antipyretic action but poor anti-inflammatory Gastric irritation and pain at the site of injection are side effects.

Analgin inj	**KAPL**
Comp	0.5 g/ml Analgin
Adm.	IM/ IV
@	LA 20-40 ml SA 5-10 ml
Pres.	30 ml

Banipin inj	**Brihans**
Comp	0.5 g/ml Analgin
Adm.	IM/ IV
@	LA 20-40 ml SA 5-10 ml
Pres.	30 ml

Cemizol inj	**IDPL**
Comp	0.5 g/ml Analgin
Adm.	IM/ IV
@	LA 20-40 ml SA 5-10 ml
Pres.	30 ml

Inflagin inj	**Neospark**
Comp	0.5 g/ml Analgin
Adm.	IM/ IV
@	LA 20-40 ml SA 5-10 ml
Pres.	30 ml

Novalgin inj	**Novartis (Hoechst)**
Comp	0.5 g/ml Analgin
Adm.	IM/ IV
@	LA 20-40 ml SA 5-10 ml
Pres.	30 ml

Ronalgin inj	**Ranbaxy**
Comp	0.5 g/ml Analgin
Adm.	IM/ IV
@	LA 20-40 ml SA 5-10 ml
Pres.	30 ml

Vetalgin inj	Intervet
Comp	0.5 g/ml Analgin
Adm.	IM/ IV
@	LA 20-40 ml SA 5-10 ml
Pres.	30 ml

Analgin Plus Combination

Valginate inj	TTK
Comp	Each ml Analgin 500 mg Valethamine bromide 2 mg
Adm.	IM
@	LA 8 ml/100 kg B.wt, SA 5-10 ml
Pres.	10 ml, 30 ml

Valgin inj	Cipla
Comp	Analgin 0.5 g/ml + 1% Lignocaine
Adm.	IM
@	LA 8 ml/100 kg B.wt, SA 5-10 ml
Pres.	30 ml, 100 ml useful in abdominal pain

Oxalgin Bol	Cadila Healthcare
Comp	Analgin 2.5 g + Oxyphenylbutazone 500 mg
Adm.	Oral
@	LA 2 Bol bid SA 1/4 -1/2 Bol bid
Pres.	Strip of 4

Bolin inj	Merial
Indi.	It acts as antipyretic and analgesic
Comp	Analgin 150 mg + Paracetamol 150 mg in each ml
Adm.	IM or IV
@	LA 25-60 ml SA 5-10 ml
Pres.	10 ml, 30 ml

Bolin Bol	Merial
Comp	Analgin 1.5 Paracetamol 1.5g
Adm.	Oral
@	LA 1-2 Bol SA 1/2 -1 Bol
Pres.	Strip of 4

Esgipyrin inj	**Zydus**
Comp	5 ml contains Analgin 750 g Phenylbutazone 750 mg Lignocaine hydrochloride 50 mg
Adm.	IM
@	LA 5-15 SA 1-5 ml
Pres.	5 ml

Baralgan inj	**Novartis**
Indi	Urogenital pain, swelling
Comp	Each ml contains Analgin 200 mg + Pitofinone hydrochloride 2 mg Fenpivenrinium bromide 0.02 mg
Adm.	IM
@	LA 20-50 ml SA 5-15 ml
Pres.	30 ml

Pitofin inj	**Marc**
Indi	Urogenital pain, swelling
Comp	Each ml contains Nimesulide 100 mg + Pitofinone hydrochloride 2 mg Fenpivenrinium bromide 0.02 mg
Adm.	IM
@	LA 20-50 ml SA 5-15 ml
Pres.	30 ml

Polygesic inj	**Cargill (Unichem)**
Indi	Urogenital pain, swelling
Comp	Each ml contains Analgin + Pitofinone hydrochloride 2 mg Fenpivenrinium bromide 0.02 mg
Adm.	IM
@	LA 20-50 ml SA 5-15 ml
Pres.	10 ml, 30 ml

Ridalpin inj	**KAPL**
Indi	Urogenital pain, swelling

Comp	Each ml contains Analgin 200 mg + Pitofinone hydrochloride 2 mg Fenpivenrinium bromide 0.02 mg
Adm.	IM
@	LA 20-50 ml SA 5-15 ml
Pres.	10 ml, 30 ml

Diclofenac Sodium/ Potassium

It has powerful anti-inflammatory action besides pain killer and antipyretic action. It inhibits diuretics. It should not be given to old animals. It inhibits PG synthesis. It is well absorbed orally. Side effects can be gastric ulceration, nausea etc. this is indicated in acute muscle- skeletal disorders, Rheumatoid arthritis, sprains and dislocation, painful post-operative conditions, painful inflammatory gynecological conditions, soft tissue injuries, High fever and as adjuvant to antibiotic therapy and hyper pyrexia.

3D Vet inj	**Intas**
Comp	Diclofenac sodium 25 mg/ml
Adm.	IM
@	1-2 mg/kg B.wt or 1ml/25 kg B.wt
Pres.	30 ml, 100 ml

Butagesic inj	**Concept**
Comp	Diclofenac sodium 25 mg/ml
Adm.	IM
@	1-2 mg/kg Bwt or 1ml/25 kg B.wt
Pres.	10 ml, 30 ml

Catlogenac inj	**Cattle Remedies**
Comp	Diclofenac sodium 25mg/ml
Adm.	IM
@	1-2mg/kg Bwt or 1ml/25 kg B.wt
Pres.	30 ml, 100 ml

Ciclogen D inj	**Cadila Pharma**
Comp	Diclofenac sodium 25 mg/ml
Adm.	IM
@	1-2 mg/kg Bwt or 1ml/25 kg B.wt
Pres.	30 ml

Clogil inj	**G. Loucatas**
Comp	Diclofenac sodium 25 mg/ml
Adm.	IM
@	1-2 mg/kg Bwt or 1ml/25 kg B.wt
Pres.	30 ml

Diclocare inj	**Vetcare**
Comp	Diclofenac sodium 25 mg/ml
Adm.	IM
@	1-2 mg/kg Bwt or 1ml/25 kg B.wt
Pres.	30 ml, 100 ml

Diclodin inj	**Indian Immunology**
Comp	Diclofenac sodium 25 mg/ml
Adm.	IM
@	1-2 mg/kg Bwt or 1ml/25 kg B.wt
Pres.	30 ml

Diclopyrin inj	**Carevet Pharma**
Comp	Diclofenac sodium 25 mg/ml
Adm.	IM
@	1-2 mg/kg Bwt or 1 ml/25 kg B.wt
Pres.	30 ml, 100 ml

Dicloven inj	**Vets Pharma**
Comp	Diclofenac sodium 25 mg/ml
Adm.	IM
@	1-2 mg/kg Bwt or 1ml/25 kg B.wt
Pres.	30 ml, 100 ml

Diclofen inj	**Marc**
Comp	Diclofenac sodium 25 mg/ml
Adm.	IM
@	1-2 mg/kg B.wt or 1 ml/25 kg B.wt
Pres.	10 ml, 30 ml, 100 ml

Diclofenac Sod inj	Sushima
Comp	Diclofenac sodium 25 mg/ml
Adm.	IM
@	1-2 mg/kg B.wt or 1 ml/25 kg B.wt
Pres.	30 ml, 100 ml

Diclovet inj	Alembic
Comp	Diclofenac sodium 25 mg/ml
Adm.	IM
@	1-2 mg/kg B.wt or 1ml/25 kg B.wt
Pres.	30 ml

Digesic inj	Vest
Comp	Diclofenac sodium 25 mg/ml
Adm.	IM
@	1-2 mg/kg B.wt or 1 ml/25 kg B.wt
Pres.	30 ml, 90 ml

Fenac inj	Tineta
Comp	Diclofenac sodium 25 mg/ml
Adm.	IM
@	1-2 mg/kg B.wt or 1 ml/25 kg B.wt
Pres.	30 ml, 90 ml

Feverdon inj	Vets Farma
Comp	Diclofenac sodium 25 mg/ml
Adm.	IM
@	1-2 mg/kg B.wt or 1 ml/25 kg B.wt
Pres.	30 ml, 90 ml

Proxyvet inj	Wockhardt
Comp	Diclofenac sodium 25 mg/ml
Adm.	IM
@	1-2 mg/kg B.wt or 1ml/25 kg B.wt
Pres.	30 ml, 100 ml

Nufenac inj	**KAPL**
Comp	Diclofenac sodium 25 mg/ml
Adm.	IM
@	1-2 mg/kg B.wt or 1 ml/25 kg B.wt
Pres.	30 ml

Restamin inj	**Century**
Comp	Diclofenac sodium 25 mg/ml
Adm.	IM
@	1-2 mg/kg B.wt or 1 ml/25 kg B.wt
Pres.	30 ml

Ulfenac inj	**Neospark**
Comp	Diclofenac sodium 25 mg/ml
Adm.	IM
@	1-2 mg/kg B.wt or 1 ml/25 kg B.wt
Pres.	30 ml

Verastan inj	**Ranbaxy**
Comp	Diclofenac sodium 25 mg/ml
Adm.	IM
@	1-2 mg/kg B.wt or 1 ml/25 kg B.wt
Pres.	30 ml, 100 ml

Zobid inj	**Zydus**
Comp	Diclofenac sodium 25 mg/ml
Adm.	IM
@	1-2 mg/kg B.wt or 1 ml/25 kg B.wt
Pres.	30 ml

Briclogen inj	**Brihans**
Comp	Diclofenac sodium 25 mg/ml
Adm.	IM
@	1-2 mg/kg B.wt or 1 ml/25 kg B.wt
Pres.	30 ml

Inflavet inj	Virbac
Comp	Diclofenac sodium 50 mg/ml
Adm.	IM
@	1-2 mg/kg B.wt
Pres.	30 ml

Paracetamol

It is also called Acetaminophen or Phenacetin. It belongs to Para Amino Phenol derivatives. Their action is like aspirin. It has strong antipyretic and analgesic action but poor anti-inflammatory effect. It is poor inhibitor of PG in peripheral tissue. It produces sense of relaxation. It does not cause irritation and does not stimulate respiration. It is indicated in hyperexia to restore normal body temperature. It is adjuvant with antibiotic

Paracetol inj	Cadila Healthcare
Comp	Paracetamol 150 mg/ml
Adm.	IM
@	LA 10-30 ml SA 20 mg/kg B.wt
Pres.	10 ml, 30 ml

Pyroxin Bol	Marc
Comp	Each bolus contains Paracetamol 2g
Adm.	Oral
@	LA 1-2 Bol bid SA ½ -1 Bol bid
Pres.	Strip of 4

Combinations

Diclofenac sodium + Paracetamol Inj

Combination acts synergistically and becomes very effective analgesic, antipyretic and anti-inflammatory. It is indicated in all painful conditions with fever and adjuvant to antibiotics.

A3 inj	Sushima
Comp	Each ml contains Diclofenac potassium 25 mg Paracetamol 150 mg
Adm.	IM
@	1 ml/25 kg B.wt
Pres.	30 ml

Briclogen inj	**Brihans**	
Comp	Each ml contains	
	Diclofenac potassium Paracetamol	25 mg 150 mg
Adm.	IM	
@	1 ml/25 kg B.wt	
Pres.	30 ml	

Cattlofenac Plus inj	**Cattle Remedies**	
Comp	Each ml contains	
	Diclofenac potassium Paracetamol	25 mg 150 mg
Adm.	IM	
@	1ml/25 kg B.wt	
Pres.	30 ml	

D Pgesic inj	**Vest**	
Comp	Each ml contains	
	Diclofenac potassium Paracetamol	25 mg 150 mg
Adm.	IM	
@	1ml/25 kg B.wt	
Pres.	30 ml	

Feverdon Plus inj	**Vets Farma**	
Comp	Each ml contains	
	Diclofenac potassium Paracetamol	25 mg 150 mg
Adm.	IM	
@	1 ml/2 5kg B.wt	
Pres.	30 ml	

Inigesic inj	**Indian Immunology**	
Comp	Each ml contains	
	Diclofenac potassium Paracetamol	25 mg 150 mg
Adm.	IM	
@	1 ml/25 kg B.wt	
Pres.	30 ml	

Lydic P inj	**Sequent (Lyka)**	
Comp	Each ml contains	
	Diclofenac potassium	25 mg
	Paracetamol	150 mg
Adm.	IM	
@	1ml/25 kg B.wt	
Pres.	30 ml	

Oxalgin DS inj	**Zydus**	
Comp	Each ml contains	
	Diclofenac potassium	25 mg
	Paracetamol	150 mg
Adm.	IM	
@	1 ml/25 kg B.wt	
Pres.	30 ml	

Proxyvet Plus inj	**Wockhardt**	
Comp	Each ml contains	
	Diclofenac potassium	25 mg
	Paracetamol	150 mg
Adm.	IM	
@	1 ml/25 kg B.wt	
Pres.	30 ml	

Restamin Plus inj	**Century**	
Comp	Each ml contains	
	Diclofenac potassium	25 mg
	Paracetamol	150 mg
Adm.	IM	
@	1 ml/25 kg B.wt	
Pres.	30 ml	

Sterlflam D Vet inj	**Sterling Lab**	
Comp	Each ml contains	
	Diclofenac potassium	25 mg
	Paracetamol	150 mg
Adm.	IM	
@	1 ml/25 kg B.wt	
Pres.	30 ml	

Verstan Plus inj	**Ranbaxy**	
Comp	Each ml contains Diclofenac potassium Paracetamol	 25 mg 150 mg
Adm.	IM	
@	1 ml/25 kg B.wt	
Pres.	30 ml	

Vetpyrin inj	**Carevet Pharma**	
Comp	Each ml contains Diclofenac potassium Paracetamol	 25 mg 150 mg
Adm.	IM	
@	1 ml/25 kg B.wt	
Pres.	30 ml	

Zosmac SP Bol	**Macnor**	**136**
Comp	Each bolus contains Aceclofenac Paracetamol Serratiopeptidose	 400 mg 2000 mg 60 mg
Adm.	Oral	
@.	LA 2 Bolus bid SA ½-1 Bolus bid	
Pres.	2 bol stip	

Diclofenac + Pitofenon + Fenpiverinium

It is effective in Visceral Pain and Swelling

Spasdic inj	**Sushima**	
Comp	Each ml contains Diclofenac sodium Pitofenon hydrochloride Fenpiverininum bromide	 25 mg 2 mg 0.02 mg
Adm.	IM	
@	1ml/25 kg B.wt	
Pres.	30 ml	

Diclofenac + Paracetamol Bolus

3D vet Plus Bol	**Intas**
Comp	Each Bol contains Diclofenac sodium 250 mg Paracetamol 1500 mg
Adm.	Oral
@	LA 1-2 Bol bid SA ½ -1 Bol bid
Pres.	Strip of 3 Bol

A 3 Bol	**Sushima**
Comp	Diclofenac sodium 200 mg Paracetamol 1500 mg
Adm.	Oral
@	LA 1-2 Bol bid SA ½ -1 Bol bid
Pres.	Strip of 4

Alfenac P Forte Bol	**Alved**
Comp	Diclofenac sodium 300 mg Paracetamol 1500 mg
Adm.	Oral
@	LA 1-2 Bol SA ½ -1 Bol
Pres.	Strip of 4

Diclovet Bol	**Alembic**
Comp	Each Bol contains Diclofenac sodium 250 mg Paracetamol 1500 mg
Adm.	Oral
@	LA 1-2 Bol bid SA ½ -1 Bol bid
Pres.	Strip of 3 Bol

Ciclofen Bol	**Cadila Pharma**
Comp	Each Bol contains Diclofenac sodium 200 mg Paracetamol 1500 mg
Adm.	Oral
@	LA 1-2 Bol bid SA ½ -1 Bol bid
Pres.	Strip of 4

Inigesic Bol	**Indian Immunology**	
Comp	Each Bol contains	
	Diclofenac sodium	250 mg
	Paracetamol	1500 mg
Adm.	Oral	
@	LA 1-2 Bol bid SA ½ -1 Bol bid	
Pres.	Strip of 2	

Molgesic Bol	**Anmark**	
Comp	Each Bol contains	
	Diclofenac sodium	250 mg
	Paracetamol	1500 mg
Adm.	Oral	
@	LA 1-2 Bol bid SA ½ -1 Bol bid	
Pres.	Strip of 4	

Briclofen Bol	**Brihans**	
Comp	Each Bol contains	
	Diclofenac sodium	250 mg
	Paracetamol	1500 mg
Adm.	Oral	
@	LA 1-2 Bol bid SA ½ -1 Bol bid	
Pres.	Strip of 4	

Proxyvet DS Bol	**Wockhardt**	
Comp	Each Bol contains	
	Diclofenac sodium	250 mg
	Paracetamol	1500 mg
Adm.	Oral	
@	LA 1-2 Bol bid SA ½ -1 Bol bid	
Pres.	Strip of 2	

Oxalgin DS Bol	**Zydus**	
Comp	Each Bol contains	
	Diclofenac sodium	200 mg
	Paracetamol	1500 mg
Adm.	Oral	
@	LA 1-2 Bol bid SA ½ -1 Bol bid	
Pres.	Strip of 4	

Pyrenil Bol	**Concept**	
Comp	Each Bol contains	
	Diclofenac sodium	200 mg
	Paracetamol	1500 mg
Adm.	Oral	
@	LA 1-2 Bol bid SA ½ -1 Bol bid	
Pres.	Strip of 4	

Restamin Bol	**Century**	
Comp	Each Bol contains	
	Diclofenac sodium	200 mg
	Paracetamol	1500 mg
Adm.	Oral	
@	LA 1-2 Bol bid SA ½ -1 Bol bid	
Pres.	Strip of 4	

Inflavet Bol	**Virbac**	
Comp	Each Bol contains	
	Diclofenac potassium	500 mg
	Paracetamol	1 g
Adm.	Oral	
@	LA 1 Bol od SA ½ Bol od	
Pres.	Strip of 2	

Pecorex Bol	**Pranav**	
Comp	Each Bol contains	
	Dicyclomine hydrochloride	100 mg
	Diclofenac sod	250 mg
	Paracetamol	1500 mg
Adm.	Oral	
@	LA ½ -1 Bol SA ½ -1 Bol	
Pres.	Strip of 4	

Diclopyrin Forte Bol	**Carevet Pharma**	
Comp	Each Bol contains	
	Diclofenac sod	250 mg
	Paracetamol	1625 mg
	Ibuprofen	2000 mg
Adm.	Oral	
@	LA 1 Bol tds SA ½ Bol tds	
Pres.	Strip of 2	

Aspirin or Acetyl Salicylic Acid

It is one of the oldest and safest NSAID. It has analgesic, antipyretic and anti-inflammatory action. It acts by inhibiting PG synthesis and blocks the sensitization of pain, pyretic symptomatic relief of pain, pyrexia and swelling of musculoskeletal origin.

Aspirin Tab	**Generic**
Comp	Aspirin 325 mg and 650 mg
Adm.	Oral
@	10 mg/kg B.wt bid
Pres.	325 mg, 650 mg

Sodium Salicylates

It is used as supportive treatment of pyrexia in acute respiratory disease in combination with antibiotics. It acts by inhibiting PG synthesis. Action is peripheral and central.

Oral Pro Sodium Salicylate Pow	**Generic**
Comp	Sodium salicylate 48.6%
Adm.	Oral with drinking water
@	250 g in 5 L of water, 25 mg/kg B.wt daily in calves
Pres.	250 g, 500 g

Sodium Salicylate Pow	**Generic**
Comp	400 mg/g of Sodium salicylate
Adm.	Oral
@	LA 15-25 g bid SA 2-5 g bid
Pres.	100 g, 200 g/kg

Pyrosan Pow	**Ballown Pharma**
Comp	Sodium salicylate 40% Ginger Powder 20%
Adm.	Oral
@	LA 70 g od, SA 15-20 g od
Pres.	200 g, 1 kg

Ibuprofen

It is NSAID and a derivative of propionic acid. It has analgesic, antipyretic and anti-inflammatory effect. It also acts by inhibiting PG synthesis. It is indicated to relieve pain, fever, and inflammation of musculoskeletal organ.

Aniprofen Bol	**Anivet Healthcare**
Comp	Ibuprofen 2 g + Paracetamol 1625 mg
Adm.	Oral
@	1-2 Bol bid
Pres.	Strip of 4

Vetpyrin Forte Bol	**Carevet Pharma**	**162**
Comp	Each Bol contains Ibuprofen Paracetamol Serratiopeptidase	 2000 mg 1500 mg 75 mg
Adm.	Oral	
@	2 Bol bid	
Pres.	Strip of 4	

Meloxicam

It is NSAID. It inhibits the PG synthesis through cyclooxygenase enzyme and effects as anti-inflammatory, analgesic, antipyretic and antioxidation. It is usually indicated in condition associated with Pneumonia, Pleuritis, uterine prolapse, mastitis and arthritis. It should not be given to animals with GI tract problems.

Melonex inj	**Intas**
Comp	Meloxicam 5 mg/ml
Adm.	IM
@	LA 0.5 mg/kg B.wt SA 0.2-0.3 mg/kg B.wt
Pres.	15 mg, 30 ml

A3 Vet inj	**Brihans**
Comp	Meloxicam 5 mg/ml
Adm.	IM
@	LA 0.5 mg/kg B.wt SA 0.2-0.3 mg/kg B.wt
Pres.	30 ml, 100 ml

Melaxone inj	**Venky**
Comp	Meloxicam 5 mg/ml
Adm.	IM
@	LA 0.5 mg/kg B.wt SA 0.2-0.3 mg/kg B.wt
Pres.	30 ml, 100 ml

Meloxyvet 20	**Carrus**
Comp	Meloxcam 20 mg/ml
Adm.	IM
@	0.5 mg/kg B.wt
Pres.	30 ml

Painkind	**Vetkind**
Comp	Meloxicam 5 mg/ml
Adm.	IM
@	LA 0.5 mg/kg B.wt SA 0.2-0.3 mg/kg B.wt
Pres.	30 ml

Diclovet M	**Alembic**
Comp	Meloxicam 5 mg/ml
Adm.	IM
@	LA 0.5 mg/kg B.wt SA 0.2-0.3 mg/kg B.wt
Pres.	30 ml, 100 ml

Meloximof	**Zydus** **253**
Comp	Meloxicam 5 mg Paracetamol 150mg in 1ml
Adm.	IM
@	15 ml/300 kg B.wt
Pres.	30 ml, 100 ml

Meloxicam Combination Bol.

A3 Vet Bol	**Brihans**
Comp	Meloxicam 100 mg + Paracetamol 1500 mg
Adm.	Oral
@	LA 2 Bol od
Pres.	Strip of 4

Melonex Plus Bol	**Intas**
Comp	Meloxicam 100 mg + Paracetamol 1500 mg
Adm.	Oral
@	LA 2 Bol od
Pres.	Strip of 4

Zobid M Bol	**Zydus**	**256**
Comp	Bolus contains 100 mg Meloxicam	
Adm.	Oral	
@	LA 2 Bol bid SA ½ -1 Bol bid	
Pres.	Blister of 4	

Meloxicom Injectables in Combination

A3 Vet Plus inj	**Brihans**
Comp	Each ml contains Meloxicam 5 mg Paracetamol 150 mg Lignocaine 1%
Adm.	IM
@	LA 15-30 ml daily
Pres.	30 ml, 100 ml

Melobest P inj	**TTK**
Comp	Each ml contains Meloxicam 5 mg Paracetamol 150 mg Lignocaine 1%
Adm.	IM
@	LA 15-30 ml daily
Pres.	15 ml, 30 ml, 100 ml

Melonex Plus inj	**Intas**
Comp	Each ml contains Meloxicam 5 mg Paracetamol 150 mg Lignocaine 1%
Adm.	IM
@	LA 15-30 ml daily
Pres.	30 ml, 100 ml

Zobid MP inj	**Zydus**	**255**
Comp	1 ml contain Meloxicam 5 mg Paracetamol 150 mg Lignocian hydrochloride 1%	
Adm.	IM	
@	15-20 ml in 300 kg B.wt	
Pres.	100 ml vial	

Piroxicam

It is NSAID. Its action and indications are same as for other NSAID. This is rapid acting NSAID and starts its action within 15 minutes. It lasts for about 24 hours due to its higher half life.

Pyrecalm inj	**Carevet Pharma**
Comp	Piroxicon 20 mg/ml
Adm.	IM
@	1 ml/kg B.wt
Pres.	30 ml, 100 ml

ROC inj	**Macwell**
Comp	Piroxicon 20 mg/ml
Adm.	IM
@	1 ml/kg B.wt
Pres.	30 ml, 100 ml

Vetzone S	**Avivet**
Comp	Piroxicon 20 mg/ml
Adm.	IM
@	1 ml/20 kg B.wt
Pres.	30 ml, 100 ml

Piroxicam Combination

Pyrecalm Plus inj	**Carevet Pharma**
Comp	Each ml contains Piroxicam 20 mg Paracetamol 75 mg

Adm.	IM
@	1 ml/20 kg B.wt
Pres.	30 ml, 100 ml

ROC Plus inj	**Macwell**
Comp	1 ml contains Piroxicam 20 mg Paracetamol 75 mg
Adm.	IM
@	1 ml/20 kg B.wt
Pres.	30 ml, 100 ml

Pecorex DD Bol	**PAIL**
Comp	Each Bol has Piroxicam 200 mg Pitofenone Hydrochloride 25 mg Fenpiverininum bromide 0.2 mg
Adm.	Oral
@	2 Bol bid
Pres.	Strip of 4

Painac D inj	**Phoenix**	**45**
Comp	Piroxiam 20 mg Paracetamol 150 mg DMSO 25%	
Adm.	IM	
@	1ml/25 kg B.wt	
Pres.	30 ml, 100 ml	

Pentavet	**Libra**	**100**
Comp	Piroxicam 20 g Paracetamol 150 mg DMSO q.s	
Adm.	IM	
@.	1ml/20 kg B.wt	
Pres.	100 ml	

Pan + Bolus	**Libra**	**113**
Comp	Bolus contains Piroxicam 200 mg Paracetamol 1500 mg Cetirizine 25 mg Magnesium trisilicate 50 mg	
Adm.	Oral	
@.	LA 2 Bol SA 1 Bol bid	
Pres.	Stip of 2	

Painac – D Bol	**Phoenix**
Comp	Piroxicam 100 mg, Paracetamol 1500 mg DMSO 25%
Adm.	Oral
@	LA 2 Bol od SA ½ -1 Bol od
Pres.	Strip of 4

Spasmoroc inj	**Macwell**
Comp	Piroxicam 10 mg Fenpivirium 0.02 mg Pitofenone hydrochloride 2 mg per ml
Adm.	IM
@	LA 20-30 ml SA 8-15 ml
Pres.	30 ml

Spasmac inj	**Macnor**
Comp	Each contains Piroxican 100 mg Petofenone 2 mg Fenfiverium 0.1 mg
Adm.	IM
@.	LA 20-30 ml SA 8-15 ml
Pres.	30 ml

Nimesulide

It is one of NSAID and has got all three properties of antipyretic, anti-inflammatory and analgesic action. It is as good as Diclofenac, Ibuprofen. It has strength of anti-infections and disorders associated with pain and swelling.

Nimpyrin inj	**Carevet Pharma**
Comp	Nimesulide 200 mg/ml
Adm.	IM
@	1 ml/20 kg B.wt
Pres.	15 ml, 30 ml, 90 ml

Nimesulide Combination Inj

Nimesulide + Paracetamol

Kemolide inj	Kepler
Comp	Each ml contains Nimesulide 100 mg Paracetamol 150 mg
Adm.	IM
@	1 ml/20 kg B.wt or 15-20 ml in LA
Pres.	30 ml, 100 ml

ROCNP Plus inj	Macwell
Comp	Each ml contains Nimesulide 100 mg Paracetamol 150 mg
Adm.	IM
@	1 ml/20 kg B.wt or 15-20 ml in LA
Pres.	20 ml, 100 ml

Protrio inj	Wellcon
Comp	Each ml contains Nimesulide 100 mg Paracetamol 150 mg
Adm.	IM
@	1 ml/20 kg B.wt or 15-20 ml in LA
Pres.	20 ml, 100 ml

Rest inj	PAIL
Comp	Each ml contains Nimesulide 100 mg Paracetamol 150 mg
Adm.	IM
@	1 ml/20 kg B.wt or 15-20 ml in LA
Pres.	30 ml, 100 ml

Anip C inj	Animax Health
Comp	Each ml contains Nimesulide 100 mg Paracetamol 150 mg
Adm.	IM
@	1 ml/20 kg B.wt or 15-20 ml in LA
Pres.	30 ml, 100 ml

Spasmogun inj	**Carevet Pharma**
Comp	Each ml contains Nimesulide 100 mg Pitofenone hydrochloride 2 mg Fenpiverinium bromide 0.02 mg per ml
Adm.	IM
@	1 ml/20 kg B.wt
Pres.	10 ml, 30 ml

Pan Forte inj	**Libra**
Comp	Each ml contains Nimesulide 200 mg Lignocaine 10 mg DMSO q.s
Adm.	IM
@.	1 ml/20 kg B.wt
Pres.	100 ml

Nimesulide + Combination Bolus

ROC -S Bol	**Macwell**
Comp	Each Bolus contains Nimesulide 400 mg Paracetamol 1500 mg Serratiopeptidase 75 mg
Adm.	Oral
@	2 Bol bid
Pres.	Strip of 4

Anip C Bol	**Animax Healthcare**
Comp	Each Bolus contains Nimesulide 500 mg Paracetamol 1500 mg Chlorzoxazone 1000 mg
Adm.	Oral
@	2 Bol bid
Pres.	Strip of 4

NPC Forte	**Animax Pharma**
Comp	Each Bolus contains Nimesulide 750 mg Paracetamol 1500 mg Chlorzoxazone 1000 mg

Adm.	Oral
@	2 Bol bid
Pres.	Strip of 4

Avifen Plus Bol	**Avivet**
Comp	Each Bolus contains Nimesulide 500 mg Paracetamol 1500 mg Chlorzoxazone 1000 mg
Adm.	Oral
@	2 Bol bid
Pres.	Strip of 4

Rumilide bol	**Bovian**
Comp	Each Bolus contains Nimesulide 400 mg Paracetamol 1500 mg Serratiopeptidase 75 mg
Adm.	Oral
@	2 Bol bid
Pres.	Strip of 4

Portrio Bol	**Wellcare**
Comp	Each Bolus contains Nimesulide 400 mg Paracetamol 1500 mg Serratiopeptidase 75 mg
Adm.	Oral
@	2 Bol bid
Pres.	Strip of 4

Jospas bol	**Animax Healthcare**
Comp	Each Bolus contains Nimesulide 400 mg Fenpiverinium bromide 0.0 mg Pitofenone hydrochloride 25 mg
Adm.	Oral
@	LA 1-2 Bol bid
Pres.	Strip of 4

Nylate S Bol	Nicosia
Comp	Each ml contains Nimesulide 400 mg Paracetamol 1500 mg Serratiopeptidase 75 mg
Adm.	Oral
@	1-2 Bol bid
Pres.	5 strip of 4

Oxal Forte Bol	Zydus
Comp	Bolus contain Nimesulide 400 mg Paracetamol 1500 mg Serratiopeptidase 75 mg
Adm.	Oral
@	LA 2 Bol bid SA ½ - 1 Bol bid
Pres.	Blister of 2

Rely NP Bol	Alivira
Comp	Each ml has Nimesulide 400 mg Paracetamol 1500 mg
Adm.	Oral
@	1-2 Bol bid
Pres.	4 Bol strip

Flunixin Meglumine

A NSAID and potent action with analgesic, antipyretic and anti-inflammatory properties. It has more action on tissues of visceral organs reducing swelling. It is indicated in all type of infections of system or organs as a supportive. It can be given IM and IV. It acts rapidly within 15 minutes. Its half life is 8-9 hours so action remains for longer period. It comforts the animal.

FM 50 Inj	Macwell
Comp	Flunixiin meglumine 83 mg provides 50 mg of Flunixin/ml
Adm.	IM or IV
@	1.1-2.2 mg/kg B.wt or 10-20 ml in LA
Pres.	20 ml

Kepflu inj	Kepler
Comp	Flunixiin meglumine 83 mg provides 50 mg of Flunixin/ml
Adm.	IM or IV

@	1.1-2.2 mg/kg B.wt or 10-20 ml in LA
Pres.	20 ml

Unixin inj	**Hester**
Comp	Flunixiin meglumine 83 mg provides 50 mg of Flunixin/ml
Adm.	IM or IV
@	1.1-2.2 mg/kg B.wt or 10-20 ml in LA
Pres.	20 ml

Neglodyne inj	**Nicosia**
Comp	Flunixin megluine 50mg/ml
Adm.	IM/IV
@	1.1-2.2 mg/kg B.wt
Pres.	20 ml, 10 ml

Megxin inj	**Agilis**
Comp	1ml contains 50 mg Flunixin meglumine
Adm.	IM/ IV
@	1.1-2.2 mg/kg B.wt
Pres.	20 ml, 100 ml

Cadifur inj	**Cadila Pharma**
Comp	Flunixin 50 mg/ml
Adm.	IM
@	2 ml/45 kg B.wt
Pres.	20 ml

Flunimeg inj	**Zydus**
Comp	Flunixin 50 mg/ml
Adm.	IM
@	2 ml/45 kg B.wt
Pres.	10 ml, 30 ml

Flizik inj	**Alivira**
Comp	Flunixin 50 mg/ml
Adm.	IM/ IV
@	1.1-2.2 mg/kg B.wt or 1ml/25 kg B.wt
Pres.	20 ml, 100 ml

Flunixin Combination

Jospas inj	**Animax Health**
Comp	Each ml contains Flunixin meglumine 20 mg Pitofenone hydrochloride 20 mg Fenipiverinium bromide 0.02 mg
Adm.	IM
@	LA 1 ml/20 kg B.wt SA 1 ml/10 kg B.wt
Pres.	30 ml, 100 ml

Fluniximol inj	**Carevet Pharma**
Comp	Flunixiin meglumine 83 mg and Paracetamol 150 mg/ml
Adm.	IM or IV
@	1 ml/20 kg B.wt
Pres.	20 ml

Ketoprofen

It is NSAID and has all three properties of anti-inflammatory, analgesic and antipyretic action. It is indicated IM and IV.

Ketop inj	**Alembic**
Comp	Each ml contains ketoprofen 100 mg
Adm.	IM or IV
@	2-4 mg/kg B.wt od for 3-5 days
Pres.	15 ml, 100 ml

Neoprofen	**Zoetis**
Comp	Each ml contains ketoprofen 100 mg
Adm.	IM or IV
@	2-4 mg/kg B.wt od for 3-5 days
Pres.	15 ml, 100 ml

Vetoprofen	**Merial**
Comp	Each ml contains Ketoprofen 100 mg
Adm.	IM or IV
@	2-4 mg/kg B.wt od for 3-5 days
Pres.	15 ml, 100 ml

Neoprofen inj	Zydus
Comp	Ketoprofen 100 mg/ml
Adm.	IM, IV, SC
@	3 mg/kg B.wt
Pres.	Vial of 15 ml, 100 ml

Phenylbutazone

This drug is used in non-visceral traumatic inflammatory conditions involving musculoskeletal system in clinical cases of lameness and posterior weakness. It is contraindicated in anaemia and cases of gastric problems. Bio-availability is very good in horses and canines. It also acts by inhibiting PG synthesis. It is indicated in Pyrexia, symptomatic treatment of inflammatory and painful conditions.

Algesin	Alembic
Comp	Each ml has Phenylbutazone sod 200 mg and Lignocaine 10 mg
Adm.	IM
@	LA 3-12ml SA 1-3ml
Pres.	3 ml ampoule

Phenylbutazone Combination

Artizone S inj	Alved
Comp	Each ml contains Phenylbutazone 200 mg Sodium salicylate 20 mg
Adm.	IM
@	LA 10-20 ml
Pres.	30 ml

Esgipyrin N	Zydus
Comp	Each ml contains Phenylbutazone 750 mg Analgin 750 mg Lignocaine hydrochloride 50 mg
Adm.	IM
@	LA 5-15 ml SA 1-5 ml
Pres.	5 ml

Nylate inj	**Nicosia**
Comp	Phenyl butazone 200 mg sodium salicylate 20 mg/ml
Adm.	IM
@	1 ml/25 kg B.wt
Pres.	30 ml, 100 ml

Artizone S inj	**Zydus**
Comp	Phenylbutazone 200 mg Sod. Salicylate 20 mg in 1ml
Adm.	IM
@	LA 20-30 ml SA 5-10 ml
Pres.	30 ml, 100 ml

Steroidal Anti / Inflammatory Drugs (SAID)

Corticosteroids are used as SAID. These are glucocorticoids. Adrenal cortex secretes steroidal hormones which include glucocorticoids, mineral corticoids and their synthetic analogues. These maintain skeletal muscular, nervous hemostasis functions normal. These prepare animals to withstand effects of external noxious stimuli. They have direct and permissible action. Irrespective in injury or cause inflammatory response is suppressed by these. It is their clinical use. This includes reduction of local exudation, phagocytic activity, fibroblastic activity and ultimalety scar formation. Action is direct and local so can be used topically. Action is by enhancing carbohydrate, protein metaboliom, increasing haemoglobin. These also suppress all types of hypersensitization and allergic phenomenon.

Various steroids are available:

(I) Short Acting: When the duration of action is less than 24 hrs. e.g. Hydrocortisone, Cortisone, Prednisolone, Methylprednisolone.

(II) Intermediate Acting: Duration of action is 24-48 hrs. e.g. Triamcinolone.

(III) Long Acting: Duration of action is around 48 hrs. e.g. Dexamethasone, Betamethasone, Isoflupredone.

Side Effects: These agents impair immunological competence, Osteoprosis, peptic ulceration, muscular weakness and growth retardation are adverse effects.

Betamethasone

It is a glucocorticoid or corticosteroid. It is indicated in acute inflammation, arthritis, allergic skin conditions, hypersensibility, stressin pregnancy. It can be used intra-ocular injection, in rheumatoid arthritis as Periarticular injection.

Betacortril inj	Pfizer
Comp	Each ml contains Betamethasone acetate 8 mg/ml
Adm.	IM/ IV
@	LA 2-4 ml SA 0.5-1 ml
Pres.	2 ml

Betavet	Pfizer
Comp	Each ml contains Betamethasone acetate 4 mg
Adm.	IM/ IV
@	LA 4-8 ml SA 1-2 ml
Pres.	5 ml

Betnesol inj	Virbac
Comp	Each ml contains Betamethasone acetate 4 mg
Adm.	IM/ IV
@	LA 4-8 ml SA 1-2 ml
Pres.	1 ml

Librabet inj	Libra
Comp	Betamethasone 2 mg/ml
Adm.	IM/ IV
@.	LA 4 ml SA 1ml
Pres.	10 ml, 30 ml, 90 ml

Dexamethasone

It is potent and long acting SAID. It meets any emergency with rapid action. Indicated as other SAID. It is a glucocorticoid.

Brisone inj	Brihans
Comp	Dexamethasone 4.4 mg/ml
Adm.	IM/ IV
@	LA 10-30 mg SA 2-5 mg
Pres.	5 ml
Can be given for induction of parturition 40 mg IV	

Cadex inj	**Cattle Remedies**
Comp	Dexamethasone 4.4 mg/ml
Adm.	IM/ IV
@	LA 10-30 mg SA 2-5 mg
Pres.	5 ml
Can be given for induction of parturition 40 mg IV	

Curadex inj	**Concept**
Comp	Dexamethasone 4.4 mg/ml
Adm.	IM/ IV
@	LA 10-30 mg SA 2-5 mg
Pres.	2 ml, 5 ml
Can be given for induction of parturition 40 mg IV	

Dexamethasone	**Alved Lyka**
Comp	Dexamethasone 4.4 mg/ml
Adm.	IM/ IV
@	LA 10-30 mg SA 2-5 mg
Pres.	5 ml
Can be given for induction of parturition 40 mg IV	

Dexasone inj	**Cadila Pharma**
Comp	Dexamethasone 4.4 mg/ml
Adm.	IM/ IV
@	LA 10-30 mg SA 2-5 mg
Pres.	2 ml, 5 ml
Can be given for induction of parturition 40 mg IV	

Dexavet inj	**Wockhardt**
Comp	Dexamethasone 4.4 mg/ml
Adm.	IM/ IV
@	LA 10-30 mg SA 2-5 mg
Pres.	5 ml
Can be given for induction of parturition 40 mg IV	

Ketocart inj	**Intas**
Comp	Dexamethasone 4.4 mg/ml
Adm.	IM/ IV
@	LA 10-30 mg SA 2-5 mg
Pres.	5 ml, 10 ml
Can be given for induction of parturition 40 mg IV	

Marcodex inj	Marc
Comp	Dexamethasone 4.4 mg/ml
Adm.	IM/ IV
@	LA 10-30 mg SA 2-5 mg
Pres.	2 ml, 6 ml
Can be given for induction of parturition 40 mg IV	

Rancortin inj	Ranbaxy
Comp	Dexamethasone 4.4 mg/ml
Adm.	IM/ IV
@	LA 10-30 mg SA 2-5 mg
Pres.	5 ml
Can be given for induction of parturition 40 mg IV	

Vetcort inj	Alembic
Comp	Dexamethasone 4.4 mg/ml
Adm.	IM/ IV
@	LA 10-30 mg SA 2-5 mg
Pres.	5 ml
Can be given for induction of parturition 40 mg IV	

Vetodex inj	Indain Immunology
Comp	Dexamethasone 4.4 mg/ml
Adm.	IM/ IV
@	LA 10-30 mg SA 2-5 mg
Pres.	50 ml
Can be given for induction of parturition 40 mg IV	

Dexona inj	Zydus
Comp	Dexamethasone 4.4 mg/ml
Adm.	IM/ IV
@	LA 10-30 mg SA 2-5 mg
Pres.	5 ml
Can be given for induction of parturition 40 mg IV	

Cipdex inj	Cipla
Comp	Dexamethasone 4.4 mg/ml
Adm.	IM/ IV
@	LA 10-30 mg SA 2-5 mg
Pres.	5 ml
Can be given for induction of parturition 40 mg IV	

Hydrocortisone

It is a natural corticosteroid and short acting SAID. Its action is like other corticosteroid. It is used for allergy, anaphylactic shock etc.

Hydrovet	**Cipla**
Comp	Hydrocortisone acetate 25 mg/ml
Adm.	IM/ IV
@	LA 1-1.5 g total dose IM or 50 mg/kg B.wt IV SA 1-3 mg/kg B.wt
Pres.	5 ml

Prednisolone

It is also a short duration acting SAID. It has a typical metabolic effects of natural corticosteroid. It has very good anti-inflammatory effect. It is indicated in inflammation, allergic bronchitis, asthma, food allergy. It can be given intra articular route.

Prednisolone inj	**Wockhardt**
Comp	Prednisolone acetate 10 mg/ml
Adm.	IM
@	LA 0.5 mg/kg B.wt Total dose 10-20 ml SA 2.5-5 ml Total dose Locally Intra articular LA 2.5-7.5 ml total dose SA 0.5-2 ml
Pres.	10 ml

Hostacortin H	**Hoechst**
Comp	Prednisolone acetate 10 mg/ml
Adm.	IM
@	LA 0.5 mg/kg B.wt Total dose 10-20 ml SA 2.5-5 ml Total dose Locally Intra articular LA 2.5-7.5 ml total dose SA 0.5-2 ml
Pres.	10 ml

BV Cort	**Venky**
Comp	Prednisolone acetate 10 mg/ml
Adm.	IM
@	LA 0.5 mg/kg B.wt Total dose 10-20 ml SA 2.5-5 ml Total dose Locally Intra articular LA 2.5-7.5 ml total dose SA 0.5-2 ml
Pres.	10 ml

Triamcilone

It is one of SAID and a corticosteroid which acts for 24-48 hours. It has anti-inflammatory and anti allergic property. It is indicated in arthritis and Ketosis.

Vetalog	**Zydus**
Comp	Triamcinolone acetate 6 mg/ml
Adm.	IM/ SC
@	LA 12-20 mg (total dose) SA 0.05 mg/kg B.wt
Pres.	5 ml

BV Log	**Venky**
Comp	Triamcinolone acetate 6 mg/ml
Adm.	IM/ SC
@	LA 12-20 mg (total dose) SA 0.05 mg/kg B.wt
Pres.	5 ml

Isoflupredone

It is latest corticosteroid SAID. Its action lasts for 24-48 hrs. Its action is higher than Hydrocortisone, Prednisolone and Betamethasone. No milk withholding is required. It is safe in pregnant and lactating animals. It is useful in local deposition in joint. It can be given in inflammatory conditions and Ketosis.

Isopred inj	**Phoenix**
Comp	Each ml contains Isoflupredone acetate 2 mg/ml
Adm.	IM
@	LA 5-10 ml SA 0.5-1 ml/kg B.wt
Pres.	10 ml

Isomax inj	**Animax Health**
Comp	Each ml contains 2 mg/ml of Isoflupredone
Adm.	IM
@	LA 5-10 ml SA 0.5-1 ml/10 kg B.wt
Pres.	10 ml with syringe and needle

Isodan inj and Bolus	**Libra**
Comp	Bol. Isoflupredane 10 mg + Serritopeptidase 25 mg Inj 2mg/ml of Isoflupredane
Adm.	Inj IM and Bolus oral
@.	Inj 5-10 ml od Bol 2 Bol od x 3 days
Pres.	10 ml, 50 ml inj, strip of 4 Bolus

Nicofluid inj	**Nicosia**
Comp	Isoflupredone acetate 2mg/ml
Adm.	IM
@	5-10 ml od
Pres.	10 ml, 30 ml

Isofluid inj	**Zydus**
Comp	Isoflupredone acetate 2 mg/ml
Adm.	IM
@	5-10 ml in LA
Pres.	5 ml, 10 ml, 30 ml

Topflud TR Bol	**Herstel**
Comp	Isoflupredone 10 mg Serriatio peptidase 25 mg
Adm.	Oral
@	1 Bol od x 5 days
Pres.	1 Bol

Skeletal Muscle Relaxants

These are drugs that act peripherally at neuro-muscular junction/ muscle fibres and centrally in cerebrospinal axis to reduce muscle tone. These are of 2 types:

(i) Neuromuscular blocking agent e.g. Gallamine succinyl choline, Benzoquinonium, Metocurine, Baclofen, etc.

(ii) Directly acting which act by depolarization of muscle membranes e.g. Dantrolene.

These are also centrally acting muscle relaxants which acts through CNS e.g. Meprobamate, diazepam, Chlorzoxazone. Side effects of Muscle relaxants are sedation, weakness, fatigue and light headcheeses

Succinyl Choline

It acts by depolarizing neuromuscular blocking agents by interfering with ACH mediated depolarization of post synaptic membrane and induce prolonged depolarization of region around muscle. It is short acting. It is indicated in all types of surgery with pre-disposition. It is used in casting and restraining the animal for clinical examination and orthopaedic manipulation.

Scoline inj	**Glaxo**
Comp	Succinylcholine 50 mg/ml
Adm.	IV
@	LA 0.08 mg/kg B.wt SA 0.02 mg/kg B.wt
Pres.	2 ml

Chlorzoxazone

A muscle relaxant which acts at the spinal cord and such critical levels of brain to inhibit multisynaptic reflex arcs involved in producing muscles spasms. It acts as centrally acting muscle relaxant with sedative properties. It is indicated in symptomatic treatment of muscle spasm. It blocks pain sensation. There can be skin rash or itching or redness by its excessive use. It is used orally. It is added in Bolus with other NSAIDS as it has synergistic action with them.

Miscellaneous

Proxyvet Bol.	**Wockhardt**
Comp	Each Bolus contains Acetaminophen 1500 mg Dextropropoxyphone hydrochloride 97.5 mg
Adm.	Oral
@	LA 4 Bolus bid SA ½ -1 Bolus bid
Pres.	Strip of 4

Karpofen inj	**Zydus**
Comp	Carpropin 50 g per ml
Adm.	IM/IV/SC
@	1ml/35 kg B.wt
Pres.	Vial of 10 ml, 30 ml

Catgall Ointment			**Cattle Remedies**
Indications: Sprain, Arthritis, Filrohi, Jointillness, chronicinflamation			
Composition: 1.00 g contains			
Aloebarbadensis	20 g	Curcummaamadirox	20 g
SodiumTetraborate	20 g	Oleumricini	40 ml
Dosage: To be applied gently on affected area.			
Presentation: 50 g, 100 g, 500 g Jar			

Rumalya Cream/tablets	**Himalya**
Indications: Sprain, Arthritis	
Composition: Not given	
Dosage: 8-12 tablets thrice daily Apply locally	
Presentation: 28 g tube 100 tab. pack	

Inflamin	**Himalya**
Indications: Mastitis for swelling	
Composition: Not given	
Dosage: Apply on affected part	
Presentation: 50 gm, 125 g tube	

❑❑❑

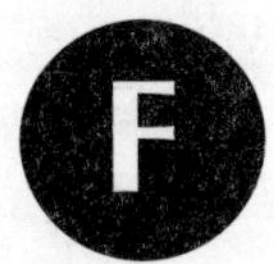

Nutrition and Metabolism

Nutrition and Nutrients

Nutrition is the sum total of processes growth, repair and maintenance of body activity. The substances found in feed material necessary for maintenance, production and health of animal is known as Nutrients. These are

I. Energy Producing Nutrients. These provide energy to animal. the are Fat, Carbohydrate, Protein.

II. Non energy Producing Nutrients. These do not provide energy but these are very essential for body functions– Water, Mineral, Vitamins.

Fat

These are fatty acids and glycerols. These are

Lipids which include Phospholipids

Steroids – Cholestrol and Sterol

These can be animal fat present there milk, cream, butter, ghee, eggyolk, mutton etc. Another source is vegetable fat present in oils like ground nut, olive oil, sunflower oil, nuts and seeds. These provide energy when needed but otherwise stored as such.

Carbohydrates

These provide energy immediately to body by process of oxidation, when present in excess these are converted into fat and when these are not available fat is converted into carbohydrate and energy. These are saccharides- fructose, glucose, maltose etc.

Proteins

These are highly complex substances. These form the major structural compounds of animal tissue. These are components of skin, hair, wool, egg, feather, nails, horns, hoofs, muscle, tendon and cartilage, connective tissue etc. these are involved in nerves, antibodies and metabolic regulation. These are utilized in building of new tissue, their maintenance, wear and tear. These have units Amino acids which are more than 300.

Essential Amino Acids	Non Essential Amino Acids
1. Arginine	Asparagine
2. Histidine	Aspartate
3. Isoleucine	Glutamate
4. Leucine	Glycine
5. Lysine	Serine

6. Methionine	Tyrosine
7. Phenylalamine	
8. Threonine	
9. Tryptophen	
10. Valine	

Essential Amino acids are not synthsized in body.

Some others are conditional Essential

1. Cysteine
2. Glutamine
3. Hydroxyproline
4. Proline, Taurine

Non Energy Producing Nutrient

Minerals

There are more than 100 minerals available but about 18-20 are important for animal body. These help to play important role in vital processes, balance of body fluids. They give rigidity and strength to bones and activate enzymes. These are constituents of protein, lipids etc.

Vitamins

These are chemical compound required to maintain growth and normal metabolism. Most of them can not be synthesized in body and hence should be supplemented.

Water

Animal body is composed of two third of water. It plays very important role and animal may die due to its shortage or Dehydration. It provides rigidity and elasticity. It has solvent action and is needed in hydrochloric and Ionic reactions. It regulates heat and lubricates various parts of body. Its deficiency may cause many problems.

Use of Nutrients

Intake of any food in the body is ingestion. Breaking of food into nutrients is digestion. Passing the nutrients in blood or lymph is absorption. When carried to various organs these are utilized called assimilation. Unused matter is excreted. This whole process is metabolism.

Minerals: These are elements and are of 2 types

(i) **Macromineral:** Their requirement in body is in higher quantity. These are Calcium, Magnesium, Potassium, Sodium, Phosphorus, Sulphur.

(ii) **Micromineral:** These are required in the body in small quantities. These are Iron, Iodine, Copper, Cobalt, Zinc, Manganese, Chromium, Selenium, Molybdenum, Flourine

Calcium: Indicated in hypocalcaemia or milk fever, as general tonic, in general metabolic disorders, debility, exhaustion and support for treating sterlity, bone formation, increase milk production and growth.

Magnesium: Indicated for general metabolic disorders particularly when protein deficiency is observed. hypomagnesaemia, hypoglycaemia, nervous irritability, paraplegia, muscular weakness, twitching & tetany.

Phosphorus: Indicated in general metabolic disorders, debility, fatigue, exhaustion, anorexia, depressed appetite, Pica, ricket, Osteomalacia, tetany andparesis, post parturient haemoglobinuria, infertility, anoestrus and repeat breeding and general tonic. Used to increase milk production & growth, in haemoglobinuria.

Potassium: Indicated in anorexia, depressed growth, dull and coarse hair or wool, Pica, hypogalactia, lethargy, muscular weakness, stiffness or paralysis and neurologic dysfunctions. For high milk yielding its requirement goes up specially in early lactation.

Sodium: Indicated in lethargy, anorexia, weight loss, hypogalactia, neuromuscular and cardiovascular dysfunction and depraved appetite. Helps in affecting feed intake, feed efficiency, basic amino-acid metabolism. Requirement increases with lactation.

Sulphur: Helps in rumen for microflora to function normally. But the requirement is usually obtained from amino acids & vitamin combinations.

Fluorine: It helps in preventing dental caries and is beneficial in reducing bone demineralization. Animals are more sensitive, to Fluorine toxicity so levels should be controlled.

Chromium: it is essential for growth and immune functions. Requirement is increased during infections.

Cobalt: It helps in impaired reproductive functions, reduced appetite, decreased growth rate and reduced milk production. It is essential for vitamin B. synthesis in rumen. Helps in anaemia and emaciation.

Copper: Essential for the activity of various enzymes and haemglobin formation. Dificiency causes depigmentation of skin, enlarged hoofs, steely wool, anaemia, haemoglobinuria due to nutritional imbalance, stiffleg syndrome, unthriftiness & infertility. Also helps in weight gain and milk production.

Iodine: Essential for hormone secretion by thyroid gland. Added for better metabolic activity of body and overall genital cycle. Indicated for better growth, Anoestrous, repeater, muscular strength, higher milk production and pregnants. Also used to treat actinobacillosis and actinomycosis.

Iron: Essental for haemoglobin formation. Indicated in general growth, anoestrus, Pica, repeat breeders, pregnants and high lactating animals. Used as haematinic.

Manganese: Its deficiency is relatively uncommon in domestic animals to control deformities, enlarged joints and twisted limbs. It helps in cartilage formation also.

Molybdenum: No deficiency is documented. Because of excessive availability leads to toxicity specially chronic diarrhea. So it should not be supplemented till there is excess of copper.

Selenium: Indicated in nutritional muscular dystrophy due to vit.E deficiency. Helps in strong bones. It helps in reproductive disorders like retained placenta, abortion, & stillbirth.

Zinc: It helps in stimulating immune system of body and provides resistance to body to fight infections.

Vitamins

There are 6 vitamins. These are of 2 types

1. Fat soluble vitamins – **A, D, E, K**
2. Water soluble vitamins- **B, C**

Fat soluble vitamins. These are not soluble in water but soluble in fat.

These are 4 :

Vitamin A: Infertility associated with vit.A deficiency. Night blindness, xeropthalmia, keratomalacia. To maintain healthy pregnancy. As a supportive in treatment of respiratory tract, GI tract, urinary tract infections, mastitis, metritis. FMD and sterility.

Vitamin D (cholecalciferol): Dificiency leads to Ricket, Osteomalacia and normal matrix biosynthesis. It stimulates calcium and Phosphorus absorption and helps in fractures, deformity of bones. Helps in parturient paresis i.e, milk fever. Helps in milk increase due to better utilization of calcium & Phosphorus. Also used to reduce neoplastic proliferation and enhance the immunity to fight infections.

Vitamin E (Tocoferol): It has an antioxidant effect which modulate several physiological processes. It helps in reproductive functions, immune competency, blood coagulation etc. it reduces the incidence of retained placenta, metritis and cystic ovary. It promotes anticancer sentinel activity of immune system.It helps in healing process and protection of cells. Acts as antisterility vitamin. Supportive in mastitis and genital tract infetions.

Vitamin K (Menadione): As the requirement of vitamin K is greatest during pregnancy, lactation and rapid growth. Vit K deficiency result due to abnormal fat digestion and absorption, injuries and anaemicas of various etiology.

Water soluble vitamins. They are soluble in water. So these are less stored in body

Vitamin C (Ascorbic acid): Requirement is increased in post injury period. So helpful in accelerating healing process of Sores and ulcers. It enhances iron absorption so useful in anaemia. Severity of cold is reduced. It increase working capacity. It increases immunity. It is antioxidant.

Vitamin B: It has 12 versions. So it is called vitamin B complex.

(i) Vitamin B_1 (Thiamine): Thiamine is indicated in weakness, paresis, anorexia and diarrhea. It is helpful in convulsion and paralysis. In horses can be given in muscle tremor and weight loss, ataxia, cardiac arrhythmias. As a supportive very helpful in chronic sick animal. It activates nerves of movement.

(ii) Vitamin B_2 or Riboflavin: Acts as coenzyme for the metabolism of carbohydrates fats. Indicated in anorexia, poor growth, metabolism, loss of hair, excessive lacrimation and salivation.

(iii) Vitamin B_3 or Niacin: Indicated in inappetance, poor growth, non-regenerative, anaemia, stomatitis, vomiting, diarrhea, dermatitis and alopecia or deficiency symptoms.

(iv) Pantothenic acid or vit B_5: Indicated in anorexia, poor growth, haemorrhagic diarrhea, rough hair coat particularly scaly dermatitis around the eyes and muzzle and locomotive disorders like spasticity and an exaggerated gait.

(v) Vitamin B_6 (Pyridoxine): It is essential for protein and amino acid metabolism. It helps in the formation of RBC's and WBC's. Indicated in diarrhea, poor growth, microcytic hypochromic anaemia & nervous disorders.

(vi) Vitamin B_{12} (cyanacobalamine): It is synthesized in the rumen by microflora and cobalt. Its supplement action can improve feed efficiency growth & reproduction. It is also useful in anaemic condition and hind leg paralysis. It protects nervous system. it helps in blood formation.

(vii) Biotin or B_7 or vitamin H: Indicated in cases with integumentary changes-especially dryness, roughness, ulceration, inflammation of oral mucosa and cracking soles and top of hooves.

(viii) Folic acid: Helps in formation of RBC. Indicated in hypochromic anaemia and glossitis to increase weight gain, feed efficiency and blood haemoglobin concentration.

(ix) Choline: It effects lipid metabolism. Indicated in growth or lactational demand. It increases milk production. The greater the level of production greater will be the need of choline. Helps in combating stress and G.I. diseases.

Other three have less importantance

Supplements

These are feed stuffs used to improve the value of basal feeds. These are

Mineral supplement: Proper ratio of mineral elements used to improve feed valve

Vitamin supplement: Addition of vitamin or mixture of vitamins depending upon the need of animals

Additive: Substances that is added to basic feed usually in small quantities for fortifying with nutrients or medicines.

Feed additives: Non nutrient product that affects the utilization of feed or productive performance of animal.

Probiotic: Seprations containing live microorganism used for the growth of microflora in GI tract.

Prebiotic: Food ingredients that benefit by stimulating the growth and/ or activity of one or number of microorganism in intestine.

Bye Pass Product: these are products specially designed are directly passed to intestine for absorption avoiding any change in rumen. These can be Bye Pass fat, Bye pass Proteins etc.

Various types of Supplements are formulated in Veterinary Practice apart from single nutrients. These are available as Powder, Bolus, Liquid, Injectables.

Mineral mixture: combination of major macro and micro- mineral indicated in non-specific infertility, anoestrus, healthy growth of foetus during pregnancy. To increase milk production, body resistance and against disease. Helpful in reducing calcium- Phosphorus deficiency such as Osteomalacia stunted growth, PICA, milk fever and general weakness.

Mineral Plus vitamins: Combinations of major and microminerals with various vitamins are indicated for better health, maintenance and increased milk production. This ensures balanced nutrition. Highly useful in calves as well as pregnant animals. Indicated in anoestrous, mineral and vitamin deficiency of animals, retention of placenta, prolapse, repeat breeders and general weakness.

Mineral Plus amino acids: Regular supplementation of minerals and amino acids, helps to maintain healthy growth and higher productivity and fertility.

Minerals Plus Amino acids Plus Vitamins: These combination products are supplemented for overall growth, production and reproduction. Deficiency of minerals, vitamins and amino acids is overall by these to provide optimum growth, milk production with higher fat percentage.

Liquid Calcium + Phosphorus and vit. D + B_{12}: Calcium Phosphorus deficiency conditions to prevent milk fever, to improve growth, production and stamina. Given to increase milk production, healthy pregnancy and better growth.

Vitamins and Amino acids: Indicated in deficiency of Vitamins and amino acids in general stress, uneven growth and decreased production. Helpful in birds after vaccination and deworoning. For better growth, production and hatchability. It also effects FCR.

Bye Pass Fat & Bye Pass Protein

Probiotics

Probiotics & Prebiotics combined

Supplement with Mineral Vitamin, Amino Acid, Probiotic- Prebiotics.

Amino Acid

These are building blocks of protein. There are about 300 amino acids in nature. 20 of these occur in proteins of all forms of life. But of these some are essential Amino Acid. These cannot be formed in our body and these have to be supplemented. These synthesise cell, help in synthesis of hormones, enzymes and bile acids. They repair the wear and tear in body. They synthesise milk protein and antibodies. They supply energy.

Vubimeth RP	Jubilant lifesciences
Comp	Rumen protected Methionine 50%
Adm.	In feed or oral
@	500 g/ MT of feed or 5-10 g od
Pres.	1 kg, 5 kg

Jubilys RP	Jubilant lifesciences
Comp	Contains 70% Lysine hydrochloride
Adm.	Oral
@	15-30 g od 1-1.5 kg 1 Ton of feed
Pres.	1 kg, 10 kg

Metabolic Diseases

Acetonaemia: (Also Ketosis) Insufficient intake of carbohydrates specially in pregnancy or excessive loss of carbohydrates through milk. There is formation of Ketone bodies

Avitaminosis A: Caused by vit A deficiency symptoms of night blindness, muscular incoordination, staggering gait, stillborn calves in cows and abortions.

Beri-Beri: Disease caused by B1or Thiamine deficiency.

Big Neck: Enlarged thyroid accompanied by hairlessness and high mortality caused due to Iodine deficiency. Also called as Goitre.

Bran Disease: Caused by diet rich in Phophorous and deficient in calcium.

Cannibalism: Eating of own body part or from same species.

Crazy Chick Disease: nervous disease caused by deficiency of vitamin E.

Curled toe paralysis: Paralysis in birds caused by B2(Riboflavin) deficiency.

Dehydration: Disturbance of body water balance in which more fluid is lost from the body than is absorbed and results in reduction in circulating volume of blood.

Downer Cow syndrome: Inability to rise. Reduced food intake.

Enzootic ataxia: Affects unweaned lambs characterised by incoordination of hind legs. Respiratory and cardiac rates are also accelerated by exertion caused by copper deficiency.

Fluorosis: Stunted growth, lameness, mottled and irregular teeth, thickening of jaws, bones, ribs and limbs. Decreased production and impaired fertility.

Haemoglobinuria: Disease in buffaloes and high producing diary cows occurring soon after calving. Can occur in severe hypophosphataemia, hypocuremia or selenium deficiency. Red urine with haemoglobin.

Hypercalcaemia: Excess of calcium.

Hypobiotinosis: Deficiency of Biotin.

Hypocalcaemia: Deficiency of calcium leads to many different symptoms.

Hypocholinosis: Deficiency of Choline.

Hypocyanocobalaminosis: Deficiency of vit B12.

Hypofolicosis: Deficiency of Folic acid.

Hypomagnesaemia: Deficiency of Magnesium leads to muscular tetany.

Hyponiacinosis: Deficiency of nicotinic acid.

Hypopentothenosis: Deficiency of Pentothenic acid.

Hypophosphataemia: Deficiency of Phosphorus.

Hypopyridoxinosis: Deficiency of Pyridoxia or B6.

Hyporiboflavinosis: Deficiency of riboflavin or B2.

Hypothermia: Temperature below normal body temperature.

Hypothiaminosis: Deficiency of thiamine or B1.

Hypvitaminosis: Deficiency of any vitamin.

Ketosis: Occurs in female adults during pregnancy or around parturition. Hypoglycaemia, Ketonuria and low level of hepatic glycogen, temperature, pulse. Respiratory rates are normal, ruminal movement reduced. Woody appearance, decrease in milk yield and appetite. Body wt. is lost. Sweet odour in breath and milk. Staggering gait & moderate tremor, aimless movement. Nervous signs if not treated.

Kumree: Unable to get up insidious lameness of hindlegs, tenderness of loin with swaying action of hindquarter. Cause not known but mineral deficiency is there.

Malnutrition: Deficit, excess or imbalance of one or more essential nutrients.

Milk fever: Occurs mostly about time of parturition in adult females and is characterized by hypocalcaemia, muscular weakness, circulatory collapse and depression of consciousness. Hindlegs are stuck out stiffy. Sternal recumbency. Muzzle is dry & no fever. Ruminal stasis and constipation.

Night blindness: Inability to see in dim light due to vit. A deficiency.

Osteomalacia: Disease of mature animals affecting bones. In earlier stages there is low productivity, fertility & loss of condition. Lameness shifting from leg to leg. Crackling sounds while walking and an arched back. In extreme cases deformities of bone can occur.

Peat Scour: Persistent diarrhea with passage of watery yellow green to black faeces with an inoffensive odour. It is due to molybdenum poisoning in grazing cattle.

Pica: Ingestion of material other than normal food & varies from licking to actual eating.

Pine of calves: Stilted gait affecting hindlimbs followed by progressive emaciation.

Ricket: Disease of young growing animals characterised by defective calcification of growing bones. There is stiffness in gait, enlargement of limbs, joints specially in forelegs. Long bones show abnormal curvature.

Swayback: Unable to stand and suck. Occurs at birth or in first few weeks of life. Inco-ordination and erratic movements are more marked caused by Hypocuporosis (deficiency of copper).

White muscle disease: Or Nutritional muscular dystrophy. Symptoms are muscular weakness. Animal can not stand, youngones cannot suckle the mother, loss of weight and death, cause in deficiency of nutrients specially selenium.

Xeropthalmia: In dogs and calves thickening and clouding of cornea due to vit.A deficiency.

Infusion

It includes essential nutrients to be given direct in the blood for immediate availability in serious diseases or conditions when these are needed instantly.

Amino Acid Infusions

These are indicated in hyproteinaemia malnutrition, post surgical nutrient supplementation for parental nutrient supply or where feeding is not possible.

Aminodrop	**Wockhardt**			
Comp	100 ml contains			
	L Isoleucine	106.8 mg	L Threonine	129.3 mg
	L Aspartic acid	360.0 mg	L Lencine	756.75 mg
	L Tryptopnan	0.5 mg	L Cystein	5.6 mg
	L Lysine	1229.25 mg	L Valine	157.5 mg
	L Glutamic acid	450 ml	L Methionine	316.8 mg
	L Alanine	675 mg	L Histidine	33.75 mg
	L Phenylalanine	253.05 mg	L Arganine	495 mg
	L probine	345 mg	L Serine	165 mg
	L Tyrosin	56.25 mg	Glycine	1650 mg
	L Hydroxyprolines	315 mg	Sodium	8.7 m
	Pottasium	1.5 m		
Adm.	IV			
@	300-500 ml			
Pres.	200 ml, 500 ml			

Hermin	**Alembic**			
Comp	Each ml contains			
	L Lysine	19.2 mg	L Isoleucine	6.6 mg
	L Threonine hydrochloride	7 mg	L Phenyl alanine	9.6 mg
	L Methionine	6.8 mg	L Valine	6.4 mg
	L Tryptopnan	3 mg	L Arginine hydrochloride	10.9 mg
	L Leucine	10 mg	L Histidine hydrochloride	4.7 mg
	Glycine	6 mg	Sorbitol	50 mg
Adm.	IV			
@	As per need			
Pres.	200 ml			

VetPlasma	**Zydus**
Comp	100 ml contains Hydroxyethyl starch 6 g Sodium chloride 0.9 gm + water
Adm.	IV
@	20 ml/kg B.wt
Pres.	500 ml bottle

Calcium Borogluconate

It is indicated in Milk fever, Hypocalcaemia, uterine involution etc.

Borocal	**Sarabhai**
Comp	Calcium 1.86% Boric acid 4.2%
Adm.	IV SC
@	As per need
Pres.	200 ml, 450 ml

Brical	**Brihans**
Comp	Calcium 1.86% Boric acid 4.2%
Adm.	IV SC
@	As per need
Pres.	450 ml

Calcicat	**Cattle Remedies**
Comp	Calcium 1.86% Boric acid 4.2%
Adm.	IV SC
@	As per need
Pres.	450 ml

Calborol	**Novartis**
Comp	Calcium 1.86% Boric acid 4.2%
Adm.	IV SC
@	As per need
Pres.	450 ml

Calcium Borogluconate	**Wockhardt/ Glaxo**
Comp	Calcium 1.86% Boric acid 4.2%
Adm.	IV SC
@	As per need
Pres.	450 ml

Calgonate	**Indian Immunology**
Comp	Calcium 1.86% Boric acid 4.2%
Adm.	IV SC
@	As per need
Pres.	450 ml

Calmex	**Ranbaxy**
Comp	Calcium 1.86% Boric acid 4.2%
Adm.	IV SC
@	As per need
Pres.	450 ml

Fevimil	**HAL**
Comp	Calcium 1.86% Boric acid 4.2%
Adm.	IV SC
@	As per need
Pres.	450 ml

Intacal	**Intas**
Comp	Calcium 1.86% Boric acid 4.2%
Adm.	IV SC
@	As per need
Pres.	450 ml

Calciboro	**Virbac**
Comp	Calcium 1.86% Boric acid 4.2%
Adm.	IV SC
@	As per need
Pres.	450 ml

Calup IV	**Vetcare – Cargill**
Comp	Calcium 1.86% Boric acid 4.2%
Adm.	IV SC
@	As per need
Pres.	200 ml, 450 ml

Calvit	**Glaxo**
Comp	Calcium gluconate 20.75% Boric acid 4.25%
Adm.	IV SC
@	As per need
Pres.	200 ml, 450 ml

Lactaid	**Intervet**
Comp	Calcium 1.86% Boric acid 4.2%
Adm.	IV SC
@	As per need
Pres.	200 ml, 450 ml

Calcium Sandozin	**Novartis**
Comp	Cal glubionate 1.375 g Calcium gluconate 10%
Adm.	IV
@	LA 30-50 ml
Pres.	10 ml

Qualidrops liq	**Zydus**
Comp	Calcium gluconate- calcium 1.86% Bori acid calcium 2.26 to 1
Adm.	IV
@	450 ml
Pres.	450 ml

Calcium Magnesium

Boromag	**Zydus**	
Comp	Calcium gluconate Magnesium hypophoshite Proportion of Boric acid in calcium Dextrose anhydrous	20.75% 5% 2.26% 20%
Adm.	IV	
@	As per need	
Pres.	450 ml	

Calbim	**Virbac**	
Comp	Calcium gluconate Calcium hypophosphite Boric acid Dextrose Magnesium chloride	16.6% 2.4% 3.4% 20% 1.33%
Adm.	IV	
@	As per need	
Pres.	450 ml	

Calmex M	**Ranbaxy**	
Comp	Calcium 1.86 Magnesium hypophosphite 5%	Boriacid 4.2% Dextrose 20%
Adm.	IV	
@	As per need	
Pres.	450 ml	

Lactomag	**Virbac**	
Comp	Calcium gluconate 20.75% Magnesium hypophosphite 5%	Boric acid 4.2% Dextrose 20%
Adm.	IV	
@	As per need	
Pres.	450 ml	

Magical	**Cadila Pharma**	
Comp	100 ml contains Calcium gluconate 20.80% Magnesium hypophosphite 5g	 Boric acid 4.2% Dextrose 20 g

Adm.	IV
@	As per need
Pres.	450 ml

Mifex	**Novartis**	
Comp	Calcium borogluconate Magnesium hypophosphite Dextrose	25% 5% 20%
Adm.	IV	
@	As per need	
Pres.	450 ml	

Miphocal	**Indian Immunology**	
Comp	Calcium 1.86% Magnesium hypophosphite 5%	Boriacid 4.2% Dextrose 20%
Adm.	IV	
@	As per need	
Pres.	450 ml	

Pfizer Milk fever formula	**Pfizer**	
Comp	Calcium gluconate Magnesium hypophosphite Boric acid Dextrose 4.2 g in	1.859 g 20.8 g 5 g 100 ml
Adm.	IV	
@	As per need	
Pres.	450 ml	

Thiacal	**Wockhardt**	
Comp	Calcium gluconate 20% Dextrose 15%	Boric acid 5% Vit B_1 300 mg
Adm.	IV	
@	As per need	
Pres.	450 ml	

Calcium Magnesium Borogluconate	Sarabhai	
Comp	Calcium gluconate Dextrose Boric acid Magnesium hypophosphite	18% 18.1% 1.85% 4%
Adm.	IV	
@	As per need	
Pres.	450 ml	

Mifical	Cadila	
Comp	Calcium gluconate 29.8 g Magnesium hypophosphite 5 g	Boric acid 4.2 g Dextrose 20 g
Adm.	IV	
@	As per need	
Pres.	450 ml	

Dextrose

It is indicated in bovine ketosis, hypoglycemia, weakness conditions in which oral feeding is impossible. Amount and rate of infusion depends on the severity of the condition.

Dextrose 5%	Wockhardt
Comp	Dextrose Anydrous 5 g in 100 ml
Adm.	IV
@	As per need
Pres.	540 ml

Wocktrose 25	Wockhardt
Comp	Dextrose Anhydrous 25%
Adm.	IV
@	As per need
Pres.	540 ml

Dextrose + Sodium Chloride

It is indicated in hypoglycaemia complicated with dehydration or fluid loss due to infections, trauma surgery, burns, debility etc. in which supplementation orally is impossible. Amount and rate of infusion depends on severity of condition.

Dextrose and Sodium chloride	**Alembic**
Comp	Dextrose Anhydrous 5% Sodium chloride 0.9%
Adm.	IV
@	As per need
Pres.	540 ml

Dextrose Saline	**Wockhardt**
Comp	Dextrose Anydrous 5 g in 100ml
Adm.	IV
@	As per need
Pres.	540 ml

Electrolyte Infusion

These are indicated for instant replenishment of electrolytes and energy in conditions associated with fluid and electrolyte loss or unbalance Amount and rate of infusion depends on severity of condition.

Intalyte	**Intas**
Comp	100 ml contains Dextrose 20 g Sodium chloride 0.6 g Potassium chloride 0.04 g Calcium chloride 0.027g Sodium lactate 0.312 g
Adm.	IV
@	As per need
Pres.	500 ml

Lacrivet	**Brihans**
Comp	100 ml contains Dextrose 20 g Sodium chloride 0.6 g Potassium chloride 0..04 g Calcium chloride 0.027 g Lactic acid 0.24 g Sodium hydroxide 0.116 g
Adm.	IV
@	As per need
Pres.	500 ml

Rintose	**Wockhardt**	
Comp	100 ml contains	
	Dextrose	20 g
	Sodium chloride	0.6 g
	Potassium chloride	0.04 g
	Calcium chloride	0.027g
	Sodium lactate	0.312 g
Adm.	IV	
@	As per need	
Pres.	500 ml	

Sodium chloride or Normal Saline

It is indicated in dehydration, shock, fluid loss due to haemorrhage, vomiting, diarrhea to restore circulatory volume.

Sodium chloride 0.45%, 0.9%	**Generic**
Comp	Sodium chloride 0.45% or 0.9%
Adm.	IV
@	As per need
Pres.	500 ml

Normal Saline 5%	**Generic**
Comp	Sodium chloride 5%
Adm.	IV
@	As per need
Pres.	500 ml

Dextrose Combination

Dextrobex V	**Sterling**
Comp	100 ml contains Dextrin 50% Vit B_1 100 mg B_2 4 mg B_6 50 mg Niacinamide 160 mg
Adm.	IV
@	As per need
Pres.	540 ml

Vitamins Injectable

Vitamin A

It is indicated in infertility cases associated with vit A deficiency, night blindness, xerophthalmia, dermatological disorders and other hypovitaminosis A conditions. It is also used in stunted growth, debility, staggering gait, running nose and eyes. It is indicated as supportive therapy- in Respiratory, Gastro intestinal or urogenital tract infections.

Alvit A inj	**Alembic**
Comp	Each ml contains Vit A 600000 IU
Adm.	IM
@	LA 10-12 ml each week SA 5-10 ml each week
Pres.	2 ml, 5 ml

Preplin Forte inj	**Virbac**
Comp	Each ml contains Vit A 600000 IU
Adm.	IM
@	LA 10-12 ml each week SA 5-10 ml each week
Pres.	2 ml, 5 ml

Spark sol A inj	**Neospark**
Comp	Each ml contains Vit A 600000 IU
Adm.	IM
@	LA 10-12 ml each week SA 5-10 ml each week
Pres.	2 ml, 5 ml

Veta A	**TTK**
Comp	Each ml contains Vit A 600000 IU
Adm.	IM
@	LA 10-12 ml each week SA 5-10 ml each week
Pres.	2 ml, 5 ml

VIT A inj	**Generic**
Comp	Each ml contains Vit A 600000 IU
Adm.	IM
@	LA 10-12 ml each week SA 5-10 ml each week
Pres.	2 ml, 5 ml

Solvit A Forte	**Vetcare**
Comp	Each ml contains Vit A 600000 IU
Adm.	Oral
@	LA 10 ml od SA 5 ml od
Pres.	2 ml, 5 ml

Vitamin B_1

It is indicated in weakness, paresis, anorexia and diarrhea. It activates neurons of muscular activity so can be injected in all sick animals for movement, muscle tremor, incoordination etc.

Beriwin inj	**Carevet Pharma**
Comp	Each ml contains 100 mg Thiamine hydrochloride
Adm.	IM
@	LA 10 ml
Pres.	10 ml

Vitamin B_1 and B_{12}

It is indicated in Anaemia, weakness, convalsence of Thiamine deficiency. Combination helps nervous system to restore normal muscular activity.

Vibijex inj	**(Pfizer) Ranbaxy**
Comp	Each ml contains Vit B_1-50 mg Vitamin B_{12}500 mcg
Adm.	IM
@	LA 5-10 ml SA 3-5 ml
Pres.	10 ml, 30 ml

Vitamin B_1, B_6 and B_{12}

This combination is indicated in neurological disorders neuritis, paralysis, fatigue, debility and parturient paresis.

Clorubra	**Sarabhai**
Comp	Each ml contains Vit $B_1$50 mg $B_6$25 mg B_{12}500 mcg
Adm.	IM
@	LA 4-5 ml od, SA 1-2 ml od
Pres.	30 ml

Neuroxin inj	**Sarabhai**		
Comp	$B_1$30 mg	$B_6$13.75 mg	B_{12}500 mcg
Adm.	IM		
@	LA 4-5 ml od, SA 1-2 ml od		
Pres.	30 ml		

Vibejex Forte inj	**Ranbaxy**		
Comp	$B_1$50 mg	$B_6$25 mg	B_{12}500 mcg
Adm.	IM		
@	LA 4-5 ml od, SA 1-2 ml od		
Pres.	30 ml		

Zeactive inj	**Cadila Pharma**		
Comp	$B_1$30 mg	$B_6$1.75 mg	B_{12}500 mg
Adm.	IM		
@	LA 4-5 ml od, SA 1-2 ml od		
Pres.	30 ml		

Neoroxin	**Cadila**		
Comp	$B_1$30 mg	$B_6$13.75 mg	B_{12}500 mcg
Adm.	IM		
@	LA 4-5 ml od, SA 1-2 ml od		
Pres.	30 ml		

Tribivet	**Intas**		
Comp	$B_1$50 mg	$B_6$50 mg	B_{12}500 mcg per ml
Adm.	IM		
@	LA 4-5 ml, SA 1-2 ml od		
Pres.	10 ml, 30 ml		

Vitamin B_{12}

It is given for neuralgia, formation of RBC, anaemia better absorption of folic acid.

Wika XL inj	**Macwell Pharma**
Comp	each ml contains Methyl cobalamin 2500 mcg
Adm.	IM/ IV
@	LA 3-5 ml alternate days
Pres.	10 ml, 30 ml

Cobiliv inj	**Sushima Pharma**
Comp	Each ml contains Liver crude 0.6 ml having B_{12} activity 2 mcg per ml
Adm.	IM
@	5-10 ml
Pres.	10 ml, 30 ml

Vitamin E Inj

It is indicated in muscular dystrophy sterility, abortion, anoestrus, poor breeding performance, exudative diathesis and Vit E deficiency conditions. It can be given to potentiate immune mechanism, build resistance to infection and healthy skin.

E Care Se	**Cargill (Vetcare)**
Comp	Each ml contains Tocopherol 50 mg Selenium 1.5 mg
Adm.	IM
@	1ml/25 kg B.wt
Pres.	10 ml

Repronol	**Cadila Pharma**
Comp	Vit E 50 mg Selenium 1.5 mg
Adm.	SC
@	1 ml/25-50 kg B.wt
Pres.	10 ml

Esenium inj	**Zydus**
Comp	Vit E 50 mg Selenium 1.5 mg in 1ml
Adm.	IM
@	1 ml/25 kg B.wt weekly
Pres.	10 ml

Other Combinations of Vitamins

Adecilin inj	**Virbac (Glaxo)**
Comp	Each ml contains Vit A 250000 IU Vit $D_3$25000 IU Vit E 150 mg
Adm.	IM

@	LA 5 ml and SA 2 ml in infertility LA 10 ml and SA 2-5 ml in Hypovitaminosis LA 10 ml and SA 5 ml in Pregnancy
Pres.	10 ml, 30 ml

Intavita	**Intas**
Comp	Each ml contains Vit A 250000 IU Vit $D_3$25000 IU Vit E 100 mg
Adm.	IM
@	LA 10-20 ml/ week, SA 5-10 ml/ week
Pres.	5 ml, 10 ml

Vet ADE inj	**Concept**
Comp	Each ml contains Vit A 250000 IU Vit $D_3$25000 IU Vit E 100 mg
Adm.	IM
@	LA 10-20 ml/ week, SA 5-10 ml/ week
Pres.	5 ml, 10 ml

Vitacept	**Concept**
Comp	Each ml contains Vit A 250000 IU Vit $D_3$25000 IU Vit E 100 mg
Adm.	IM
@	LA 10-20 ml/ week, SA 5-10 ml/ week
Pres.	5 ml, 10 ml

Wokantol	**Wockhardt**
Comp	Each ml contains Vit A 6 Lakh IU Vit D 60000 IU Vit E 200 mg in each ml
Adm.	IM
@	LA 12 ml per week
Pres.	2 ml

Vetade inj	**Zydus**
Comp	Each ml contains Vit A 2.5 Lac $D_3$25000 IU E 100 IU

Adm.	IM
@	LA 6-10 ml SA 2-4 ml
Pres.	10 ml

Adevet	**Vets Farma**
Comp	Each ml contains Vit A 250000 IU Vit $D_3$25000 IU Vit E 100 mg
Adm.	IM
@	LA 10-20 ml/ week, SA 5-10 ml/week
Pres.	5 ml, 10 ml

Multivet inj	**Dosch**
Comp	Each ml contains Vit A 2000 IU $D_3$2000 IU Niacinamide 10 mg $B_1$10 mg B_2 1 mg Pyridoxine hydrochloride 5 mg D Panthenol 1 mg B_{12}10 mcg Calcium glycerol phosphate 10 mg Vit E 4 mg Biotin 10 mcg
Adm.	IM/ IV
@	As per need
Pres.	30 ml

IH5 inj	**Nicosia**
Comp	Each ml contains Vit A 250000 IU D_3 2500 IU Vit E 100 IU Biotin 125 mg with 150 mg/ml iodine
Adm.	IM
@	LA 5 ml SA 1-2 ml
Pres.	5 ml with needle and syringe

Vitamin B Complex

It is indicated in B complex deficiency and for supportive therapy in all sick animals

Alviplex Forte inj	**Alved**
Comp	Each ml contains Vit B_1 100 mg Vit B_2 5 mg Vit B_6 7 mg Vit B_{12} 100 mcg Niacinamide 25 mg Biotin 10 mcg D pathenol 25 mg Choline chloride 5 mg Lysine Hcl 50 mg
Adm.	IM
@	LA 10 ml od SA 5 ml od
Pres.	10 ml, 30 ml

Pinkojet inj	**Brihans**
Comp	Each ml contains Vit B_1 20 mg Vit B_6 20 mg B_2 1 mg Vit B_{12} 200 mcg Nicotinamide 20 mg D pathenol 10 mg Choline chloride 3 mg
Adm.	IM
@	LA 10 ml od SA 5 ml od
Pres.	30 ml

Libraliv inj	**Libra**
Comp	Thiamine 25 mg Ribiflavin 1.37 mg Nicotinamide 100 mg D panthenol 5 mg Pyridoxine 5 mg B_{12}30 mcg Liver extract 5 g Choline chloride 15 mg Lignocaian 1% in 1ml
Adm.	IM
@.	LA 10-15 ml SA 2-5 ml
Pres.	99 ml

Livoguard inj	**Carevet Pharma**
Comp	Each ml contains $B_1$25 mg $B_2$1.37 mg $B_3$100 mg $B_5$5 mg $B_6$5 mg B_{12}30 mcg Choline chloride 15 mg Lignocaine 1%
Adm.	IM

@	5-10 ml bid
Pres.	10 ml, 30 ml, 50, 100 ml

Vibelan inj	**Glaxo**
Comp	Each ml contains Vit B_1 25 mg Vit B_2 4.1 mg Vit B_6 2.5 mg Nicotinamide 100 mg D pathenol 50 mg
Adm.	IM
@	LA 10 ml od SA 5 ml od
Pres.	30 ml

Nutriliv inj	**Cargill (Vetcare)**
Comp	Each ml contains Vit B_1 25 mg Vit B_2 1.37 mg Vit B_{12} 32 mcg Nicotinamide 100 mg Vit B_6 5 mg Choline chloride 15 mg
Adm.	IM
@	LA 10 ml
Pres.	30 ml, 10 ml

Multivitamin with Mineral / Amino Acid

It is indicated in Anorexia of any etiology, sterility, anoestrus, stress of any origin, debility, convalscances, anaemia, growth, muscular dystrophy, infertility, osteomalacia and deficiency disease conditons due to hypvitaminosis.

Hitone inj	**Lyka**
Comp	Each ml contains Vit A_1 2000 IU D_3 2000 IU E 4 mg B_1 10 mg Pyridoxine 5 mg B_2 1mg B_{12} 10 mcg Panthenol 1 mg Biotine 10 mcg Niacinamide 10 mg Calcium 10 mg
Adm.	IM/ IV
@	1 ml/ 10-15 kg B.wt
Pres.	30 ml

Hivit inj	**Ranbaxy**
Comp	Each ml contains Vit A_1 2000 IU $D_3$2000 IU E 4 mg $B_1$10 mg Pyridoxine 5 mg $B_2$1 mg B_{12}10 mcg Panthenol 1 mg Biotine 10 mcg Niacinamide 10 mg Calcium 10 mg
Adm.	IM/ IV
@	1 ml/ 10-15 kg B.wt
Pres.	30 ml

X Liplex Forte inj	**Zydus**
Comp	Each ml contains Vit 100 mg $B_1B_2$5 mg $B_6$7mg B_{12}100 mcg Nictinamide 25 mg Biotin 10 mcg D panthenol 25 mg Lysine 50 mcg
Adm.	IM/IV
@	LA 10 ml SA 5 ml
Pres.	30 ml

Lipzed inj	**Alivira**
Comp	Each ml contains Choline chloride 15 mg B_{12}20 mcg Glycine 30 mg
Adm.	IM/ IV
@	10-15 ml 3 to 5 days
Pres.	100 ml

Multivet inj	**Merial (Dosch)**
Comp	Each ml contains VitA_1 2000 IU $D_3$2000 IU E 4 mg $B_1$10 mg Pyridoxine 5 mg $B_2$1 mg B_{12}10 mcg Panthenol 1 mg Biotine 10 mcg Nacinamide 10 mg Calcium 10 mg

Adm.	IM/ IV
@	1 ml/ 10-15 kg B.wt
Pres.	30 ml

Iveplex inj	**Alved**
Comp	Each ml contains Vit 100 mg B_1B_2 5 mg $B_6$5 mg Niacinamide 100 mg Inositol 5 mg O panthenol 10 mg Choline chloride 10 mg Methionine 10 mg
Adm.	IM/ IV
@	2-5 ml od
Pres.	1 ml, 10 ml

Caldee 12 inj	**Wockhardt**
Comp	Each ml contains Calcium levulinate 76.4mg Vit D_3 5000 IU B_{12}50 mcg
Adm.	IM
@	LA 10-15 ml alternate days SA 1-3 ml alternate days
Pres.	30 ml

Suplements Powder/Liquid

Nutrimac Forte Pow	**Macnor**
Comp	1 kg contains Calcium 25% Phosphorus 13% Magnesium 6 g Iodine 325 mg Copper 1200 mg Manganese 1500 mg Sodium 5.9g Vit A 70000 IU $D_3$7000 IU E 250 mg Niacinamide 1g
Adm.	Oral
@	LA 50 g od SA 25 g od
Pres.	1 kg, 5 kg, 20 kg

Livophoria liq	**Zydus**

Comp	100 ml contains Liver extract 50 mg Choline chloride 200 mg Silymarine 10 mg Copper sulphate 100 mg Ferric ammonium citrate 100 mg Methionine 20 mg Lysine 20 mg Glycin 10 mg Zinc 10 mg Biotic 6 mg B_{12} 1 mcg Sorbitol 1500 mg Protein hydrosylate 100 mg
Adm.	Oral
@	50 ml od
Pres.	500 ml, 1 L, 5 L

CRS Pow (chelated Ranmix Shakti)	**Zydus**
Comp	Chelated minerals Zinc Copper Manganese Macro minerals Vitamins and by pass methionine
Adm.	Oral
@	30 g od
Pres.	1 kg, 2.5 kg, 5 kg

Prolimin Forte Pow	**Agilis**
Comp	1 kg contains Iron 980 mg Manganese 1.5 mg Yeast culture 6 g Iodine 156 mg Calcium 240 g (Sc 47) Copper 312 mg Phosphorus 120 g Cobalt 45 mg Magnesium 4 g Zinc 4.26 g L lysine 6 g DL methionine 2 g
Adm.	Oral
@	LA 50 g od SA 15 g od
Pres.	1 kg, 10 kg

Haem up Pow	**Cadila Pharma**	
Comp	20 g contains	
	Malt extract	5.2 g
	Vit D_3	400 IU
	Calcium gluconate	380 mg
	Niacinamide	75 mg
	Ferric ammonium citrate	800 mg (160 mg)
	Biotin	275 mcg
	Ferric sulphate	335 mg (100 mg)
	Folic acid	1.5 mg
	Copper sulphate	120 mg
	B_{12}	20 mcg
	Cobalt sulphate	1.5 mg
	Magnesium sulphate	200 mg
	Total iron	260 mg
Adm.	Oral	
@	LA 30-50 g od SA 10-15 g od	
Pres.	500 g, 2.5 g	

Cal Dmin Forte chelaled Pow supreme	**Cadila Pharma**			
Comp	1 kg contains			
	Vit A	150000 IU	Phosphorus	127.5 g
	Cobalt	150 mg	D_3	230000 IU
	Magnesium	6 g	Iodine	325 mg
	E	230000 IU	Sodium	6 mg
	Iron	1.5 g	Nicotinamide	1 g
	Potassium	100 mg	Manganese	2.4 g
	Calcium	255 g	Copper	4.5 g
	Zinc	9.6 g		
Adm.	Oral			
@	40 g od for high milker 60 g od or 1kg in 100 kg feed			
Pres.	1 kg, 5 kg, 25 kg			

CMEV gold Pow	**Boehringer Ingelheim**			
Comp	1 kg contains			
	Calcium	230 g	Phosphorus	115 g
	Copper	4.5 g	Manganese	3.9 g
	Cobalt	300 mg	Iron	2 g
	Iron	2 g	Iodine	500 mg
	Sulphur	0.85%	Magnesium	6 g
	Chromium	100 mg	Potassium	150 mg
	Vit A	1500000 IU	E	1000 IU
	D_3	1500000 IU	Niacin	1 g
	Liver yeast	10 g		
Adm.	Oral			
@	LA 50 g od SA 15 g od			
Pres.	1 kg, 5 kg			

Mincham Forte Pow	**Boehringer Ingelheim**			
Comp	1 kg contains			
	Calcium	240 g	Phosphorus	120 g
	Zinc	9.6 g	Copper	1.2 g
	Manganese	1.5 g	Cobalt	150 ml
	Iron	1.5 g	Iodine	300 mg
	Magnesium	6 g	Chromium	100 mg
	Vit A	750000 IU	E	250 IU
	Niacin	1 g	D_3	750000 IU
	Live yeast	20 g		
Adm.	Oral			
@	LA 100 g od SA 30 g od or 1-2% in feed			
Pres.	1 kg, 5 kg			

Calcibo Bolus	**IHC (International Health Care)**
Comp	Calcium and Vitamins with trace minerals
Adm.	Oral
@	1 Bol od for 10 days then gap of 10 days
Pres.	2 Bol blister

Trace Bolus	**IHC (International Health Care)**
Comp	Multivitamins, minerals and trace elements
Adm.	Oral
@	1 Bol od
Pres.	4 Bol blister

Boviprash Pow	**Herstel**			
Comp	21 g contains			
	Malt extract	4.5 g	Calcium gluconate	360 mg
	Ferric ammonium citrate	300 mg	Copper sulphate	100 mg
	Cobalt chloride	1.5 mg	Vit D_3	3500 IU
	Niacinamide	45 mg	Biotin	75 mcg
	Folic acid	1.5 mg	B_{12}	15 mcg
Adm.	Oral			
@	LA 50 g od Sa 15 g od			
Pres.	450 g			

Vitaron syp	**Natural Herbs**
Comp	Each 100 ml contains Vit A 25000 IU D_3 5000 IU E 1500 IU C 500 mg IU Energy 500 cl Protein 4% Mineral 90% + Extract of Ashvgandha, Draksh, shatavar, Panernav, Bidasikand, Bhringraj, Kaunch, Sudh shilagit, Musli safed, Inderjava, Amla, Manjth, Urab, Saptpam, Hantaki, Kesar, Wheatgramal, Apple conic
Adm.	Oral
@	LA 100 ml od SA 20 ml od
Pres.	250 ml, 500 ml, 1L

Vitamix AF Plus	**Natural Herbs**			
Comp	Each kg contains			
	Calcium	240 g	Copper	312 mg
	Zinc	2.13 g	Phosphorus	120 g
	Iodine	156 mg	L lysine	4.4 g
	Maganesium	45 mg	Chromium	65 mg
	DL methionine	1.92 g	Iron	979 mg
Adm.	Oral			
@	LA 80-100 g od SA 25-30 g od			
Pres.	1 kg, 2.5 kg, 5 kg			

Vitamix AF Gold	Natural Herbs			
Comp	Each 1.2 kg contains			
	Calcium	Iron	Sulphur	Vit D_3
	Phosphorus	Iodine	Potassium	Vit E
	Magnesium	Copper	Selenium	Chromium
	Manganese	Cobalt	Vit A	
	Saccharomyle acidophilus 2x10		Lactolacillus acidophilus 2x10	
Adm.	Oral			
@	LA 50 g od SA 25 g od			
Pres.	1.2 kg, 2.5 kg, 5 kg			

Venlyte Pow	Venky	
Comp	100 g contains	
	Sodium 1 g	Calcium lactate 1.1 g
	Calcium gluconate 1.1 g	Magnesium sulphate 0.9 g
	Potassium chloride 3 g	Sodium citrate 2.5 g
	Sodium bicarbonate 1 g	Vit C 1 g
Adm.	Oral	
@	LA 50 g qid SA 10 g qid	
Pres.	250 g, 1 kg	

Vitosel Pow	Brihans	
Comp		
100 g contains		
Sodium chloride 24 g	Potassium chloride 2.5 g	
Sodium bicarbonate 9.4 g	Magnesium sulphate 11 g	
Calcium gluconate 4.71 g	Magnesium chloride 1.72 g	
Vit B_1 281. 8mg	$B_2$340.4 mg	
B_6 157 mg	B_{12}1.43 mg	
E 340.4 mg	Niacin 1.05 g	
Folic acid 81.6 mg	Inositol 877.5 mg	
Rutoside 1.77 mg	Choline chloride 510.3 mg	Dextrose qs
Adm.	Oral	
@	LA 25 g qid SA 10 g qid	
Pres.	25 g, 100 g, 250 g, 2.5 kg	

Oral Vitamin A

It is indicated to- Stimulate growth and milk production.

Cadisol Liq	**Cadila**
Comp	Vit A 100000 IU/ml
Adm.	Oral
@	LA 7.5-10 ml od SA 5 ml od
Pres.	30 ml, 500 ml

Retisol Liq	**Vets Farma**
Comp	Vit A 100000 IU/ml
Adm.	Oral
@	LA 5 ml od SA 5 ml od
Pres.	500 ml

Solvit A Forte	**Vetcare**
Comp	Vit A 100000 IU/ml
Adm.	Oral
@	LA 5 ml od SA 5 ml od
Pres.	500 ml

Vitamin E Oral

It is indicated for anoestrus, sterility and potentiate immune system.

Alvisol E Liq	**Alved**
Comp	Each ml contains Vit E 150 mg
Adm.	Oral
@	LA 2 ml SA 1 ml od
Pres.	100 ml, 250 ml, il

E care Se Forte	**Cargill (Vetcare)**
Comp	Vit E 20% Selenium 440 ppm
Adm.	Oral
@	250 g /ton of feed in LA
Pres.	250 g, 1 kg

E care Se Pow	**Cargill (Vetcare)**
Comp	Vit E 10% Selenium 200 ppm
Adm.	Oral
@	5-10 g od
Pres.	200 g

Vitamin K

It is indicated as supportive in Coccidiosis or haemorrhagic syndrome.

Alvisol K 20% Pow	**Alved**
Comp	Vit K (Menadione Sod. Bisulphate) 200 mg/g
Adm.	Oral
@	LA 2.5 g od SA 0.75 g od
Pres.	100 g, 500 g, 1 kg

Vitamin C

It is indicated as antioxidant, supportive therapy in all infections and other disorders for early recovery as well as immune booster and enhance animal resistance to disease.

CMac inj	**Macnor**
Comp	Each ml contains Ascorbic acid 250 mg
Adm.	IM, IV
@	LA 20-30 ml SM 2.-5 ml
Pres.	30 ml, 100 ml

Vit C inj	**Animax Healthcare**
Comp	Each ml contains Ascorbic acid 250 mg
Adm.	IM, IV
@	LA 20-30 ml SM 2.-5 ml
Pres.	30 ml, 100 ml

Ascorvet inj	**Phoenix**
Comp	Each ml contains Ascorbic acid 250 mg
Adm.	IM, IV
@	LA 20-30 ml SM 2.-5 ml
Pres.	30 ml, 100 ml

Pail C inj	PAIL
Comp	Each ml contains Ascorbic acid 250 mg
Adm.	IM, IV
@	LA 20-30 ml SM 2.-5 ml
Pres.	30 ml, 100 ml

Herbal C Pow	Indian Herbs
Comp	Vit C
Adm.	Infeed
@	200 g /Ton feed
Pres.	1 kg, 5 kg

Phytocee Pow	Natural Remedies
Comp	Polyphenola, with anolides and Triterpenoide
Adm.	In feed
@	200 g/Ton of feed
Pres.	5 kg

Vitamin D

Dicirol granules	Cadila Pharma
Comp	Vit $D_3$600000 IU/g
Adm.	In feed
@	2 g /Ton of feed
Pres.	5 g, 10 g

Dilvit D_3 200 Pow	Wockhardt
Comp	Vit $D_3$200000 IU/g
Adm.	In feed
@	10-15 g /Ton
Pres.	1 kg, 25 kg

Vitamins AD_3

Indicated for vit A & vit D deficiency conditions like night blindness, xerophthalmia, dermatological disorders, stunted growth, debility respiratory tract infection. It is also used to improve growth, fertility, production and enhance resistance of animal to infection.

Filovet liq	**Cargill (Vetcare)**
Comp	Each ml contains vit A 6000 IU D_3 600 IU
Adm.	Oral
@	LA 5 ml bid SA 5 ml od
Pres.	200 ml, 400 ml, 4.5 L

Indomix AD3 Pow	**Piramal**
Comp	Each g contains vit A 5000 IU $D_3$500 IU
Adm.	Oral
@	LA 5-10 g od SA 2-2 g od
Pres.	500 g, 1 kg

Rakshablend H	**Indian Immunology**
Comp	Each 5g contains vit A 325000 IU vit $D_3$32500 IU
Adm.	Oral
@	16-20 g /Ton of seed
Pres.	500g, 1kg

Vitablend AD_3	**Virbac**
Comp	Each g contains vit A 5000 IU $D_3$500 IU
Adm.	Oral
@	LA 5-10 g od SA 2-2 g od
Pres.	20 g, 1 kg

Vardhan	**Tineta**
Comp	Each g contains vit A 5000 IU $D_3$500 IU
Adm.	Oral
@	LA 5-10 g od SA 2-2 g od
Pres.	30 g, 1 kg

Vitamins Combination Oral

Bovital Pow	**Concept**
Comp	5 g contains Vit A 50000 IU $D_3$5000 IU E 5 mg B_{12} 50 mcg

Adm.	Oral
@	LA 25 = 50 g od 5-10 g od
Pres.	100 g, 1 kg

Brivita Pow	**Brihans**
Comp	5 g contains Vit A 50000 IU $D_3$5000 IU E 5mg B_{12} 50 mcg
Adm.	Oral
@	LA 25 = 50 g od 5 - 10 g od
Pres.	100 g, 1 kg

Vadeb Liq	**Zydus**
Comp	Each ml contains Vit A 12000 IU $D_3$6000 IU E 48 mg B_{12}20 mcg
Adm.	Oral
@	LA 10 ml od, SA 5 ml od
Pres.	30 ml , 500 ml

Vetral Liq	**Vets Farma**
Comp	Water miscible Vit A, D_3, E, B_{12}
Adm.	Oral
@	LA 20 ml od, SA 10 ml od
Pres.	100 ml , 500 ml

Vimeral Liq	**Virbac**
Comp	Water miscible Vit A, D_3, E, B_{12}
Adm.	Oral
@	LA 20 ml od, SA 10 ml od
Pres.	100 ml , 500 ml

Alviton Plus	**Alembic**
Comp	5 ml contains Vit A 250000 IU $D_3$25000 IU E 150 IU C 500 mg Selenium 0.5 mg

Adm.	Oral
@	LA 10 ml bid, SA 5 ml bid
Pres.	500 ml, il

Dhenu H liq	**Phoenix**		
Comp	Each ml contains		
	Vit A 20000 IU	Vit D_3	Vit E 50 mg
	Vit H 100 mcg	Vit C 50 mg	Selenium 8 mcg
	Zinc 18 mg	Cobalt 0.2 mg	Flex seed oil 10%
	Aloevera q.s		
Adm.	Oral		
@	LA 10 ml od SA 5 ml od		
Pres.	100 ml, 250 ml, 500 ml, 1L		

Vitto H liq	**Macwell**		
Comp	Vit A 20000 IU	$D_3$10000 IU	E 50 mg
	Biotin 12.5 mcg	C 10 mg	Selenium 8 mcg
	Flaxseed oil q.s		
Adm.	Oral		
@	LA 10 ml od x 5 days		
Pres.	120 ml, 250 ml, 1L		

Libral H Syp	**Libra**				
Comp	Vit A	Vit D	Vit E	Vit H	Vit C
	Vit B_{12}	Vit B	Vit C	Selenium	Cobalt
	Chromium	Zinc	Nicotinic acid		
Adm.	Oral				
@	LA 10 ml od x 5 days				
Pres.	500 ml, 1 L				

Uddergro H Liq	**Nicosia**		
Comp	1 ml contains		
	Vit A 25000 IU	$D_3$10000 IU	# 50 mg
	H 70 mcg	Nictoinamide 10 mg	
Adm.	Oral		
@	10 m od		
Pres.	100 ml, 250 ml, 500 ml, 1 L poly pack		

Freshmin liq	Boehringer Ingelheim		
Comp	1 ml contains		
	Vit A 12000 IU	$D_3$6000 IU	E 48 IU
	B_{12}20 mcg	Biotin 500 mcg	Selenium 0.1 mg
	Energy 0.5 cal		
Adm.	Oral		
@	10 ml od		
Pres.	240 ml, 500 ml		

Bovimust gold Bol	Herstel		
Comp	B carotene	Bioactive chromium	Vandayl sulphate
	Copper	Zinc	Selenium
	Cobalt	Iodine	Manganese
	Iron	Vit E	
Adm.	Oral		
@	LA 1 Bolus od x 7 days SA 1 Bol alternate day		
Pres.	7 Bol pack		

Bovitop CS2 liq	Alivira		
Comp	5 ml contains		
	Vit A 250000 IU	$D_3$50000 IU	E 300 IU
	Biotin 1000 mcg	Copper 500 mcg	Zinc 250 mg
	Selenium 150 mcg		
Adm.	Oral		
@	LA 5-10 ml od SA 1-2 ml		
Pres.	100 ml, 250 ml, 500 ml , 1 L		

V- Tone liq	Natural Herbs		
Comp	Vit A 12000 IU	B_{12} 20 mcg	Natural C 100 mg
	$D_3$6000 IU	E 100 mg	Selenium 0.5 mg
Adm.	Oral		
@	LA 10 ml SA 5 ml od		
Pres.	30 ml, 60 ml, 100 ml, 500 ml		

Amino Acid + Vitamin Powders

Cholymbi Powder/ Bolus	Lyka	
Comp	Powder 50 g contains Choline chloride 10 g	L lysine hydrochloride 10 g
	D methionine 10 g	D biotin 1 mg
	Vit B_{12} 15 mg, [composition of Bolus not given]	
Adm.	Oral	
@	LA 25 g bid, SA 10g bid LA 2-4 Bolus od SA 1-2 Bolus od	
Pres.	500 g, strip of 4	

LMG Pow	Sterling		
Comp	100 g contains Lysine 33 g	Methionine 16.5 g	Glycine 16.5 g
Adm.	Oral		
@	LA 10 g od SA 5 g od		
Pres.	100 g, 500 g		

Vitamins and Trace Minerals

Vitto H Liq	Macwell			
Comp	Each ml contains Vit A 20000 IU	$D_3$10000 IU	E 50 mg	H 12.5 mcg
	C 10 mg	Selenium 8 mcg	Flaxseed oil q.s.	
Adm.	Oral			
@	LA 10 ml od			
Pres.	120 ml, 250 ml, 1L			

Alvitone Plus Liq	Alembic		
Comp	5 ml contains Vit A 250000 IU	$D_3$25000 IU	E 150 IU
	C 500 mg	Selenium 0.5 mg	
Adm.	Oral		
@	LA 10 ml bid SA 3-5 ml bid		
Pres.	100 ml, 500 ml, il		

Amvitone Liq	Pranav
Comp	5 ml contains Vit A 62500 IU $D_3$25000 IU E 150 mg C 500 mg
Adm.	Oral
@	LA 20 ml SA 5-10 ml od
Pres.	500 ml, IL

Capovit LIq	Indian Immunology
Comp	5 ml contains Vit A 12000 IU $D_3$6000 IU B_{12}20 mcg E 48 mg
Adm.	Oral
@	LA 10-20 ml od SA 5 ml od
Pres.	30 ml, 500 ml

Capsitone Liq	Ranbaxy
Comp	Each 20 ml contains Vit A 120000 IU $D_3$60000 IU E 10 mcg Zinc 80 mg Cobalt 180 mg Selenium 1 mg
Adm.	Oral
@	LA 10 ml od SA 5-10 ml od
Pres.	100 ml, 500 ml

Lactivet Pow	Alvet
Comp	100 g contains Vit A 1.25 Lac IU $D_3$12500 IU E 50 IU Calcium 25.2 g Phosphrous 10 g Copper 0.5 g Iodine 0.05 g Manganese 0.2 g Cobalt 0.02 g Zinc 0.1 g
Adm.	Oral
@	LA 30 g od SA 10 g od
Pres.	2.5 kg

Lavitone Liq	TTK
Comp	5 ml contains Vit A 60000 IU $D_3$25000 IU E 150 mg C 200 mg B_{12}25 mcg Selenium 10 ppm
Adm.	Oral
@	LA 20 ml od SA 5 ml od
Pres.	100 ml, 500 ml

Mega brick Bol	**Natural Remedies**
Comp	107 g contains Copper 16500 mg Manganese 880 mg Zinc 13500 mg Iodine 250 mg Cobalt 240 mg Selenium 240 mg Vit A 5 Lac IU $D_3$1 Lac IU E 1000 IU Iron q.s.
Adm.	Oral
@	LA 1 Bol od
Pres.	107 g Bol

Recovit	**Brihans**
Comp	Each ml contains Vit A 50000 IU, $D_3$1500 IU E 50 mg C 100 mg B_{12}25mcg
Adm.	Oral
@	LA 5 ml od SA 2 ml od
Pres.	120 ml, 500 ml, ilc

Beekom forte Pow	**Wockhardt**
Comp	Each g contains Vit $B_1$11.25 mg $B_2$3.75 mg $B_5$4.3 mg $B_6$1.86 mg B_{12}18.75 mcg Naicinamide 112.5 mg
Adm.	Oral
@	LA 5-10 od SA 1.25-2.5 g od
Pres.	100 g

Supplosol B Pow	**Sarabhai**
Comp	Each g contains Vit $B_1$18 mg $B_6$3 mg B_{12} 26 mcg $B_2$6 mg Cal pantothenate 7.5 mg Naicinamide 152 mg
Adm.	Oral
@	LA 5-10 od SA 2-3 g od
Pres.	100 g

Vetsol B Pow	Vets Farma
Comp	Each g contains Vit B_1 3.75 mg B_2 1.25 mg B_6 0.62 mg B_{12} 6.25 mcg Cal pantothenate 1.25 mg Naicinamide 36.5 mg
Adm.	Oral
@	Dissolve 100 g in il of water LA 80-100 ml SA 30-50 od
Pres.	100 g

Plexa BC Pow	Concept
Comp	Each g contains Vit $B_1$10 mg $B_2$5 mg $B_6$10 mg B_{12}10 mcg Naicinamide 40 mg Calcium pantothenate 5 mg Vit C 10 mg Sodium 74 mg Chloride 110 mg
Adm.	Oral
@	LA 15 g od SA 10 g od
Pres.	250 g

Vitamin + Iodine + Selenium

V5 inj	Carevet Pharma
Comp	Each ml contains Vit A 250000 IU $D_3$25000 IU E 100 IU Biotin 125 mcg Each ml provide Iodine equivalent to 150 mg/ml
Adm.	IM
@	LA 5 ml
Pres.	5 ml, 10 ml

Vitto H inj	Macwell
Comp	Each ml contains Vit A 250000 IU $D_3$25000 IU E 100 IU Biotin 125 mcg Each ml provide Iodine equivalent to 150 mg/ml
Adm.	IM
@	LA 5 ml
Pres.	10 ml

Libral H inj	Libra
Comp	1ml contains Iodine 150 mg Vit A 250000 IU $D_3$25000 IU E 100 IU Biotin 12.5 mcg
Adm.	IM

@.	LA 5 ml SA 1-2 ml
Pres.	5 ml, 10 ml with syringe and needle

Mineral Prepations

Copper Preparations

Copper is very important trace mineral. Its deficiency leads to nutritional haemoglobinuria. Overgrown hoofs, depigmentation of skin, stiff leg syndrome, chronic diarrhea, anaemia, temporary infertility and unthriftiness. Copper glycinate injections are available.

Copper glycinate Inj: Organic preparations as suspension or emulsion. One treatment is sufficient for 60-90 days.

Curan 9	**Carevet Pharma**
Comp	Copper glycinate 75 mg/ml
Adm.	SC
@	0.5 mg/kg B.wt
Pres.	2 ml, 3 ml, 20 ml vial

Curan BH	**Carevet Pharma**
Comp	Copper glycinate 500 mg
Adm.	IV in normal Saline
@	1.5 mg/kg B.wt
Pres.	Vial of 500 mg

If temperatue of animal is normal it can be given in Dextrose saline. Should be given when immediately needed.

Iodine Preparations

Iodine preparations containing elemental Iodine an integral part of thyroid are used for Iodine deficiency. Iodine deficiency is exhibited by Hypothermia, Reproductive failure, Calf mortality, poor body growth & poor milk production.

I Fer H	**Carevet Pharma**
Comp	Elemental iodine 375 mg/ml 2ml vial
Adm.	SC
@	2.5 mg/kg B.wt or 2 ml
Pres.	2 ml

Copper Cobalt Preprations

Copper and cobalt preprations are given for treating irregular heat, late maturity due to deficiency of copper and cobalt. These are given in anaemia and loss of appetite or copper deficiency syndrome. These are available as Capsule and Tablets

Vets cuco Tab	Vets Farma
Comp	Each tablet contains Copper sulphate 200 mg Cobalt sulphate 20 mg
Adm.	Oral
@	LA 4 Tab for 3-4 weeks daily, SA 2-4 Tab for 3-4 weeks daily
Pres.	Pack of 20

Miscellaneous

Preprations of Arsenic were earlier given as General tonic in debility, helminthiasis, anaemia and chronic infections.

Acetylarsan inj	Prima Vetcare
Comp	Dimethylamine acetarsol 236 mg equal to 50 mg per ml
Adm.	IM, SC
@	LA 3.6 injection on alternate days Sa 20 ml
Pres.	2 ml, 10 ml

Trace Mineral Preprations

These are indicated in animals with delayed maturity anoestrus, repeat breeders, unhealthy skin and skeletal system, drop in production or lowered immunity and resistance to infections. It regulates oestrus cycle, helps in early conception and prevents habitual abortions.

Anmark TM	Anmarks				
Comp	Manganese 10.8%	Zinc 10.4%	Iron 4%	Copper 0.4%	Iodine 0.4%
Adm.	Oral				
@	20 gm od				
Pres.	1 kg, 10 kg				

Cocu Plus Tab/Bol	**Anmark**		
Comp		Tab	Bol
	Copper sulphate	250 mg	1250 mg
	Cobalt sulphate	20 mg	100 mg
	Manganese sulphate	12.5 mg	60 mg
	Ferrous sulphate	12.5 mg	60 mg
	Zinc sulphate	12.5 mg	60 mg
	Calcium	90 mg	450 mg
	Phosphorus	50 mg	250 mg
Adm.	Oral		
@	LA 5 Tab od or 1-2 Bol od SA 1-2 Tab od or ½ -1 Bol od		
Pres.	100 Tab, strip of 4 Bolus		

Tone up	**Novartis**
Comp	Copper 50 mg Cobalt 100 mg Iron 30 mg Methionine 40 mg Yeast 1.5 g Ginger 50 mg Sodium biocarbonate q.s
Adm.	Oral
@	LA 2 Bol bid
Pres.	Strip of 4

Cyclomin Bol	**Alved**
Comp	Each Bolus contains Cobalt 56 mg Copper 700 mg Iodine 40 mg Iron 140 mg Manganese 560 mg Selenium 4 mg Zinc 280 mg
Adm.	Oral
@	1 Bol/week
Pres.	Strip of 4

Repromax Bol	**Dosch**
Comp	Each Bolus contains Cobalt 80 mg Copper 100 mg Iodine 20 mg Iron 200 mg Manganese 80 mg Selenium 0.5mg Zinc 40 mg
Adm.	Oral
@	LA 1 Bol od SA ½ Bol od
Pres.	Strip of 4

Repromin Bol	Novartis		
Comp	Each Bolus contains		
	Cobalt 80 mg	Copper 100 mg	Iodine 20 mg
	Iron 200 mg	Manganese 80 mg	Selenium 0.5 mg
	Zinc 40 mg		
Adm.	Oral		
@	LA 1 Bol od SA ½ Bol od		
Pres.	Strip of 4		

Stalmin Bol	Stallen		
Comp	Each Bolus contains		
	Cobalt 5 6 mg	Copper 700 mg	Iodine 140 mg
	Iron 400 mg	Manganese 560 mg	Selenium 4 mg
	Zinc 280 mg		
Adm.	Oral		
@	LA 1 Bol od weekly		
Pres.	Strip of 4		

Tracemin Pow	Venky		
Comp	Copper 0.1%	Iodine 0.001%	Iron 0.08%
	Manganese 12%	Zinc 0.12%	Selenium 0.001%
Adm.	Oral		
@	500 g to 1 kg /Ton of feed		
Pres.	5 kg		

Vets Trace mineral Pow	Vets Farma		
Comp	Each kg contains		
	Copper 16 g	Cobalt 3 g	Iodine 6 g
	Zinc 30 g	Manganese 20 g	Iron 100 g
Adm.	Oral		
@	500 g- 1 kg/ Ton of feed		
Pres.			

Cofecu Plus Tab	Indian Herbs
Comp	Copper, Cobalt, Iron, Manganese
Adm.	Oral
@	LA 1 Tab od SA ½ Tab od
Pres.	20's, 100's

CRS Pow (chelated Ranmix Shatki)	**Zydus**		**260**
Comp	Chelated minerals		
	Zinc	Copper	Manganese
	Macro minerals	Vitamins and by pass methionine	
Adm.	Oral		
@	30 g od		
Pres.	1 kg, 2.5 kg, 5 kg		

Macro Minerals

Calcium Injections

Gilcal	**G Longtos**
Comp	Each ml contains Calcium gluconoloctobionate 137.5 mg Vit $D_3$5000 IU B_{12}50 mcg
Adm.	IM
@	LA 15 ml alternate day SA 2 ml alternate day
Pres.	30 ml

Sanical Vet inj	**Novartis**
Comp	Each ml contains Calcium gluconoloctobionate 137.5 mg Vit $D_3$5000 IU B_{12}50 mcg
Adm.	IM
@	LA 15 ml alternate day SA 2 ml alternate day
Pres.	30 ml

Capsola inj	**Zydus**
Comp	Each ml has Calcium gluconalactobionate 137.5 mg $D_3$500 IU B_{12}50 mcg
Adm.	IM
@	LA 5-25 ml SA 5-12 ml
Pres.	30 ml, 100 ml

Calcium Bolus

Leptocal Bol	**Phoenix**
Comp	Tribasic calcium phosphate 4.8 g Vit A 50000 IU D3 20000 IU Vit E 25 mg Vit H 100 mcg B12100 mcg Lysine 125 mg Jivanti 350 mg Shatavari 2000 mg Copper 50 mg Manganese 25 mg Zinc 500 mg
Adm.	Oral
@	1 Bol bid
Pres.	Strip of 1 Bol

Pawas Forte Bol	**Libra**
Comp	Herbs and Vit A, D, E, H_1, B_{12}, lactic acid and Saccharomyces with Protein, calcium and Phosphorus
Adm.	Oral
@.	4 Bol 2 hours before milking bid
Pres.	Stirp of 4

MD3 Mac Bol	**Macnor**
Comp	Each Bolus has Tribasic calcium phosphate 4.8 g Magnesium 20 mg Vit D_3 10000 IU Vit B12 100 mcg Vit E 25 mg L Lysine 125 mg Shatavari 350 mg Jiwanti 2500 mg
Adm.	Oral
@.	1 Bol bid for 10 days
Pres.	1 Bol strip

Phosphorus Preparations

Phosphorus occurs in the blood in both organic and inorganic form and continuous interchange takes place. Most of the Phosphorus is found in organic combination. Inorganic phosphates are in process of ossification. This is a macromineral and its deficiency leads to many problems including anoestrous, reduced milk, milk fever disease, stunted growth, haemoglobinuria, ketosis, pica and even Indigestion.

Fertophos inj	**Virbac (Glaxo)**
Comp	Contains Salt of 4, Dimethylamino 2, Methyl phosphinic acid 20%
Adm.	IM, IV, SC
@	LA 5-25 ml SA 1-3 ml
Pres.	30 ml

Alphos 40 inj	**Alved**
Comp	Each ml contains Sodium acid phosphate 400 mg which Provides 79.4 mg of elemental Phosphorus
Adm.	IM, IV, SC
@	LA 7.5-10 ml SA 2.5-5 ml
Pres.	10 ml, 20 ml

Phosphine inj	**Primavet**
Comp	Each ml contains Sodium acid phosphate 400 mg which Provides 79.4 mg of elemental Phosphorus
Adm.	IM, IV, SC
@	LA 7.5-10 ml SA 2.5-5 ml
Pres.	10 ml, 20 ml

Tonegil inj	**G Loucatos**
Comp	Contains Salt of 4, Dimethylamino 2, Methyl phosphinic acid 20%
Adm.	IM, IV, SC
@	LA 5-25 ml SA 1-3 ml
Pres.	30 ml

Tonophosphan inj	**Intervet**
Comp	Contains Salt of 4, Dimethylamino 2, Methyl phosphinic acid 20%
Adm.	IM, IV, SC
@	LA 5-25 ml SA 1-3 ml
Pres.	30 ml

Tonoricin inj	**Wockhardt**
Comp	Contains Salt of 4, Dimethylamino 2, Methyl phosphinic acid 20%
Adm.	IM, IV, SC
@	LA 5-25 ml SA 1-3 ml
Pres.	30 ml

Urimin inj	Virbac (Glaxo)
Comp	Sodium acid phosphate 40.3% equivalent to Elemental Phosphorus 8.0%
Adm.	IM, IV, SC
@	LA 5-10 ml SA 1-3 ml
Pres.	30 ml

Sodaphos Sol	Ranbaxy
Comp	Sodium acid phosphate 79% provide Phosphorus 19%
Adm.	Oral
@	LA 60 ml od x 5 days
Pres.	500 ml

T Phos inj	Zydus
Comp	Contains Salt of 4, Dimethylamino 2, Methyl phosphinic acid 20%
Adm.	IM, IV, SC
@	LA 5-25 ml SA 1-3 ml
Pres.	30 ml

Libraphos inj	Libra
Comp	Sodium acid phosphate 40% or 80 mg/ml of of phosphorus
Adm.	IM/ SC/ IV
@.	LA 1 ml
Pres.	30 ml, 100 ml

Alphos 40	Zydus
Comp	Sodium acid Phosphate 400 mg per ml
Adm.	IM, SC, IV
@	LA 5 ml SA 1ml
Pres.	30 ml

Phosfovet	Boehringer Ingelheim
Comp	Butaphosphan 100 mg B_{12} 50 mcg/ml
Adm.	IM/IV/SC
@	LA 10-25 ml SA 2.5-5 ml
Pres.	90 ml

Alviphos inj	Alivira
Comp	Butaphosphan 100 mg B_{12}0.05ml
Adm.	IM/ IV/ SC
@	LA 10-25 ml SA 5-12 ml
Pres.	30 ml, 100 ml

Phosphorus with Vit B_{12}

It is indicated to improve metabolism, strengthen resistance as tonic to improve muscular efficiency and as a supportive therapy in hypocalcaemia, paresis, anoestous and other infections.

Alphos 20+B12	Alved
Comp	Each ml contains Sodium acid phosphate 200 mg, Vit B_{12}50 mcg
Adm.	IM
@	LA 15-20 ml SA 5 ml
Pres.	100 ml

Cobaphos inj	Virbac (Glaxo)
Comp	Each ml contains Sodium salt of oxybenzyl phospinate 125 mg Sodium dihydrogen phosphate 9 mg vit B_{12}50 mcg
Adm.	IM
@	LA 10-25 ml od SA 2.5-3 ml od
Pres.	30 ml, 100 ml

Cobaphos Forte inj	Virbac (Glaxo)
Comp	Each ml contains Sodium salt of oxybenzyl phospinate 125 mg Cynocobalmine 50 mcg
Adm.	IM
@	LA 10-25 ml od SA 2.5-3 ml od
Pres.	5 ml, 30 ml

Injectophos	Pfizer
Comp	Each ml contains Toldimphos sodium 200 mg Cyanocobalamine 50 mcg
Adm.	IM, IV, SC
@	LA 10-25 ml od SA 5-10 ml od
Pres.	30 ml, 100 ml

Vetphos	Cipla
Comp	Each ml contains Sodium acid phosphate 200 mg Vit B_{12} 50 mcg
Adm.	IM
@	LA 15-20 ml SA 5 ml
Pres.	100 ml

Cynophos	Primavetcare
Comp	Each ml contains 4 Dimethylamino 2 Methylphemylphosphine Sodium 200 mg Vit B_{12} 50 mcg
Adm.	IM IV
@	LA 10-25 ml SA 2.5-3 ml od
Pres.	10 ml, 30 ml

Catosan inj	Bayer
Comp	Each ml contain Butaphosphan 100 mg Vit B_{12} 50 mcg
Adm.	IM IV
@	LA 10-25 ml SA 5-12 ml od
Pres.	30 ml, 100 ml

Phosvet M inj	Phoenix	47
Comp	Sodum acid Phosphate 400 mg Methyl cobalamin 100 mcg	
Adm.	IM/ IV/ SC	
@	15-30 ml	
Pres.	30 ml	

Libraphos M inj / Bol	Libra	115
Comp	Inj 1 ml contains Sodium acid phosphate 400 mg Methyl cobalamin 100 mcg Bolus contains sodium acid phosphate 1.2 g Methyl cobalamin 1.5 mg	
Adm.	Inj 1m/Sc Bolus oral	
@.	10-30 ml injection or 1-2 Bol od	
Pres.	Inj 30 ml, 100 ml, Bolus strip of 2	

Cadiphos inj	**Cadila Pharma**	**212**
Comp	Butaphosphan 100 mg	Cyanocobalmin 0.05 mg
Adm.	IM/SC/IV	
@	LA 10-25 L	
Pres.	30 ml, 100 ml	

Vitamin AD_3 + Trace Minerals

It is indicated to assure Calcium and Phosphorus utilization, repeat breeder, pregnancy, lactation and stress.

Capsitone	**Ranbaxy**
Comp	20 ml contains Vit A 120000 IU $D_3$60000 IU E 10 mcg Zinc 180 mg Cobalt 180 mg Selenium 1 mg
Adm.	Oral
@	LA 10 ml od SA 2 ml od
Pres.	50 ml, 100 ml, 500 ml

Combination of Vitamins/ Amino Acids

This combination is indicated to improve appetite for betterment of liver function and for improvement of skin and indicated. It is also used for growth of calves and pregnancy.

Viselam Liq	**Brihans**
Comp	Each 5 ml contains Vit A 60000 IU D3 30000 IU E 15000 IU B_{12}2500 mcg C 1000 mg Folic acid 250 mg Methionine 1250 mg Lysine 2500 mg Tryptophan 500 mg Selenium 10000 mcg
Adm.	Oral
@	LA 15 ml od SA 7 ml od
Pres.	200 ml, 500 ml, il

Vitatone LM liq	**Zydus**
Comp	Each 5 ml contains Vit A 2.5 Lac IU $D_3$25000 IU C 500 mg E 150 mg Lysine 25 mg Methionine 10 mg
Adm.	Oral
@	LA 5 ml Sa 2 ml
Pres.	100 ml, 500 ml, il

XL Plex Forte inj	Alved
Comp	Each ml contains Vit $B_1$7mg; $B_2$2.5 mg $B_6$1 mg; B_{12}12.5 mcg Biotin 2 5 mcg; Calcium pantothenate 2.5 mg Niacin 75 mg; Choline chloride 10 mg Methionine 10 mg; Lysine 10 mg
Adm.	Oral
@	LA 30-50 ml od SA 10-20 ml od
Pres.	60 ml, 120 ml, 500 ml, il, 5 L

B care sol	Cargill (Vetcare)
Comp	Each 5 ml contains Vit $B_1$3.75 mg; $B_2$1.25 mg; B_{12}6.25 mcg Niacin 37.5 mg; D L Methionine 5 mg; Calcium gluconate 2.73 mg Dextrose monohydrate 95.83 mg
Adm.	Oral
@	Reconstitute 5 mg in 100 ml, LA 20 ml bid SA 10 ml bid
Pres.	250 g

Bivinal Liq	Alembic
Comp	Each 5 ml contains Vit $B_2$1.25 mg; $B_6$0.62 mg; B_{12} 6.25 mcg Methionine 5 mg; Niacin 37.5 mg; D Panthenol 1.25 mg Choline chloride 5 mg; Lysine 5 mg
Adm.	Oral
@	LA 50 ml od SA 10-20 ml od
Pres.	1 L, 5 L

Cadiplex L Liq	Sarabhai
Comp	Each 5 ml contains Vit $B_2$1.25 mg; $B_6$0.62 mg; B_{12}6.25 mcg D Panthenol 0.62 mg; Choline chloride 10 mg Lysine 5 mg
Adm.	Oral
@	LA 10-20 ml od SA 3-5 ml od
Pres.	1 L, 5 L

Groviplex Liq	**Glaxo**
Comp	Each 5 ml contains Vit $B_1$3.75 mg $B_2$1.25 mg B_{12}6.25mg Niacin 37.5 mg Methionine 5 m
Adm.	Oral
@	LA 40-60 ml SA 10-20 ml
Pres.	500 ml, 5 L

Lykoplex Liq	**Lyka**
Comp	Each 5 ml contains Vit $B_1$3.75 mg $B_2$1.25 mg B_{12}6.25 mg Niacin 37.5 mg Methionine 5 m
Adm.	Oral
@	LA 40-60 ml SA 10-20 ml
Pres.	500 ml, 5 L

Bonnysol AD3 ECB12 liq	**Neospark**
Comp	Each 5 ml contains Vit A 250000 IU $D_3$25000 IU E 150 IU B_{12}100 mcg C 500 mg Protein hydrolysate 20 mg Sodium 1967me Cobalt 5 mg
Adm.	Oral
@	10-15 ml od
Pres.	500 ml, 1 L

Briplex Pow	**Brihans**
Comp	Each g contains $B_1$8 mg $B_2$4 gm $B_6$16 mg B_{12}80 mcg Niacinamide 120 mcg Calcium pantothenate 80 mg Vit E 80 mg
Adm.	In feed
@	LA 100 g/ ton of feed
Pres.	1 kg

Lyvim liq	**Cadila Pharma**
Comp	Each g contains Vit A250000 IU $D_3$25000 IU C 500 mg E 150 mg Lysine 25 mg Methionine 10 mg
Adm.	Oral
@	LA 5 ml od SA 2 ml od
Pres.	500 ml, 1 L

Vitamins, Amino Acid and Minerals

Gesta Forte Bol	**TTK**		
Comp	Each Bolus contains		
	Calcium 55 mg	Phosphorus 25 mg	Copper 31 mg
	Cobalt 6 mg	Zinc 11.3 mg	Iodine 19 mg
	Iron 50 mg	Selenium 0.9 mg	
	Fortfied with herbal ingredients		
Adm.	Oral		
@	LA 2 Bol od		
Pres.	Strip of 4		

Gowala Pow	**Zydus**		
Comp	Each Bolus contains		
	Calcium 28%	Phosphorus 12%	Iron 0.55%
	Cobalt 0.013%	Copper 0.077 g	Manganese 0.12%
	Iodine 0.026%	Zinc 0.18%	
	DL methionine 0.19%	Lysine 0.44%	
Adm.	Oral		
@	LA 25 g SA 5-15 g or 1 kg /Ton feed		
Pres.	1 kg, 10 kg		

Groblend Pow	**Virbac**		
Comp	2 kg contains		
	Vit A 50 Lac IU	$B_2$2 g	B6400 mg
	B_{12}5600 mcg	$D_3$625000 IU	E 800 IU
	Calcium pantothenate 4 g	Choline chlorid 10 g	Copper 2 g
	Manganese 27.5 g	Iron 7.5 g	Zinc 15 g
	Calcium 27.25%	Phosphorus 7.45%	Iodine 1 g
Adm.	Oral		
@	LA 25 g od SA 10 g od		
Pres.	2 kg		

Grogold Pow	**Vets Farma**
Comp	Vitamins, Minerals, Proteins, Linoleic acid, Enzymes
Adm.	Oral
@	LA 40 g od Sa 20 g od
Pres.	400 g, 800 g

Gromin Mineral Mixture	**Vets Farma**
Comp	Minerals in appropriate combination
Adm.	Oral
@	LA 50 g od SA 15 g od
Pres.	1 kg, 25 kg, 50 kg

Gromin SE Pow	**Vets Farma**
Comp	Mcrofined and balanced calcium, phosphorus with Iron, Copper, cobalt, Selenium and vit A, D, EB_{12}
Adm.	Oral
@	LA 50 g od SA 15 g od
Pres.	500 g, 1 kg, 2 kg, 5 kg

Kalmin L Pow	**KAPL**		
Comp	Calcium 18%	Phosphorus 9%	Magnesium 5%
	Iron 0.4%	Iodine 0.02%	Copper 0.06%
	Manganese 0.1%	Cobalt 0.009%	Zinc 0.3%
	Salt 22%	Sulphur 0.4%	Fluorine 0.05%
	Moisture 5%		
Adm.	Oral		
@	LA 28 g od SA 8 g od		
Pres.	1 kg		

Kalvimin Forte	**KAPL**		
Comp	2.5 kg contains		
	Calcium 800 g	Phosphorus 150 g	Manganese 27.5 g
	Iodine 1 g	Iron 7.5 g	Zinc 15 g
	Copper 2 g	Vit A 50 Lac IU	B_2 2 mg
	D_3 10 Lac IU	E 800 IU	B_{12} 6 mg
	Calcium pantothenate 4 g		
Adm.	Oral in feed		
@	2.5 kg /Ton of feed		
Pres.	2.5 kg, 5 kg		

Kalmin without salt	**KAPL**		
Comp	2.5 kg contains		
	Calcium 23%	Phosphorus 12%	Magnesium 6.5%
	Iron 0.5%	Iodine 0.026%	Copper 0.077%
	Manganese 0.12%	Cobalt 0.012%	Zinc 0.38%
	Sulphur 0.5%	Flourine 0.07%	Moisture 5%

Adm.	Oral
@	LA 28 g od SA 8 g od
Pres.	1 kg

Ayumin V Pow	**Ayurvet**
Comp	250 g contains Vit A 5 Lac IU; Vit D_3ilac IU $B_2$200 mg; E 75 IU K 100 mg; Calcium pantothenate 250 mg Nicotinamide 1g; B_{12}0.6mg Choline chloride 15 g; Calcium 75 g Manganese 2.75 g; Iodine 100 mg Iron 750 mg; Zinc 1.5 g Copper 200 mg Cobalt 45 mg
Adm.	Oral
@	LA 30 g od SA 15-20 g od
Pres.	250 g, 2.5 kg, 5 kg

Bovivita Special Pow	**Zydus**
Comp	5 g contains Vit A 50000 IU; $D_3$5000 IU E5 mg; Fortified with calcium phosphorus
Adm.	Oral
@	LA 5 g od SA 2 g od
Pres.	100 g

Cadfeed Bol	**Zydus**
Comp	Each Bol contains Nicotinamide 100 mg; Copper sulphate 250 mg Cobalt chloride 40 mg; Dibasic sodium phosphate 100 mg Ferrous sulphate 500 mg; Sodium bicarbonate 600 mg Magnesium trisilicate 800 mg; Piper nigrum 100 mg Zingiber officinalis 20 mg; Andographis paniculata 210 mg Apium graveolens 100 mg; Dried yeast 700 mg Lysine 20 mg; Methionine 20 mg Dextrose 500 mg
Adm.	Oral
@	LA 4 Bol od x 3 day 1 Bolus for 20 days in Anoestus SA 1 Bol od x 3 days
Pres.	Strip of 4

Calmin Powder	**Cattle Remedies**
Comp	1 kg contains Calcium 310 g Phosphorus 120 g Copper 1 g Cobalt 150 mg Manganese 1.2 g Iron 3 g Zinc 2.15 g Iodine 260 mg D L methionine 1.92 g L. lysine monohydrochloride 4.4 g
Adm.	Oral
@	LA 25 g od SA 5-10 g od
Pres.	1 kg, 5 kg, 10 kg

Centromin Powder	**Century**
Comp	Each 1kg contains Calcium 30% Phosphorus 8.25% Zinc 2.13 g Magnesium 2.11 g Cobalt 45 mg Copper 312 mg D methionine 1.92 mg Iodine 156 mg Iron 9.79 mg L lysine 4.4 g
Adm.	Oral
@	LA 30 g od SA 15 g od
Pres.	1 kg, 10 kg

Concimin Pow	**Concept**
Comp	250 g contains Calcium 70 g Phosphorus 20 g Cobalt 45 mg Copper 200 mg Iodine 100 mg Iron 750 mg Manganese 2.75 g Zinc 1.5 g Vit A 5Lac IU D3 ilac B2 200 mg E 750 IU K 100 mg B12 600 mg Calcium pantothnate 250 mg Nicotinamide 1 g Cholinechloride 15 g
Adm.	Oral
@	LA 20 g od SA 10 g od
Pres.	1 kg, 2.5 kg

Concitone Liq	**Concept**
Comp	5 ml contains Vit A 60000 IU $D_3$30000 IU E 240 mg C 5 mg $B_2$5 mg $B_4$5 mg B_{12}125 mcg Nicotinamide 35 mg D panthenol 10 mg Elemental sodium 10 mg Elemental potassium 1.1 mg Elemental chloride 1 mg

Adm.	Oral
@	LA 20 ml od SA 5 ml od
Pres.	100 ml, 500 ml

Dosmin Pow	**Dosch**
Comp	Each kg contains Calcium 30% Phosphorus 9% Cobalt 59 mg Magnesium 2150 mg Copper 406 mg Zinc 2130 mg Selenium 40 mg Live yeast culture 5000 mg DL methionine 2000 mg L lysine 4400 mg
Adm.	Oral
@	LA 30 g od SA 10 g od or 1 kg/ 100 kg feed
Pres.	1 kg, 10 kg, 50 kg

Ecotas Bol	**Intas**
Comp	Each Bolus contains Biotin 10 mg DL methionine 1g Zinc sulphate 200 mg Cobalt 40 mg Copper 100 mg *Saccharomyces cerevisiae* 25 x 10^9 *Lactobacillus sprogenes* 20 x 10^8 *Aspergillus oryzae* 20 x 10^8 *Fructo oligosaccharide* 250 mg
Adm.	Oral
@	2 Bol od x 4 days
Pres.	Strip of 4

Metabolite	**Virbac**
Comp	Not given but nutritional supplement
Adm.	Oral
@	LA 50 g bid for 20 days during last month of pregnancy
Pres.	50 g pouch

Milkmin Pow	**Zydus**
Comp	Calcium 24% Phosphorus 9% Manganese 0.12% Iodine 0.1% Iron 0.6% Copper 0.1% Cobalt 0.02% Sodium chloride 30% Fluorine below 0.03%

Adm.	Oral
@	LA 28 g od SA 15 g od
Pres.	1 kg

Milkmin without Salt	**Zydus**	
Comp	Calcium 28%	Phosphorus 20%
	Iron 0.5%	Iodine 0.026%
	Copper 0.077%	Manganese 0.12%
	Cobalt 0.013%	Zinc 0.18%
	Fluoric below 0.04%	Ash below 2.5%
Adm.	Oral	
@	2-3% infeed	
Pres.	1 kg	

Minal Forte Pow	**Alembic**		
Comp	100 g contains		
	Calcium 30 g	Phosphorus 12 g	Manganese 0.12 g
	Iodine 0.1 g	Iron 0.6 g	Cobalt 0.02 g
	Zinc 0.215 g	Lysine 0.45 g	Methionine 0.2 g
	Copper 0.1 g		
Adm.	Oral		
@	LA 28 g od SA 8g od		
Pres.	1 kg, 10 kg		

Minamil Pow	**Brihans**		
Comp	125 g contains		
	Calcium 80 g	Phosphorus 5 g	Manganese 3 g
	Iodine 0.1 g	Iron 0.8 g	Zinc 2 g
	Copper 0.25	Cobalt 0.05 g	Vit A 5Lac IU
	$D_3$100000 IU	E 80 IU	K 0.1 g
	$B_2$0.3 g	$B_6$0.1 g	B_{12}1 mg
	Calcium pantothenate 3 g	Nicotinamide 2 g	Choline chloride 15 g
Adm.	Oral		
@	LA 20 g od SA 5-10 g od		
Pres.	250 g, 1 kg, 5kg, 25 kg		

Minarex Pow/ Bol	Rakesh		
Comp	Each 1 kg contains		
		Bolus	Powder
	Calcium	25%	30%
	Phosphorus	14%	8.25%
	Salt	12%	Nil
	Iron	0.6%	0.01%
	Iodine	0.1%	0.014%
	Copper	0.1%	0.035%
	Cobalt	0.02%	0.005%
	Zinc	0.6%	0.2%
	Mag sulphate	0.4%	0.2%
	Manganese	0.12%	Nil
	Lysine	0.2%	0.44%
	Methionine	0.12%	0.192%
Adm.	Oral		
@	Pow LA 30 g od Bol 4 od , SA Pow 10 g od		
Pres.	1 kg, 20 Bol pack		

Minotas Bol	Brihans	
Comp	Contains	
	Zinc sulphate 280 mg	Copper sulphate 700 mg
	Manganese chloride 2 g	Cobalt suphate 5 mg
	Potassium iodate 30 mg	Sodium selenite 2 mg
	Ferrous sulphate 1400 mg	Yeast 500 mg
Adm.	Oral	
@	LA 4 Bol od	
Pres.	Bol 4 strip	

Nutrimilk Pow	Pfizer		
Comp	Each kg contains		
	Vit A 625000 IU	$D_3$62500 IU	E250 IU
	Nicotinamide 1 g	Calcium 280 g	Phosphorus 120 g
	Cobalt 0.2 g	Selenium 0.01g	Zinc 2 g
Adm.	Oral		
@	LA 40-50 g od SA 15-25 g od		
Pres.	1 kg		

Nutrisacc Bol	**Vetcare**
Comp	Each kg contains Vit A 5750 IU, D_3 1150 IU, E 650 IU B_3 5 mg, Calcium 150 g, Copper 5 mg Cobalt 0.225 g, Iron 14.8 mg, Iodine 2.5 mg Magnesium 30 mg, Manganese 94.5 mg, Zinc 5 mg Phosphorus 120 mg, Selenium 5 mg Bioactive chromium 1 mg
Adm.	Oral
@	LA 2 Bol bid SA 2 Bol bid
Pres.	Pack of 30

Nutrisacc Powerpack Pow	**Vetcare**
Comp	Each kg contains Yeast culture 100 x 10^9 CFU CFU vit A 115000 IU, D_3 23000 IU E 13000 IU, B_3 100 mg Calcium 76 g, Copper 100 mg Cobalt 5 mg, Iron 313 mg Iodine 50 mg, Magnesium 600 mg Manganese 840 mg, Phosphorus 24 mg Selenium 10 mg, Zinc 100 mg Sustained release protein 280 g, Bypass protein 133 g By pass fat 80 g, Energy 2000 k cal
Adm.	Oral
@	LA 100-200 g SA 50-75 g
Pres.	1 kg, 20 kg

Ossomin Susp	**TTK**
Comp	10 ml contains Calcium 66 mg, Phosphorus 30 mg, Magnesium 15 mg Zinc 200 mg, Manganese 300 mg, Iron 50 mg Iodine 7 mg, Selenium 1 mg
Adm.	Oral
@	LA 30 ml od , 10 ml od
Pres.	200 ml, 450 ml, 4.5 L

Ostophos FS graules	**Neospark**
Comp	Calcium 165 mg, Phosphorus 75 mg Hydroxy apatite 1g bone extract

Adm.	Oral
@	LA 20g od SA 10g od
Pres.	100 g 500g

Promix Y Tab	**Alembic**
Comp	Tab contains Protein 35% Carbohydrate 30% Mineral salt 8% Vit $B_1$0.0 3 mg $B_2$0.012 mg Nicotinic acid 0.09 mg
Adm.	Oral
@	LA 4-6 Tab bid SA 2-4 Tab bid
Pres.	150's, 1000's

Ranmix Pow	**Ranbaxy**
Comp	Each kg contains Calcium 30% Phosphorus 8.25% Copper 312 mg Cobalt 45 mg Magnesium 2.114 g Iron 979 mg Zinc 2.13 g Iodine 156 mg D L methionine 1.92 g L lysine 4.4 g
Adm.	Oral
@	LA 35 g od SA 15 g od
Pres.	1 kg, 10 kg, 25 kg

Sharkoferol Liq	**Alembic**
Comp	15 ml contains Calcium gluconate 300 mg Ferric ammonium citrate 100 mg $D_3$400 IU Naicinamide 45 mg Folic acid 1.5 mg B_{12}15 mcg Malt extract 4.52 g
Adm.	Oral
@	LA 50 ml od SA 10 ml od
Pres.	500 ml IL

Supplevite M Pow	**Zydus**
Comp	250 ml contains Calcium 75 g Manganese 2.75 g Iodine 0.1 g Iron 0.75 g Zinc 1.5 g Copper 0.2 g Cobalt 0.045 g Vit A 5 Lac IU $D_3$100000 IU E 75 IU $B_2$0.2 g K 0.1 g Nicotinamide 1g Calcium pantothente 0.25 g B_{12}0.6 mg Choline chloride 15 mg

Adm.	Oral
@	LA 30 g od SA 8 g od
Pres.	250 g, 2.5 kg

Ultra min Pow	**Neospark**
Comp	Each kg contains Calcium 30% Phosphorus 9% Copper 312 mg Cobalt 45 mg Magnesium 2.114 g Iron 979 mg Zinc 2.13 g Iodine 1.56 mg Methionine 1.929 g Lysine 4.4 g
Adm.	Oral
@	LA 30 g od SA 15 g od
Pres.	1 kg, 20 kg

Calcium Oral

It is indicated to increase milk yield, maintain calcium and Phosphorus balance in blood for improving skeletal and muscular strength.

Ascal Liq	**Alembic**
Comp	Each ml contains Calcium phosphate 240 mg Chole calciferol (D_3) 500 IU Vit B_{12} 7.5 mcg
Adm.	Oral
@	LA 50 ml od SA 10 ml od
Pres.	500 ml, il, 5L

Cal D Rubra	**Cadila**
Comp	Each 5 ml contains Calcium gluconate 416 mg Vit $D_3$600 IU B_{12} 8.38 mcg Ferric ammonium citrate 83.5 mg Stomach extract 16.5 mg
Adm.	Oral
@	LA 50 ml bid SA 25 ml bid
Pres.	100 ml, 500 ml, 1 L, 5 L

Caldhan Susp	**Ayurvet**
Comp	Each 20 ml contains Calcium 325 mg Phosphorus elemental 168 mg

Adm.	Oral
@	LA 50 ml bid SA 20 ml bid
Pres.	500 ml, 1 L, 5 L

Calcicare liq	**Brihans**
Comp	Each 5 ml contains Calcium gluconate 500 mg Calcium lactobionate 5mg Vit B_{12}10 mcg Vit D_{12}600 IU
Adm.	Oral
@	LA 30-50 ml od SA 10-20 ml od
Pres.	120 ml, 500 ml, 1L, 5L

D P Calplus Susp	**Century**
Comp	Each ml contains Trical phosphate 0.24 g Vit D_3 500 IU Vit B_{12} 7.5 mcg
Adm.	Oral
@	LA 100 ml od SA 20 ml od
Pres.	120 ml, 1 L, 5L

Leptamilk Forte	**Concept**
Comp	Each 100 ml contains Calcium phosphate 7.5 g Elemental calcium 2.2 g Elemental phosphorus 1.7 g Vit B_{12}100 mcg Vit D_3 10000 IU and Herbal aqueous extract
Adm.	Oral
@	LA 30-40 ml bid SA 15-30 ml bid
Pres.	1 L, 5 L

Nutrical	**Pfizer (SKF)**
Comp	Each ml contains Elemental calcium 100 mg Elemental phosphorus 50 mg Vit $D_3$400 IU Vit B_{12}5 mcg
Adm.	Oral
@	LA 50-100 ml bid SA 10-20 ml bid
Pres.	1 L, 5 L

Osteocalcium or Ostovet	**Virbac (Glaxo)**
Comp	Each 20 ml contains Calcium 325.6 mg Phosphorus 167.7 mg Vit $D_3$1600 IU Vit B_{12}20 mcg

Adm.	Oral
@	LA 100 ml od SA 20 ml od
Pres.	150 ml, 500 ml, 1 L, 5 L

Ravical Sus	**Gybro**
Comp	Each 20 ml contains Calcium 325.6 mg Phosphorus 167.7 mg Vit $D_3$1600 IU Vit B_{12}20 mcg
Adm.	Oral
@	LA 100 ml od Sa 20 ml od
Pres.	150 ml, 500 ml, 1 L, 5 L

Recalp 12	**Stallen**
Comp	Each 0 ml contains Elemental calcium 100 mg Phosphorus 50 mg Vit $D_3$400 IU Vit B_{12}5 mcg
Adm.	Oral
@	LA 100 ml od SA 20 ml od
Pres.	5 L

Solvical	**Venky**
Comp	Each ml contains Elemental calcium 100 mg Elemental phosphorus 50 mg Vit $D_3$400 IU Vit B_{12}5 mcg
Adm.	Oral
@	LA 50-100 ml bid SA 10-20 ml bid
Pres.	1 L, 5 L

Stercalvet	**Sterling**
Comp	Each 20 ml contains Calcium 340 mg Phosphorus 170 mg Vit D_3 1600 IU Vit B_{12}20 mcg
Adm.	Oral
@	LA 100 ml od SA 20 ml od
Pres.	500 ml

Tinacal DS	**Tineta**
Comp	Each 20 ml contains Calcium 625.2 mg Phosphorus 335.4 mg Vit $D_3$3200 IU Vit B_{12} 40 mcg

Adm.	Oral
@	LA 50 ml od SA 10 ml od
Pres.	500 ml, 1 L, 5 L

Tinacal Sus	**Tineta**
Comp	Each 5 ml contains Calcium 325.6 mg Phosphorus 167.7 mg Vit D_3 600 IU Vit B12 20 mcg
Adm.	Oral
@	LA 100 ml od SA 20 ml od
Pres.	500 ml, 1 L, 2 L, 5 L

Vetcal B_{12}	**Sarabhai**
Comp	Each 20ml contains Calcium 325.6 mg Phosphorus 167.7 mg Vit $D_3$1600 IU Vit B_{12}20 mcg
Adm.	Oral
@	LA 100 ml od SA 20 ml od
Pres.	200 ml, 1 L, 5 L

Lactomix AD_3	**Arosol**
Comp	20 ml contains Calcium 325.6 mg Phosphorus 167.7 mg Vit A 9000 IU $D_3$1600 IU B_{12}20mcg
Adm.	Oral
@	LA 100 ml od SA 20-40 ml od
Pres.	500 ml, 1 L, 5 L

Lactin Bol	**Tineta**
Comp	Bolus contains Calcium elemental 2000 mg Phosphorus elemental 1000 mg $D_3$1200 IU B_{12}50 mcg Asparagus racemosus 500 mg
Adm.	Oral
@	LA 1-2 Bol od
Pres.	Strip of 4

Vetkal Plus granule	**Sarabhai**
Comp	Each 100 g contains Calcium 25 g Phosphorus 12.5 g Magnesium 21 mg Enzymes 1 g

Adm.	In feed
@	1 kg /Ton
Pres.	1 kg

Caldivet	**Ranbaxy**
Comp	Each ml contains Cal. Lactate 250 mg Cal. Gluconate 200 mg $D_3$500 IU B_{12}5mcg Cobalt chloride 5 mg
Adm.	Oral
@	LA 50-75 ml bid, SA 20-50 ml bid
Pres.	1 L, 5 L

Calpar Liq	**Cadila Pharma**
Comp	Each 20 ml contains Calcium 350 mg Phosphorus 170 mg Vit B_{12}20 mcg $D_3$1600 IU
Adm.	Oral
@	LA 100 ml od SA 20 ml od
Pres.	1 L, 5 L

Capsola Liq	**Ranbaxy**
Comp	Each 20 ml contains Calcium 325.6 mg Phosphorus 167.7 mg $D_3$1600 IU B_{12}20 mcg
Adm.	Oral
@	LA 100 ml od SA 20 ml od
Pres.	500 ml, 1 L, 5 L

Doscal AL Susp	**Dosch**
Comp	Each 20 ml contains Calcium 326mg Phosphorus 168 mg $D_3$1600 IU B_{12}20 mcg Leptadina reticulata 200 mg Asparagus racemosus 60 mg
Adm.	Oral
@	LA 100 ml od SA 20 ml od
Pres.	500 ml, 1 L, 5 L

Lactomilk Chelated	**Macwell**
Comp	Each 100 ml contains Calcium 6 g Phosphorus 3 g Vit a 5000 mcg $D_3$12000 IU B_{12}100 mcg E 4500 IU Copper 500 mg Zinc 1500 mg Chromium 200 ppm Shatavari 1 g Jiwanti 1 g Bad peepali 400 mg Silymarine 450 mg

Adm.	Oral
@	LA 50 ml bid
Pres.	6 L

Prical DS Susp	**PAIL**
Comp	Each 100 ml has nutritional value of Calcium 1750 mg Phosphorus 875 mg D3 800 IU B_{12} 100 mcg Jiwanti 1.5 g Iron 100 mg Shatavari 3 g Javitri 3 g Cobalt chloride 20 mg
Adm.	Oral
@	LA 100 ml od
Pres.	1 L, 5 L

LDM	**Animax Healthcare**
Comp	Not given
Adm.	Oral
@	100 ml od
Pres.	1 L, 5 L

Agrical	**Sushima**
Comp	Each 20 ml contains Calcium 400 mg Phosphorus 200 mg D_3 1600 IU B_{12} 20 mcg Protein hydrolysate 300 mg
Adm.	Oral
@	LA 100 ml od
Pres.	1 L, 5 L

Calciliv	**Carevet Pharma**
Comp	Each 20 ml contains Calcium citrate 500 mg Sodium acid phosphate 375 mg D_3 1600 IU B_{12} 20 mcg Asparagus racemosus 5 mg Leptadenia reticulata 5 mg Carbohydrate 8000 mg
Adm.	Oral
@	LA 100 ml od
Pres.	1 L, 5 L

Inomilk	**Hester**
Comp	Micronized calcium and Phosphorus
Adm.	Oral
@	LA 100 ml od
Pres.	5 L

Lactoplus AD3 Gold	**Argano**
Comp	Not given
Adm.	Oral
@	LA 100 ml od
Pres.	5 L

Merical	**Merial**
Comp	Each 20 ml contains Calcium 350 mg Phosphorus 170 mg Vit B_{12}20 mcg $D_3$1600 IU
Adm.	Oral
@	LA 100 ml od SA 20 ml od
Pres.	500 ml, 1 L, 5 L

Vitacal D_3 liq	**Unjha**
Comp	Calcium phosphate tribasic 0.24 g Vit $D_3$400 IU Vit B_{12}5 mcg
Adm.	Oral
@	LA 100 ml od
Pres.	500 ml, 5 L

Inomilk Gold	**Hester**
Comp	Double strength cal, Phasphorus, Vit D_3, Vit B_{12}, Biotin, Jiwanti and shatavari
Adm.	Oral
@	LA 50 ml od bid SA 20 ml bid
Pres.	1 L, 5 L

Amcal Forte Bol	**Pranav**
Comp	Each Bolus contains Calcium 1700 mg Phosphorus 850 mg $D_3$8000 IU B_{12} 100 mg Cobalt 20 mg Iron 100 mg Lipase 10 mg Shatavari 1 g Jiwanti 300 mg
Adm.	Oral
@	1 Bol od x 10 days
Pres.	Strip of 4

Biocalcium Forte Bol	**Anmark**
Comp	Bolus contains Calcium 1700 mg Phosphorus 850 mg $D_3$50 mg Copper 50 mg Cobalt 50 mg Ferrous sulphate 100 mg Jiwanti 500 mg Shatavari 1 g

Adm.	Oral
@	1 Bol od
Pres.	Strip of 4

Doscal Bol	**Dosch**
Comp	Calcium, Phosphorus, VIt D_3, B_{12}, Enzymes, Asparagus and Leptadenia
Adm.	Oral
@	2 Bol od
Pres.	4 Bol strip

DP Cal B12 Bol	**Century**
Comp	Each Bolus contains Tribasic calcium phosphate 4.8 g $D_3$8000 IU B_{12}100 mcg
Adm.	Oral
@	LA 1 Bol bid
Pres.	Strip of 4

Milk up Bol	**Anmark**
Comp	Each Bolus contains Calcium 750 mg Phosphorus 450 mg Copper 100 mg Cobalt 20 mg Shatavari 600 mg Jiwanti 600 mg Vidarkand 600 mg Ashvgandha 600 mg
Adm.	Oral
@	LA 3-4 Bol od
Pres.	4 Bol pouch or 50 Bol container

Calci Royal Pow	**Concept**
Comp	5 g contains Elemental calcium 174 mg Elemental phosphorus 50 mg B_{12}50 mcg C 30 mg $D_3$1000 IU Citric acid 1 g
Adm.	Oral
@	10 g od
Pres.	2 kg

Orcal P Pow	**TTK**
Comp	5 g contains Microcytalline MCHC equivalent to Calcium 165 mg Phosphorus 75 mg $D_3$500 IU
Adm.	Oral
@	LA 20 g od x 10 days
Pres.	100 g, 250 g container

Tonox Pow	**Pranav**
Comp	125 g contains Calcium phosphate diabasic 45 g Magnesium sulphate 10 g Vit E 75 mg Poly herbal powder with LYC 10000 million CFU Sodium selenite 10 mg Citric acid 1g
Adm.	Oral
@	25 g od x 5 days
Pres.	125 g pouch

Vita Forte M Pow	**Anmark**
Comp	250 g contains Calcium 75 g Cal pantothende 300 mg Vit A 5 Lac IU $D_3$1 lac IU $B_2$200 mg K 100 mg B_{12}600 mcg Niacinamide 1 g Choline chloride 15 g Manganese 1.75 g Iodine 0.1g Iron 0.75 g Zinc 1.5 g Copper 200 mg Cobalt 45 mg Antioxideant q.s
Adm.	Oral
@	LA 25 g od
Pres.	25 kg

Biocalcium Forte Liq	**Anmark**
Comp	20 ml contains Calcium 325.6 mg Phosphorus 167.7 mg $D_3$1600 IU Zinc 50 mg Manganese 5 mg Cobalt 5 mg Jivanti 60 mg Shatavari 200 mg

Adm.	Oral
@	LA 500-100 ml od
Pres.	500 ml, 1 L, 5 L

Ascosol C Pow	**Neospark**
Comp	Each g contains Vit C 500 mg Casein protein 500 ppm Sodium 8.2 mg
Adm.	Oral
@	LA 250 mg/ kg B.wt
Pres.	100 g, 500 g, 1 kg

Biospur – LS bol	**Primavetcare**
Comp	Each Bolus contains Calcium 500 mg Phosphorus 350 mg Protein hydrolysate 50% 1g Lactobacillus sporogenes 20 million spores Alpha amylase 25 mg Papaine 25 mg
Adm.	Oral
@	LA 1-2 Bolus od SA ½ -1 Bolus od
Pres.	Strip of 2

Cadisol DC liq	**Zydus**
Comp	10 ml contains Calcium gluconate 889 mg Vit $D_3$1600 IU Calcium D saccharate 4 mg Ferric ammonium citrate 167 mg Vit B_{12}16.7 mcg Papaine 25 mg
Adm.	Oral
@	LA 50 ml bid SA 20 ml bid
Pres.	5 L

Cadisol Plus liq	**Zydus**
Comp	10 ml contains Calcium gluconate 833 mg Vit $D_3$1600 IU Stomach ext 3.3 mg Ferric ammonium citrate 167 mg Vit B_{12}16.7 mcg
Adm.	Oral
@	LA 50 ml bid SA 25 ml bid
Pres.	500 ml, 1 L, 5 L

Cal K	**KAPL**
Comp	10 ml contains Calcium 200 mg Phosphorus 100 mg Vit $D_3$1600 IU Vit B_{12}6 mcg Manganese 5 mg Vit C 10 mg
Adm.	Oral
@	LA 50 ml od SA 10 ml od
Pres.	500 ml, 1 L, 5 L

Calcicare C	**Brihans**
Comp	20 ml liq contains Calcium 325.6 mg Phosphorus 167.7mg Vit $D_3$1800 IU Vit B_{12}20 mcg
Adm.	Oral
@	LA 50 ml bid SA 20 ml bid
Pres.	120 ml, 500 ml, 1 L, 5L

Calcizol Liq	**Rakesh**
Comp	20 ml contains Calcium 440 mg Phosphorus 340 mg Vit D3 1600 IU Vit B_{12}20 mcg Asparagus racemosus extract 1.5 g
Adm.	Oral
@	LA 50 ml bid SA 20 ml bid
Pres.	500 ml, 1 L, 5 L

Cadlec Forte	**Wockhardt**
Comp	100 ml contains Calcium 1700 mg Phosphorus 850 mg Vit $D_3$8000 IU VitB_{12}100 mcg Shatavari 1g Cobalt chloride 20 mg Iron 100 mg Lipase 10 mg Jivanti 300 mg
Adm.	Oral
@	LA 100 ml od
Pres.	500 ml, 1 L, 5 L

Cal D Plus DS liq	**Cadila Pharma**
Comp	100 ml contains Calcium gluconate 416.5 mg Vit $D_3$800 IU Vit B_{12}8.35 mcg Stomach ext 1.65 mg Ferric ammonium citrate 83.5 mg
Adm.	Oral
@	LA 50 ml bid SA 25 ml bid
Pres.	100 ml, 250 ml, 500 ml, 1 L, 5 L

Calfos D_3 Plus Pow	**Vets Farma**
Comp	500 g contains Calcium 26% Phosphorus 16% Copper 0.5% Cobalt 0.02% Vit $D_3$30000 IU
Adm.	Oral
@	LA 50-100 g od SA 10-15 g od
Pres.	500 g, 2 kg

Calfosvet Liq	**Vets Farma**
Comp	Calcium Phosphorus Vit D_3 B_{12}
Adm.	Oral
@	LA 100 ml od SA 25 ml od
Pres.	500 ml, il, 2 L, 5 L

Calmore Liq	**Indian Herbs**
Comp	Not given but contains Calcium Phosphorus Biotin VitB_{12}
Adm.	Oral
@	LA 3-4 Bol od
Pres.	4 Bol pouch or 50 Bol container

Calmore DS Liq	**Indian Herbs**
Comp	Not given but contains Calcium Phosphorus Biotin VitB_{12}
Adm.	Oral
@	LA 50 ml SA 25 ml
Pres.	500 ml

Calsagar Plus Pow	**Indian Immunology**
Comp	50 g contains Calcium 10 g Phosphorus 5 g Vit$D_3$2000 IU Herbal galactagogue 5 g
Adm.	Oral
@	50 g od
Pres.	1 kg

Calshakti Liq	**Intas**
Comp	100 g contains Calcium 1700 mg Phosphorus 850 g Vit $D_3$8000 IU Vit B_{12}100 mcg Ext of shatavari 1000 mg Jivanti 100 mg Piper longum 400 mg
Adm.	Oral
@	LA 100 ml od SA 25 ml od
Pres.	500 ml, 1 L, 2 L, 5 L, 7.5 L

Cal Strong Liq	**Alved**
Comp	20 ml contains Calcium 400 mg Phosphorus 200 g Vit D3 1600 IU Vit B_{12}20 mcg Cobalt 20 mg Casein protein 200 ppm Elemental iron 55.2 mg
Adm.	Oral
@	LA 50 ml bid SA 25 ml bid
Pres.	500 ml, 1 L, 5 L

Casphodil Liq	**Lyka**
Comp	Each 5 ml contains Calcium 100 mg Phosphorus 50 mg VitD$_3$400 IU VitB$_{12}$ 5 mg Protein hydrolycate 75 mg
Adm.	Oral
@	LA 100 ml bid SA 50 ml bid
Pres.	1 L, 5 L

Casphodil Gold Liq	**Lyka**
Comp	Each 20 ml contains Calcium 400 mg Phosphorus 200 mg Vit D3 1600 IU Vit B12 20 mcg Shatavari 100 mg Jivanti 100 mg Piper longum 100 mg
Adm.	Oral
@	LA 100 ml od SA 50 ml od
Pres.	5 L

Goudhara Shakti	**Indian Immunology**
Comp	1 kg contains Calcium 68 mg Yeast culture 100 g Bypass fat 660 g Herbal galactagogue 100 g

Adm.	Oral
@	100 g od
Pres.	1 kg

Lactoboon Tab	**Lyka**		
Comp	Calcium 5.65%	Phosphorus 4.37%	Potassium 0.5%
	Zinc 0.5%	Iodine 0.12%	Sodium 0.2%
	Magnesium 0.1%	Iron 0.6%	Manganese 1.3%
	Copper 1.3%	Cobalt 0.12%	Shatavari 18%
	Jivanti 18%		
Adm.	Oral		
@	LA 10 Tab od SA 2 Tab od		
Pres.	100 Tab.		

Lactofat Pow	**Dosch**	
Comp	1 kg contains	
	Vit A 1000000 IU	E 300 IU
	Iron 1272 mg	Cobalt 50 mg
	Zinc 2310 mg	Copper 406 mg
	Calcium 30%	Phosphorus 9%
	Live yeast culture 5 g	Amino acid 5 g
	Lactobacillus sporogenes culture 50 million CFU	Shatavari 50 g
	Jivanti 30 g	Nardostachys jatamansi 30 g
Adm.	Oral	
@	LA 30 g od SA 20 g od	
Pres.	500 g, 10 kg	

Lactovet Powder	**Rakesh**		
Comp	500 g contains		
	Calcium 20%	Phosphorus 5.37%	Iron 0.066%
	Cobalt 0.03%	Copper 0.02%	Zinc 0.133%
	Iodine 0.09%	Magnesium 0.133%	Shatavari 13.5%
	Jivanti 13.5%	Piper longum 6%	
Adm.	Oral		
@	LA 50 g od SA 20 g od		
Pres.	500 g, 1 kg		

Merical Plus Liq	**Wockhardt**		
Comp	100 ml contains		
	Calcium 1700 mg	Phosphorus 850 mg	Vit B_{12} 100 mg
	Vit D_3 8000 IU	Cobalt 20 mg	Iron 100 mg
	Lipase 10 mg	Shatavari 1000 mg	Jivanti 300 mg

Adm.	Oral
@	LA 100 ml od SA 40 ml od
Pres.	1 L, 5L

Ossopan granules	**TTK**
Comp	Each g contains Calcium 165 mg Phosphorus 75 mg
Adm.	Oral
@	LA 10-20 g bid SA 35 g bid
Pres.	100 g, 12.5 kg, 25 kg

Ravical Sus	**Gybro**
Comp	20 ml contains Calcium 325.6 mg Phosphorus 167.7 mg Vit D_3 1600 IU B_{12} 20 mcg
Adm.	Oral
@	LA 100 ml od SA 20 ml bid
Pres.	1 L, 5 L

Recalp 12 Susp	**Stallen**
Comp	Each ml contains Elemental Calcium 100 mg Phosphorus 50 mg Vit D_3 400 IU B_{12} 5mcg
Adm.	Oral
@	LA 100 ml od SA 30 ml bid
Pres.	5 L

Sanical Vet granules	**Novartis**
Comp	Each g contains Elemental calcium 42 mg Elemental Phosphorus 50 mg B_1 10 mg C 6 mg D 400 IU Citric acid 6.27 mg
Adm.	Oral
@	LA 20 g x 5 days SA 15 g x5 days
Pres.	500 g

Ultracal D Liq	Neospark	
Comp	5 ml contains	
	Calcium gluconate 416.5 mg	$D_3$800 IU
	Ferric ammonium citrate 83.5 mg	Vit B_{12}8.35 mcg
	Casein protein 200 ppm	Iron 13.8 mg
	Cobalt 5 mg	Stomach ext 1.65 mg
Adm.	Oral	
@	LA 50 ml bid SA 25 ml bid	
Pres.	500 ml, 1 L, 5 L	

Wesimilk gold	Wesfa pharma	
Comp	1 L contains	
	Calcium 35 g	Phosphorus 17.5 g
	Vit A 50000 IU	$D_3$300000
	B_{12}2000 mcg	Copper MHA 5000 mg
	Zinc MHA 15000 IU	Cobalt 100 mg
	Potassium iodide 100 mg	Vit H 100 mcg
	Carbohydrate 180 g	
Adm.	Oral	
@	100 ml od	
Pres.	1 L, 5 L, 10 L, 20 L	

Fibrokit MRF Pow	Wesfa pharma	
Comp	Each 60 g contains	
	Trisodium citrate 35 g	Vit A 4000 IU
	Lactobacillus 200 million	Amino nitrogen 100 mg
	Vit E 1500 IU	Serratiopeptidase 120 mg
	Potassium iodide 7g	Vit K 400 IU
	Live yeast culture 7500 million	Zinc sulphate 150 mg
	Bromelian 320 mg	Ocimum sanctum 1000 mg
	Sodium selenite 10 mg	Aloe vira 100 mg
	Azadirachta indica 4000 mg	
Adm.	Oral	
@	30 gm bid	
Pres.	60 g	

Leptocal Bol	**Phoenix**
Comp	Tribasic calcium phosphate 4.8 g Vit A 50000 IU · D320000 IU · Vit E 25 mg Vit H 100 mcg · $B_1$2100 mcg · Lysine 125 mg Jivanti 350 mg · Shatavari 2000 mg · Copper 50 mg Manganese 25 mg · Zinc 500 mg
Adm.	Oral
@	1 Bol bid
Pres.	Strip of 1 Bol

Pawas Forte Bol	**Libra**
Comp	Herbs and Vit A, D, E, H_1, B_{12}, lactic acid and Saccharomyces with Protein, calcium and Phosphorus
Adm.	Oral
@.	4 Bol 2 hours before milking bid
Pres.	Stirp of 4

MD3 Mac Bol	**Macnor**
Comp	Each Bolus has Tribasic calcium phosphate 4.8 g · Magnesium 20 mg Vit $D_3$10000 IU · Vit B_{12}100 mcg Vit E 25 mg · L Lysine 125 mg Shatavari 350 mg · Jiwanti 2500 mg
Adm.	Oral
@.	1 Bol bid for 10 days
Pres.	1 Bol strip

Leptocal gold Sus	**Phoenix**
Comp	100 ml contains Calcium 3.5 g · Phosphorus 1.75 g · Vit A 45000 IU D3 16000 IU · B_{12}300 mcg · Jivanti 350 mg Shatavari 2000 mg · Carbohydrate 13 g · Protein 3 g Fat 1 g · Fibre 8 g
Adm.	Oral
@	LA 50-100 ml od SA 30-5 0ml od
Pres.	1 L, 2 L, 5L, 20 L

Doxocal Liquid	**Libra**		
Comp	100 ml contains		
	Calcium 3. 5g	Phosphorus 1.75 g	B12 400 mcg
	$D_3$20000 IU	Vit H 500 mcg	Dextrose 25%
	Shatavari	Jivanti	Vidarkand
	Jeera	Pureria mirifica	Sibymarin
Adm.	Oral		
@.	LA 100 ml od SA 50 ml od		
Pres.	5 L, 20 L		

Libracal Gold Liq	**Libra**		
Comp	100 ml contains		
	Calcium 1650 ml	Phosphorus 850 mg	$D_3$10000 IU
	B_{12}250 mcg	Cobalt 10 mg	Magnesium 150mg
Adm.	Oral		
@.	LA 100 ml od SA 25-50 ml od		
Pres.	5 L		

Phoscal AD3 liq	**Argano organic**		
Comp	Calcium	Phosphorus	Vitamins with herbs
Adm.	Oral		
@	100 ml od		
Pres.	1 L, 3 L, 5 L, 10 L, 20 L		

Agrical Liq	**Sushima Pharma**		
Comp	20 ml contains		
	Calcium 400 mg	Phosphorus 200 mg	Vit $D_3$1600 IU
	Vit B_{12}20 mcg	Protein hydro lysate 300 mg	
Adm.	Oral		
@	100 ml od		
Pres.	1 L, 5 L		

Caldhara Gold DS liq	**Agilis**			
Comp	Calcium	4 g	Manganese	72 mg
	Phosphorus	2 g	Copper glycinate	600 mg
	Vit D_3	17000 IU	Cobalt glycinate	5 mg
	Vit B_{12}	600 mcg	Chromium glycinate	8 mg
	Vit H	20 mg	Zinc glycinate	500 mg
	Potassium	18 mg	Iodin	5.9 mg
	Trisodium citrate	10 g	Shatavari	1 g
	Jivanti	1 g	Carbohydrate	28%

Adm.	Oral
@	100 ml od
Pres.	1 L, 5 L, 20 L

Calpar Gold Susp	**Cadila Pharma**
Comp	100 ml contains Calcium 1750 mg Phosphorus 859 mg Vit B_{12} 100 mcg D_3 8000 IU
Adm.	Oral
@	100 ml od
Pres.	1 L, 5 L, 20 L

CalciKal liq	**Boehringer Ingelheim**
Comp	100 ml contains Calcium 3500 mg Phosphorus 1750 mg Vit D_3 20000 IU B_{12} 200 mcg Zince 150 mg Herbal galactagogue 1%
Adm.	Oral
@	LA 100 ml od SA 20 ml od
Pres.	1 L, 2 L, 5 L

Alvical DS	**Alivira**
Comp	100 ml contains Calcium 3600 mg Phosphorus 1800 mg Iodine 5.9 mg Copper glycinate 12 mg Zinc glycinate 540 mg Chromium glycinate 8 mg Cobalt glycinate 5mg Manganese glycinate 270 mg Vit $D_3$15000 IU B_{12} 200 mcg Carbohydrate 28 g
Adm.	Oral
@	LA 50-100 ml od SA 25 ml od
Pres.	1 L, 5 L

Lactoplus AD_3 Gold	**Argano organic**
Comp	Calcium Phosphorus Vitamins Chelated mineral with herbs
Adm.	Oral
@	100 ml od
Pres.	1 L, 3 L, 5 L, 10 L, 20 L

Milkoplex Bolus.			**Rakesh Pharma**
Indi: Letting down of milk and galactogogue			
Comp: Each Bolus.			
Withaniasomnifera	1250 mg	Asparagusracemosus	500 mg
NardostackysJatamansi	500 mg	Leptadeniareticulata	1750 mg
Adm: Oral			
@ : 1-2 Bol.twice a day			
Pres: 20 Bol. 200 Bol.			

Himcal Liq.	**Himalya**
Indi: For milk production Ca+Phosp.	
Comp: Not given	
Adm: Oral	
@ : 100 ml twice daily for 3 days thenoncea day	
Pres: 500 ml, 1 L	

Calmin	**Cattle Remedies**
Indi: Tonic, Milk booster	
Comp: Not given	
Adm: Oral	
@ : 25-50 g daily	
Pres: 1 kg, 5 kg, 10 kg	

Tonical	**Cattle Remedies**
Indi: Calcium deficiency Milk fever, Ketosis	
Comp: Not given	
Adm: Oral	
@ : 50 ml daily twice a day	
Pres: 500 ml, 1 L, 5 L	

Patanjali Samvridhi Liq./Bolus	**Patanjali**
Indi: Calcuim FS	
Comp: Not given	
Adm: Oral	
@ : 100 ml daily 2 Bol.	
Pres: 1 L, 5 L, 10 L Bol.	

Calcium Gel

Calup Gel	**Cargill (Vetcare)**
Comp	In one pack calcium 43.5 g Ions
Adm.	Oral
@	1 pack in LA 6 hrly
Pres.	300 g

Milkup gel	**Libra**		
Comp	Calcium 67.6 g	Phosphorus 6.2 mg	Magnesium 2.9 g
	Potassium 1 g	Glucose 50 g	
Adm.	Oral		
@.	300 ml		
Pres.	300 ml pack		

Lactomilk gel	**Macwell**		
Comp	Calcium 43.5 g	Magnesium 200 mg	Vit $D_3$32000
	IUVit B_{12}400 mcg	Pantothenic acid 152 mg	
	Nicotinic acid 3000 mg	Silymarine 300 mg	
Adm.	Oral		
@	One pack		
Pres.	300 ml		

LDM gel	**Animax Healthcare**		
Comp	300 ml contains		
	Vit D 120000	Vit B_{12}1200 mcg	Vit A 600000 IU
	Vit E 15000 IU	Phosp 15.3 g	
	Pureria mirifico extr. 15000 IU	Calcium 30 g	
Adm.	Oral		
@	1 Bottle		
Pres.	300 ml		

Calcia gel	**Nicosia**		
Comp	300 ml contains		
	Calcium ionic 43.5 g	Nicotinic acid 300 mg	B_{12}400 mcg
	B_{12} 200 mg	Pantothenic acid 32000 IU	

Adm.	Oral
@	300 ml bid
Pres.	300 g gel

Probiotics / Prebiotics

Bioboost Bol	**Lyka**
Comp	Each Bolus has Live yeast culture 3 g Live lactobacillus sporogenes culture 20 million CFU Amino acid 2 g Liver extract 5 mg
Adm.	Oral
@	LA 2 Bol od SA ½ Bol od
Pres.	Strip of 4

Bioboost Powder	**Lyka**
Comp	100 g contains Live yeast culture 3 g Live lactobacillus sporogenes culture 20 million CFU Amino acid 2 g Liver extract 5 mg
Adm.	Infeed
@	1-1.5 kg /Ton feed
Pres.	1 kg

Bioton FS Bol /Pow	**KAPL**		
Comp	Each Bolus	500 g Powder	
	30 million	Lactoliocillus coagulans hammer	300 m
	3 g	Live yeast	30 g
	2 g	Amino acid	30 g
Adm.	Oral powder infeed		
@	LA 2-3 Bol od SA ½ -1 Bol od, all animal 50 g in 100 kg feed		
Pres.	Strip of 4, 500 g, 5 kg		

Biovet Bol	**Wockhardt**
Comp	Each Bolus contains Biological derived natural product 1 g Live yeast 3 g Liver ext 5 mg Amino acid 1g Lactobacillus 20 million CFU Albha amylase 10 mg Essential trace minerals 8 mg

Adm.	Oral
@	LA 2-4 Bol bid, SA 1-2 Bol bid
Pres.	Strip of 4

Biovet YC Pow	**Wockhardt**
Comp	Each 100 g contains Lactobacillus acidophilus 3000 million CFU Lactobacillus sporogenes 75 million CFU Live yeast culture Saccharomyces cerevisiae SC 47 2500 million CFU Alpha amylase 5 g Sewed extract 100 g
Adm.	Oral or feed
@	15-20 g / day or 200 g/100 kg feed
Pres.	100 g, 1 kg

Boost up Bol / Powder	**Dosch**
Comp	Each Bolus contains Live yeast culture 3 g Lactobacillus sporogenes culture 200 million CFU Amino acid 2 g Liver extract 5 mg Fungal diastase 50 mg **Powder 1 kg contains** Live yeast culture 25 g Lactobacillus 200 million CFU Amino acid 25 g Liver extract 500 mg Fungal diastase 5 g
Adm.	Oral
@	LA 1-2 Bol od 10-15 g od SA ½ -1 Bol od 3-5 g od
Pres.	Strip of 4, 100 g, 1 kg

Goutryl Liq	**Lyka**
Comp	Each 5 ml contains Sodium bicarbonate 1.5 mg Ammonium chloride 1 g Ascorbic 0.5 g Citosidine 1 g Halite 1 g
Adm.	Oral
@	100 ml od
Pres.	1 L

Improval Pow	**Zydus**
Comp	Sacchromyces cerevisiale 1.5 x 10^{11} Lactobacillus sporogenes 30000 million CFU Calcium Phosphorus Protein Carbohydrate Vitamin and UGF
Adm.	Oral
@	LA 20 g od SA 5 g od or 1 kg/ ton of feed
Pres.	50 g, 250 g, 1 kg, 20 kg

Provisac Bol	**Vetcare**
Comp	Each Bolus contains Yeast culture of Saccharomyces cerevisiae strain 1026 5 x10^4 cells
Adm.	Oral
@	LA 2 Bol od Sa ½ -1 Bol od
Pres.	5 g Bol

Protexin Pow	**Novartis**
Comp	Multistrain probiotic containing Live viable strains of streptococcus faecium, Bifidobacterum bifidum, Lactobacillus plantrarum, Lactobacillus bulgaricus, Streptococus thermophiles, Lactobacillus casei, Lactobacillus acidophilus, Torulopsis spp and Aspergillus oryzae
Adm.	Oral
@	LA 5 g od SA 2g od
Pres.	100 g, 10 kg

Vergest Liq	**Ranbaxy**
Comp	Contains Engymes, Complexed vitamins, Minerals and Marine algal protein
Adm.	Oral
@	LA 3 ml od SA 1 ml od
Pres.	100 ml, 1 L

Electrolyte / Energisers

These yeprations are formulated to provide essential nutrients for energy and rehydration. These can be used supportive and curative in conditions where these nutrients are instantly needed. These are concentrated electrolytes powder, liquid and feed supplements. It is indicated in dysentery, diarrhea, dewoing, haemorrhges fatigue and stress.

Amlyte Pow	**Pranav**
Comp	100 ml contains Potassium chloride 3.5 g; Magnesium sulphate 1.2 g Sodium choride 1.75 g; Sodium bicarbonate 1 g Sodium citrate 2.5 g; Calcium lactate 1.1g Calcium gluconate 1.1g; Dextrose monohydrate 40 g Vit C 1 g
Adm.	Oral
@	LA 50-100 g bid SA 10-20 g bid in drinking water
Pres.	250 g, 1 kg

E Booster liq	**Intas**
Comp	Gluconegenic precursor fortified with Nicotinamide and cynocobalamin
Adm.	Oral
@	LA 200 ml bid in first 2 days then 100ml od next two days
Pres.	il

Electrocare Plus Pow	**Cargill (Vetcare)**
Comp	100 ml contains Sodium chloride 12.3%; Potassium chloride 5.3% Sodium citrate 10.2%; Dextrose anhydros 70.2%
Adm.	Oral
@	LA 50 g 4 times a day SA 10 g 3-4 times a day
Pres.	50 g, 200 g, 1 kg

Ortiz Pow	**Novartis**
Comp	5 g contains Sodium chloride 0.25 g; Potassium chloride 0.3 g Sodium bicarbonate 0.5 g; Citric acid 1.154 g Dextrose 5.3 g
Adm.	Oral
@	LA 10 g tds SA 5 g tds
Pres.	5 g

Ultralytec Pow	**Neospark**

Comp	100 g contains Sodium chloride 1 g · Potassium chloride 5 g Sodium bicarbonate 3 g · Sodium acid phosphate 0.8 g Sodium citrate 6.5 g · Calcium lactate 1.7 g Magnesium sulphate 1 g · Vit C 1.2 g DFM CFU 330 million · Casein protein 200 ppm Elemental sodium 2.62 g · Lactose 40 g Dextrose qs
Adm.	Oral
@	LA 10 SA 5 g tds
Pres.	100 g, 250 g, 500 g, 1 kg

LDM Liq	**Animax Healthcare**
Comp	Herbs and minerals
Adm.	Oral
@	100 ml bid
Pres.	1 L, 3 L

Enermac Liq.	**Macwell**
Comp	Minerals · Vitamins · Amino acids · Probiotic Silimarin · Honey energy · 13 electrolytes
Adm.	Oral
@	100 ml od
Pres.	1 L

Ketonex Bol	**Zydus**
Comp	Bolus contains Nicotinic acid 1.5 g · Dried yeast 1.5 g Sodium hydrogen phosphate 0.375 g
Adm.	Oral
@	2 Bol bid
Pres.	4 Bolus in strip

Diakur plus Pow	**Boehringer Ingelheim**
Comp	Contains Glucose · Yeast · Hydrochloric citrus Fiber · Balanced electrolyte

Adm.	Oral
@	LA 100 g SA 10 g
Pres.	100 g sache

Vet Cool Plus Pow	**Animax Healthcare**
Comp	100 g contains Calcium lactate 1 g, Vit C 5 g Potassium chloride 4 g, Vit B1 100 mg Magnesium sulphate 4.5 g, Vit B2 100 mg Sodium chloride 800 mg, Vit B12 100 mcg Sodium bi-carbonate 700 mg Cyproheptadine Sodium citrate 3 g Water soluble carbohydrate 40 g Dextrose 40 g Lactobacillus sporogenes 1500 million
Adm.	Oral
@	LA 100-125 g od SA 10-50 g od
Pres.	1 kg

Performance Promototers

BMD Pow	**Ranbaxy**
Comp	Bacitracin methyl disalicylate 10%
Adm.	In feed
@	150-300 g/ Ton of feed
Pres.	1 kg

Flavomycin 40	**Intervet**
Comp	Flavophospholipol 40 mg/g
Adm.	Infeed
@	SA 300 g/ ton of feed Pig 125 g/ton
Pres.	1 kg

Liv52 Protec Liq/Gel	**Himalya**
Comp	Herbal growth promoter

Adm.	Oral
@	LA 50 ml bid SA 20 ml bid
Pres.	500 ml, il, 5 L, 30 L, il, 5 L Gel

Protexin	**Novartis**
Comp	Not given
Adm.	Refer probiotics
@	Refer probiotics
Pres.	Refer probiotics

Roxarsone Pow	**Wockhardt**
Comp	3 Nitro 4 Hydrophenylarsonic acid 50 g/kg
Adm.	Infeed
@	I kg/ ton of feed
Pres.	1 kg, 5 kg

TM 100	**Pfizer**
Comp	Oxytetracycline 100 g/kg
Adm.	Infeed
@	SA 150-400 g/ ton of feed
Pres.	20 kg

Doodh Dana granule	**Cadila Pharma**
Comp	Jiwanti 150 g Kambojika 100 g Calcium 1176 mg Phosphorus 910 mg Bypassfat 14 g Energy 300 kcal
Adm.	Oral
@	30g od
Pres.	300g

Cal Dmin Forte chelaled Pow supreme	**Cadila Pharma**
Comp	1 kg contains Vit A 150000 IU Phosphorus 127.5 g Cobalt 150 mg D_3 230000 IU

	Magnesium	6 g	Iodine	325 mg
	E	230000 IU	Sodium	6 mg
	Iron	1.5 g	Nicotinamide	1 g
	Potassium	100 mg	Manganese	2.4 g
	Calcium	255 g	Copper	4.5 g
	Zinc	9.6 g		
Adm.	Oral			
@	40 g od for high milker 60 g od or 1 kg in 100 kg feed			
Pres.	1 kg, 5 kg, 25 kg			

CaldhanV Liq.	**Ayurvet**
Indi: Improve, Milkyield, Mineral, Supplement	
Comp: Not given	
Adm: Oral	
@ : 50 ml bd	
Pres: 1 L, 5 L Jar	

Himilk Pow.			**Vets Farma**
Indi: Increase milk yield			
Comp:			
Tinospora cordifolia	20%	Leptadenia reticulata	5%
Luffa amara	2%	Trilbulus terrestris	10%
Asparagns racemosus	5%	Sesamum orientale	10%
Nagarmotha	10 g	Zingiber officinale	5 g
Marodfall	10 g	Phyllanthus emblica	10 g
Berberis aristata	10 g	Alum (Fitkari)	5 g
Adm: Oral			
@ : 25-40 g with rice or curd twice a day			
Pres: 100 g			

Cofecu Tablets/Cofecuplus	**Indian Herbs**
Indi: Fertility	
Comp: Not given	
Adm: Oral	
@ : 1 tab. daily for 20 days	
Pres: 20 tab. pack	

MegabrickBol.	Natural Remedies
Indi: Mineral Supplement	
Comp: Not given	
Adm: Oral	
@ : 1 Bol. daily	
Pres: 107 G Bolus	

Generalton			VetsFarma
Indi: General tonic, Anaemiaetc.			
Comp:			
Hara Kasis	10%	Smertia chirata	5%
Neela Thotha	1%	Apium graveolens	25%
Epsum salt	6%	Emblica officinalis	25%
Namak	10%	Strychnos nuxvomica	8%
		Base	qs
Adm: Oral			
@ : 50 g twice daily for 7-10 days			
Pres: 150 g. 1 kg			

Samvridhi gel	Patanjali
Indi: Mineral Supplement Ca	
Comp: Not given	
Adm: Oral	
@ : 1 Bottle daily	
Pres: 300 ml	

Anabolic Steroids

Some potent anabolic steroids with androgenic, progestogenic and erythorpoetic acitivity are used in Veterinary Practice. These stimulate erythropoiesis by direct effect on erythroprotein production. These are indicated in live stocks including cattle, horse, swine, sheep and goats. These are used when these is chronic, convalescence debility, anaemic, fracture, surgery, osteoporosis. These are given to increase the body weight in young animal and for commercial fattening.

Decaneurabol inj	Cadila Heathcare
Comp	1ml contains 25 mg of Nandrolone
Adm.	IM, SC
@	1 mg/kg B.wt in all animal
Pres.	1 ml amp

Laurabolin	Intervet
Comp	1ml contains 25 mg of Nandrolone
Adm.	IM, SC
@	1 mg/kg B.wt in all animal
Pres.	1 ml amp

Salt Bricks

These are mineralized brick shaped blocks and kept in large animal manger to lick. These are used to compensate the mineral deficiency. These are used for preventive and curative objective. Mostly companies formulate as per the guidelines and specification of Bureau of Standard (ISI).

Vetlick	Vets Farma
Comp	Mineralized salt bricks guided by ISI
Adm.	Oral for licking
@	Brick to be placed in manger
Pres.	Block of 2 kg, 5 kg

Megalick	Natural Remedies
Comp	107 g contains Copper 16.5 g Magnesium 0.88 g Zinc 13.5 g Iodine 250 mg Cobalt 240 mg Selenium 240 mg Vit A5 Lac IU D_3 ilac IU E 1000 IU Iron q.s
Adm.	Oral
@	1 Bol od
Pres.	107 g

Minchat Brick	Zydus
Comp	2 kg contains Zinc 2.6 g Copper 2.6 g Manganese 2.6 g Cobalt 0.6 g Iron 1.6 g Iodine 0.2 g Magnesium 55 g Sodium 640 g

Adm.	Oral
@	1 Block where animal congregate
Pres.	2 kg Block

Antistress

Vet Cool Plus Pow	**Animax Healthcare**
Comp	100 g contains Calcium lactate 1 g; Vit C 5g Potassium chloride 4 g; Vit B1 100 mg Magnesium sulphate 4.5 g; Vit B2 100 mg Sodium chloride 800 mg; Vit B12 100 mcg Sodium bi-carbonate 700 mg Cyproheptadine Sodium citrate 3 g Water soluble carbohydrate 40 g Dextrose 40 g Lactobacillus sporogenes 1500 million
Adm.	Oral
@	LA 100-125 g od SA 10-50 g od
Pres.	1 kg

Macool liq	**Macwell**
Comp	1ml contains Calcium lactate, Dextrose, Tri sodium citrate Niacinamide, Vit E, Vit C Selenium, Potassium iodide, Manganese chloride Amino nitrogen, Yeast extract, Live yeast culture Polysaccharides
Adm.	Oral
@	LA 100 ml od SA 50 ml od
Pres.	1L

CMac Powder	**Macnor**
Comp	60 contains Zinc sulphate 500 mg; Tri sodium citrate 25 g Amino nitrogen 16.6 mg; Iodine with TC phase 15 mg Vit A 30000 IU Leptadenia 5 g; Selenium 5 mg Lactobacillus 60 million spores

Adm.	Oral
@	30 g bid in jaggery or flour
Pres.	5 x 60 g pack

Magnipik 8 liq	**Agilis**
Comp	Each 10 ml contains Vit A 500000 IU $D_3$100000 IU E 1000 IU H 20000 mcg Chromium 5 mg Copper 50 mg Zince 500 mg Selenium 1000 mcg
Adm.	Oral
@	10 ml od
Pres.	50 ml, 100 ml, 250 ml, 500 ml, 1 L

Galactagogue

Milkoplex Bolus.	**Rakesh Pharma**
Indi: Letting down of milk and galactogogue	
Comp: Each Bolus Withania somnifera 1250 mg Asparagus racemosus500 mg Nardostackys Jatamansi 500 mg Leptadenia reticulata 1750 mg	
Adm: Oral	
@ : 1-2 Bol. twice a day	
Pres: 20 Bol. 200 Bol.	

Payapro Bol.	**Ayurvet**
Indi: ❖ Optimizes lactational yield. ❖ Restores milk yield in lactational problems	
Comp: Each Bolus Asparagus racemosus Foeniculum vulgare Pueraria tuberosea Leptadenia reticularea Glycyrrhiz aglabra Cuminum cyminum	
Adm: Oral	
@ : 4 bolus or allyonce daily for 10-15 days.	
Pres: 4 bolus in aluminium foil strip.	

Dugdh Dan	**Cattle Remedies**
Indi: Hypogalactia, Agalactia, Mastitis	
Comp: Each 5 g tab. Contains Gumacacia niloticaindica 0.8 g Leptadenia reticulata 1.4 g Asparagus racemosus 1.4 g Argyrea nervosa 1.4 g	

Adm: Oral
@ : 4 tab.twice daily for 10 days.Taper down the dose to half or next 5 days
Pres: 6 × 8 tab.

Milkvet Tab.			**Rakesh Pharma**
Indi: Galactagogue, Lactogenic			
Comp: Each Bolus			
Leptadenia reticulata	150 mg	Breynia	150 mg
Adm: Oral			
@ : 10-20 tablets twice a day			
Pres: 100 tab., 1000 tab.			

Galog Strong Bolus			**Indian Herbs**
Indi: Milk Booster, Post Mastitis, Fatpercentage of milk			
Comp: Not given			
Leptadenia reticulata	150 mg	Breynia	150 mg
Adm: Oral			
@ : 4 Bol. For10-15 days			
Pres: 4 Bol. × 12 Strip			

Milkmore Pow.	**Arosol Herbal**
Indi: Galactogogue	
Comp: Not given	
Adm: Oral	
@ : 50 g twice daily	
Pres: 300 gm,1 kg	

Milchey Tablet/Powder	**Charak**
Indi: Let down milk, agalactia	
Comp: Not given	
Adm: Oral	
@ : 10 tab. twice daily for 3 days then 4 tabs.Twice daily for 10 days	
Pres: 100, 2000 tab pack 100 g, 1 kg powder	

Lactoplex Bolus	**Unjha Formulation**
Indi: Let down of milk & galactogogue	
Comp: Each Bolus Ashwagandha 125 mg Shatavari 500 mg Jivanti 1000 mg Vidarikand 125 mg Dilseed 1000 mg	
Adm: Oral	
@ : 2-3 Bol.Twice of only for 7-10 days	
Pres: Strip of 2 Bol.	

Lactovet Pow.	**Rakesh Pharma**
Indi: Galactagogue	
Comp: Not given	
Adm: Oral	
@ : 50 gm daily	
Pres: 100 g, 500 g	

Leptamilk Forte Liq.	**Concept Pharma**
Indi: Galactagouge	
Comp: Not given	
Adm: Oral	
@ : 40 ml twice daily	
Pres: 450 ml	

Milmore Pow.	**Novartis**
Indi: Galactogogue	
Comp: Not given	
Adm: Oral	
@ : 40 g twice daily	
Pres: 500 g	

Galactin Bol.	**Himalya**
Indi	
Comp: Not given	
Adm: Oral	
@ : 4-6 Bol. for 10 day safter calving	
Pres: Strip of 4 Bol	

Mastigo Cap.			**Libra Biotech.**
Indi: Galactagogue, Utdom milk			
Comp: Each Contains			
Bhasam Parad	14%	Kachnar	7%
Bhasam Tamra	7%	Lahsoon	14%
Bhasam Shubhra	14%	Chiniakapoor	2%
Bhasam Godanti	7%	Sendha Lavan	14%
Bhasam Kashish	7%	Naushadar	7%
Bhasam Yarad	7%		
Adm: Oral			
@ : 1-2 Cap. twice a day in banana.			
Pres: 6 Cap.			

Immunomudulator

SPE 15	**Macnor**	
Comp	10 contains	
	Potassium iodide 8 g	Niacin 1. 6 g
	Sipymarin 100 mg	Serratiopeptidase 300 mg
Adm.	Oral	
@.	1 sachet for 5 days with jaggery	
Pres.	5 sachet of 10 g in pack	

Uniselit Pow.	**Ayurvet**
Indications: Improve issue, Immunity, Milk Quality	
Composition: Not given	
Dosage: 1 sachet OD for 15 days	
Presentation: 10 gm sachet	

Restobal Liq.		**Ayurvet**
Indi:		
❖ Normalizes the cortisol level of blood serum restoring normal body function sand milk production of animal.		
❖ Prevents losses due to various stress conditions.		
Comp:		
Withania somnifera	Ocimum sanctum	Mangifera indica
Phyllanthus emblica	Shilajit Shudh	

Adm: Oral
@ : 50 ml twice daily. For 5-10 days.
Pres: IL

Bioboost Forte Pow.	**Lyka**
Indi: Immunity, Performance	
Comp: 200 g contains ❖ Live yeast culture saccharomyces carevisiae 5 g ❖ Live culture Bacillus coagulans 6000 18 million CFU	
Adm: Oral	
@ : 5 g	
Pres: 200 g ton	

Multivitamin	**Patanjali**
Indi: Immunomodulator, Anoestrus	
Comp: Not given	
Adm: Oral	
@ : 100g OD	
Pres: 100 g 450 g	

❑❑❑

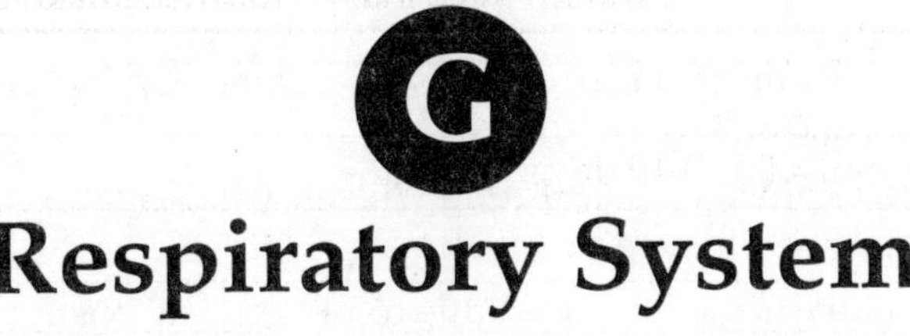

Respiratory System

Diseases of Respiratory System

Anoxia: Inadequate supply of oxygen to tissues.

Asthma: Hyper-responsiveness of tracheobronchial muscles resulting in narrowing down of air tube accompanied by increased secretion and mucosal edema.

Breathlessness: Difficulty in breathing.

Bronchitis: Inflammation of the bronchioles.

Bronchopneumonia: Inflammation of bronchioles and lungs.

Catarrh: Inflammation of the mucous membrance particularly of air passage.

Choking: Obstruction of respiratory passage.

Coryza: Respiratory disease in Poultry.

Cough: Reflex act initiated by irritation of respiratory mucosa of air passage to expel respiratory secretions or foreign particles.

Cyanosis: Bluish discolouration of skin, conjunctiva and visible mucosa caused by reduced haemoglobin in blood.

Dyspnea: Increased respiratory movement which appears to cause distress to the animal.

Emphysema: Abnormal distention of lung caused by rupture of alveolar wall with or without escape of air into interstitial tissue also called pulmonary emphysema.

Epistaxis: Nose bleed can be due to disease of mucosa of upper respiratory tract.

Haemothorax: Accumulation of whole blood in pleural sacs.

Hiccough: Sudden jerky expression of breathing.

Hydrothorax: accumulation of oedematous transudate in thoracic cavity or pleural sac.

Hypercapnia: Retention and accumulation of carbondioxide in blood and tissues.

Hyperpnoea: Increased pulmonary ventillation.

Nasal discharge: Excessive or abnormal discharge from nasal cavities and is indicative of respiratory tract disease.

Panting: Acute inflammation of pleura cause pain during respiratory movement.

Pneumonia: Inflammation of pulmonary tissue usually accompanied by inflammation of bronchioles.

Pneumothorax: Entry of air into pleural cavity.

Pulmonary congestion: Depth of respiration is increased, nostrils flared and mouth breathing. Extreme dyspnea.

Rhinitis: Inflammation of nasal cavities characterised by sneezing, difficult respiration and nasal discharge.

Sneezing: Sudden expulsion of air through the nostrils designed to expel irritating material from upper air passage.

Snoaring: Respiratory noise produced due to pharyngeal obstruction.

Tracheitis: Inflammation of Trachea.

Bronchodilators

These reverse the airways smooth muscles contraction. These also act as anti-inflammatory and relax bronchial smooth muscles.

Septilin Tab	**Himalya Drug**
Comp	Not given
Adm.	Oral with jaggery
@	16-20 Tab tds. Inacute cases 24 Tabs.
Pres.	100 Tab

Septilin tablet	**Himalya**
Indi: Respiratory infections	
Comp: Not given	
Adm: Oral	
@ : 16-20 tab. thrice daily in a cute cases 24 tabs	
Pres: 100 tab	

Catcough Electuary			**Cattle Remedies**
Indi: Respiratory stimulant, expectorant			
Comp: 100 g contain			
Pistacia interrima	16.5 g	Solanum xanthecarpum	15 g
Glycyrrhiza glabra	13 g	Adhatodazeylanica	12 g
Curcuma amadaroxb	5 g	Ammonium Chloride	10 g
Oleumlinum usitatissmum	10 g	Sodium Chloride	25 g
Treacle	20 g		
Adm: Oral			
@ : 25-30 g thrice daily for 3 day			
Pres: 100 g, 250 g, 1 kg			

Coughdon			Vets Farma
Indi: Bronchitis, Pneumonia			
Comp:			
Adhatoda vasika	15%	Ammonie Chloride	12%
Glycerrohiza glabra	10%	Yavkshar	8%
Pistacia integriima	2%	Linum usitatissimum	25%
Ephedra vulgaris	2%	Base	qs
Adm: Oral			
@ : 50 g bid for 3-4 days			
Pres: 150 g, 1 kg			

Caflon	Indian Herbs
Indi: Respiratory Infections	
Comp: Not given	
Adm: Oral	
@ : 40-50 gm 3-4 day sina day with Jaggery	
Pres: 100 g	

Expectorants

Drugs which increase fluidity of respiratory bronchial secretion or reduce its viscosity facilitating its removal by coughing. Mycolytics induce the copious secretions. These can be antihistaminic which provide relief by sedative and anti cholinergic action or antitussive which act on CNS on cough centre and act peripherally in respiratory tract to reduce tussal impulse.

Caflon	Indian Herbs
Comp	Not given
Adm.	Oral with Jaggery
@	40-50 g od for 3-4 days
Pres.	100 g

Coughdon	Vets Farma			
Comp	Adhatoda vasika	15%	Ammonium chloride	12%
	Glycerrhiza glabra	10%	Yavkshar	8%
	Pistacia interriima	2%	Linum usitatissimum	25%
	Ephedra vulgaris	2%	Base	QS

Adm.	Oral
@	50 g bid for 3-4 days
Pres.	150 g, 1 kg

Catcough Electuary	**Cattle Remedies**	
Comp	100 g contains	
	Pistacia interrima	16.5 g
	Solanum xanthocarpum	11 g
	Glycerrhiza glabra	13.0 g
	Adhatoda zeylanica	12 g
	Curcuma amadarixb	5 g
	Ammonium chloride	10 g
	Oleumlinum usitatissimum	10 g
	Sodium chloride	2.5 g
	Treacle	20 g
Adm.	Oral	
@	25-30 g tds	
Pres.	100 g, 250 g, 1 kg	

Animon	**Indian Herbs**
Comp	Not given
Adm.	Feed additive
@	2.5 kg I Tonn of feed for Prevention
Pres.	1 kg, 25 kg

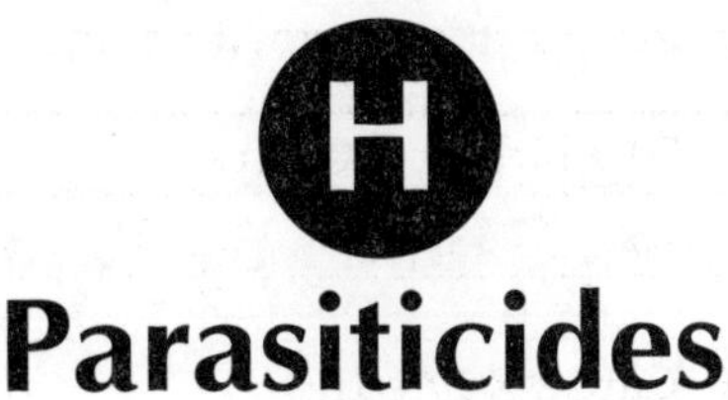

Parasiticides

Terms associated with Parasites

Parasites: These are living beings that live on or in another living one and is metabolically dependent on that

Host: The living one which harbours a parasite is called host.

Helminth: A common term for a parasite

Vectors: These are carrier that transfer infective agent from one host to another

Endo parasites: Parasites which live inside the body of host

Ecto parasites: Parasites which live on the surface of their host

Temporary parasites: Those who live only during the part of their life span on or inside their host

Permanent parasites: Those parasites which live on or in their host through-out their life

Nematodes

Endo parasites are Nematodes or round worms in different system of livestock. e.g. skin, digestive and respiratory system.

Cestodes: Found in Gastro-intestinal tract, Larval form is located outside the G.I tract

Trematodes or **Flukes**: Found in liver and blood.

Protozoa: Single celled organisims found in blood and other internal organs. During the course of life endo parasites can damage host's tissue, growth and productivity.

Ecto parasites: Live on surface of host like skin, hairs. The host blood and lymph serve as their food source. These are fly, warble, mange, mite etc

Ticks: These can bite which develop into wound where the secondary infection can occur and infested with Maggots. Ticks suck blood. These may be hard ticks or soft ticks. These can be single host or multiple host ticks.

Lice: These also suck blood or bite and cause patches of hair loss haemorrhages and damage the skin leading to anemia. There are biting lice and sucking lice.

Grubs or Warbles: These are flies cause gadding or restlessness and cause loss of production

Mange and mites: These cause lesions, itching, crustation papules, looks like allergic reaction.

Parasites cause economic losses due to growth, feed conversion ratio, mortality, loss of production and production of their host or animal.

Diseases Caused by Parasites

Amebiasis: Disease caused by infection of ameba specially with Entamoeba histolytica

Amphistomiasis: Infection of amphistomes leading to intestinal irritation, foetid diarrhea and death of animal

Ascariasis: Infestation of Ascaria Symptoms resemble with bottle jaw, foetid smell of dung, pale yellow eyes, listless skin, pot belly, general weakness, low productivity, anorexia, indigestion, tetanus death in young calues.

Coccidiosis: Infestation of coccidia characterised by unformed faeces followed by diarrhea same time mixed with bright blood coloured, soiled anal region, anaemia, loss of body weight, productivity and reproduction.

Dirofilariasis: Infestation with heart worm or Dirofilaria immitis weight loss, good appetite, excessive tiring with exercise and coughing. Ascites or odema, sudden weakness or callapse.

Ecto parasiticides: Agents effective against external parasites

Endo parasiticides: Agents effective against internal parasites

Endecto parasiticides: Agents effective against external and internal parasites

Fascioliasis: Infestation of liver fluke or Fasciola hepatica symptoms of parasitism and bottle jaw like symptoms.

Larvicidal: Agents which kill or prevent further growth of larvae

Maggots: Also called as Blowfly myiasis. The wound are infested with maggots or larvae of blow flies.

Mange: Skin infestation caused by mange and mites (ecto parasites) with sumptoms of itching and low production. They can be sarcoptic mange or psoroptic mange as per the parasitic infestation.

Nasal Bots: Adult flies deposit larvae in nostrils. Animals shake their head due to annoyance and pus containing nasal discharge which get dried to stick to nasal passage to prevent smooth inhalation. Animal graze less and lose weight

Ovicidal: Agents which destroy ova

Parasiticide: Drugs which intend to kill parasitis

Scabies: A parasitic skin disease caused by itch mite, highly contagious.

Schistosomiasis or Nasal granuloma: Caused by schistosomes characterised by nasal discharge interfering with breathing

Verminosis pneumonia: Caused by Dictyocola filaria (Lung worm) characterised by respiratory distress like frequent coughing, retarted growth, loss of weight, pyrexia, and associated symptoms and causes death

Wormicidal: Agents which kills worms

Ecotoparasiticides

Amitraz

This belongs to formidine compound of antiparasitic which is not related to any major class of parasiticides. Its major use is an acaricide. Drug act on CNS of arthropods and available in dip or spray. It controls mites and ticks. It is soluble only in organic compound and is slightly soluble in water. It is short acting parasiticide. It is lethal to arthropods such as mites, lice and ticks. It can not be used in breeding stock. Its spray is prepared on the day of treatment using clean water. Treat all infested and non-infested animals in a group at the same time. It is harmful if swallowed. It irritates eyes. Avoid working in spray mixture. Avoid contact by mouth. Wash hands and exposed skin thoroughly before eating, drinking or smoking. Avoid using in dogs and horses.

Ekodex	**Cargill**
Comp	Amitraz 5%
Adm.	For cattle, sheep, goat, prepare in clean water and spray
@	2 ml/L for liver stock and 4 ml/L for pigs
Pres.	6 ml, 60 ml

Taktic	**Novartis**
Comp	Amitraz 12.5%
Adm.	For cattle, sheep, goat, prepare in clean water and spray
@	2 ml/L for liverstock and 4 ml/L for pigs
Pres.	60 ml, 90 ml

Ridd.	**Venky**
Comp	Amitraz 5%
Adm.	For cattle, sheep, goat, prepare in clean water and spray
@	2 ml/L for liverstock and 4 ml/L for pigs
Pres.	60 ml

Qtik spray	**Phoenix**
Comp	Amitraz
Adm.	Local
@	As per need
Pres.	50 ml, 100 ml

Diptraz 12.5 E	Boehringer Ingelheim
Comp	Amitraz 12.5%
Adm.	Local
@	As per need
Pres.	15 ml, 50 ml

Carbamates

Carbaryl

These are similar to organophosphates in many properties. Some of these have significant application as parasiticides. Carboryl has been used for many years as ectoparasiticide because of its efficacy and low toxicity. These inhibit the enzyme acetylcholinestrase. These act faster than organophosphates. Detoxification in exposed animal is usually rapid. These don't accumulate in tissue and toxicity is low. If doses are exceeded toxicity is acute. It is highly biodegradable.

Notix scrub/ Talc	Venky
Comp	Carbaryl 10%, 5%
Adm.	Oral
@	In water as directed
Pres.	15 g, 150 g

Organophophates

These have less residual effect on environment and are less likely to accumulate in meat or milk and have extremely low carcinogenic potential. Many used in agriculture organophosphates are highly toxic to mammals. But some of them have been developed with margin of safety. These are coumaphos, Malathion, Diazinon, Fenthion, chloropyrophos and crotoxyphos. These are available as emulsified concentrates, wettable powders, oil base, formulations, dust, sprays and pour on solutions. These inhibit the enzyme acetylecholinestrase in nervous system and paralyse the insect. Their toxicity can be altered by the chemicals which may be either synergistic or antagonist. All are highly bio-degradable. Resistance to these need multiple treatment.

Coumaphos

It is organophosphorous anthelmintic available in powder used for control of ticks, mites, biting and sucking lice, flies etc. in all domestic animals. It is composed of 0-0- diethyl-0- phospharothioate. It may cause inappetence, diarrhea and vomition but will disappear. Its antidote is Atropine sulphate 1%. It is used for sprays and dip.

Asuntol	Bayer
Comp	Diethyl -0 phospharothioate 50%
Adm.	Spray
Dose	Dilute 1-1.4 g/L in cattle, 1 g/L in sheep 500 mg/L in horses (with water)
Pres.	15 g

Asuntol Medicated soap	Bayer
Comp	Diethyl -0 phospharothioate 50%
Adm.	To wash with
Dose	10 mg/kg B.wt
Pres.	Soap

Negasunt Pow	Bayer
Comp	Coumaphos propoxur sulfanilamide
Adm.	Wound dressing and in maggot wound
@	As per need
Dose	40 g

Malathion

It is organophosphorous ectoparasiticide act on contact and stomach poisons. This acts by combining with and neutralizing enzyme leading to spastic paralysis. It is toxic to man and animals. The handler must adopt enough protective measure. Care should be taken to avoid ingestion by animal due to licking. Avoid using in cats.

Cython	Generic AHP
Comp	50% Malathion
Adm.	Spray on application
@	10 ml/L of water
Pres.	250 ml, 500 ml, I L, 5 L

Diazinon

It is an organophosphate ectoparasiticide and acts both as contact poison and stomach poison. It also causes spastic paralysis. It is used for external parasite infestation especially flies in animals. Compound is toxic to man and animals. So care should be taken to avoid its ingestion by animal due to licking. Avoid use in cats. Antidote is atropine sulphate 1%.

Neocidol 20 EC liq	Novartis
Comp	20% Diazinon
Adm.	Wash or spray
@	60 ml in 20 L of water
Pres.	30 ml, I L, 5 L

Dichlorophos

It is an organophosphate ectoparasiticide. It also acts both as contact and as stomach poison. It also kills by spastic paralysis of parasites. All precaution using organophosphates should be taken. Antidote is Atropine sulphate 1%.

Nuvon Liq	Novartis
Comp	Dichlorovos 76%
Adm.	Wash or spray
@	100 ml in 20 L of water
Pres.	100 ml, 200 ml, I L

Chlorinated Hydro Carbons

These are contact poison. These cause spastic paralysis of parasites. These are indicated for maggot infestation and follicular mange. Licking of compound should be avoided as these are highly toxic. These are mainly solvents. Such vehicles facilitate their penetration through skin.

Benzene Hexachloride

This is one of chlorinated hydrocarbon group ectoparasiticide. Licking of the compound should be avoided as it is very toxic. It is available in cream and lotion to be applied or sprayed used in combinations as synergistic.

D Mag spray	Intas
Comp	Gammabenzone hexachloride 0.1%, Cetrimide 0.45%, Proflavin hemisulphate 0.1% with Eucalyptus oil and Turpentine oil as base
Adm.	Spray
@	As per need
Pres.	50 ml, 100 ml

Healall cream	Novartis
Comp	Gammabenzone hexachloride 0.1%, Cetrimide 0.45%, Proflavin hemisulphate 0.1% with Eucalyptus oil and Turpentine oil as base
Adm.	Spray
@	As per need
Pres.	100 g

Lorexane cream/ spray	Virbac
Comp	Gammabenzone hexachloride 0.1%, Cetrimide 0.45%, Proflavin hemisulphate 0.1% with Eucalyptus oil and Turpentine oil as base
Adm.	Spray
@	As per need
Pres.	30 g, 100 g cream 50 ml spray

M. Lorax cream	Marc
Comp	Gammabenzone hexachloride 0.1%, Cetrimide 0.45%, Proflavin hemisulphate 0.1% with Eucalyptus oil and Turpentine oil as base
Adm.	Spray
@	As per need
Pres.	25 g, 100 g

Coolmac spray	Macnor
Comp	Gammabenzone hexachloride 0.1%, Cetrimide 0.45%, Proflavin hemisulphate 0.1% with Eucalyptus oil and Turpentine oil as base
Adm.	Spray
@	As per need
Pres.	100 g

Dema cure	Pranav
Comp	Gammabenzone hexachloride 0.1%, Cetrimide 0.45%, Proflavin hemisulphate 0.1% with Eucalyptus oil and Turpentine oil as base
Adm.	Spray
@	As per need
Pres.	100 g

Methoxychlor

It is one of chlorinated hydrocarbon compound. Popularly it is known as DDT. It is used as such but now not used.

Pyrethrin and Synthetic Pyrethroids

Natural pyrethrins are obtained from flowers of chrysanthemum plants. These are being used since 1800 to control ectoparasites. Synthetic pyrethroids are with improved stability. These are effective to control variety of lice, flies, ticks, mange, mite. These effect the nervous system of parasites causing hyperexcitation as followed by convulsions and death. These have biodegradability. So their metabolites are non toxic and excreted rapidly. These are rated as safe insecticides. These have knock down effect (Quick lethal effect showing almost immediate visible results) Resistance has been reported especially where eartags have been used.

Cypermethrin

One of pyrethroids and is contact poison producing muscular excitation and convulsions by its effect on nerve cell membrane delaying depolorisation leading to rapid paralytic action on parasite. They have prolonged action to bring about knock down and kill effect. Direct contact to eyes and skin should be avoided. Licking should be prevented.

Clinar	**Virbac**
Comp	Cypermethrin 100 g/L
Adm.	To be sprayed
@	1 ml/L for body spray, 5 ml/L backline spray 20 ml/L for house spray in wate
Pres.	5 ml, 15 ml, 50 ml, I L

Cyperin 100 E C	**Merial (Wockhardt)**
Comp	Cypermethrin 100 g/L
Adm.	To be sprayed
@	1 ml/L for body spray, 5 ml/L backline spray 20 ml/L for house spray in water
Pres.	15 ml, 50 ml

Indocard	**Vets Farma**
Comp	Cypermethrin 100 g/L
Adm.	To be sprayed
@	1 ml/L for body spray, 5 ml/L backline spray 20 ml/L for house spray in water
Pres.	10 ml, 50 ml

Cutirore	Concept
Comp	Cypermethrin 100 g/L
Adm.	To be sprayed
@	1 ml/L for body spray, 5 ml/L backline spray 20 ml/L for house spray in water
Pres.	15 ml

Cisaflux	Zydus (Ranbaxy)
Comp	Cypermethrin 100 g/L
Adm.	To be sprayed
@	1 ml/L for body spray, 5 ml/L backline spray 20 ml/L for house spray in water
Pres.	100 ml, 185 ml

Ektomin	Novartis
Comp	Cypermethrin 100 g/L
Adm.	To be sprayed
@	1 ml/L for body spray, 5 ml/L backline spray 20 ml/L for house spray in water
Pres.	15 ml, 50 ml, I L

Cyprol	Intas
Comp	Cypermethrin 100 g/L
Adm.	To be sprayed
@	1 ml/L for body spray, 5 ml/L backline spray 20 ml/L for house spray in water
Pres.	15 ml, 50 ml, I L

T. Kont	Alembic
Comp	Cypermethrin 100 g/L
Adm.	To be sprayed
@	1 ml/L for body spray, 5 ml/L backline spray 20 ml/L for house spray in water
Pres.	15 ml, 50 ml, I L

Tik Kil	Indian Immunologicals
Comp	Cypermethrin 100 g/L
Adm.	To be sprayed
@	1ml/L for body spray, 5 ml/L backline spray 20 ml/L for house spray in water
Pres.	15 ml, 50 ml, 5 g, 15 g

Pectocide	**Zydus (Sarabhai)**
Comp	Cypermethrin 100 g/L
Adm.	To be sprayed
@	1 ml/L for body spray, 5 ml/L backline spray 20 ml/L for house spray in water
Pres.	15 ml, 50 ml

Deltamethrin

It is as good as cypermethrin member of pyrethroids. It has bit longer action.

Butox Sol	**Hoechst**
Comp	Deltamethrin 12.5 mg/ml
Adm.	External application
@	Dilute as per infestation Ticks 2-3 ml/L of water Mite 4-6 ml/L of water Lice 1-1.5 ml/L of water Fly 2-3 ml/L of water
Pres.	50 ml, 250 ml, I L

Almethrin	**Merial (Alved)**
Comp	Deltamethrin 12.5 mg/ml
Adm.	External application
@	Dilute as per infestation Ticks 2-3 ml/L of water Mite 4-6 ml/L of water Lice 1-1.5 ml/L of water Fly 2-3 ml/L of water
Pres.	50 ml, IL

Fenvalerate

It is also a pyrethroid and contact poison leading to paralytic action on parasite. Action, indication, precautions are same as for other pyrethroids.

Sumicidin 20%	**Novartis**
Comp	20% Fenvalerate
Adm.	External application
@	0.5 ml/L of water
Pres.	100 ml, 250 ml, 500 ml, IL

Ticomax	Zydus (Ranbaxy)
Comp	20% or 200 mg/ml Fenvalerate
Adm.	External application
@	0.5 ml/L of water
Pres.	15 ml, 50 ml, IL

Flumethrin

It is one of Pyromethroid

Baytical Pour on	Bayer
Comp	1% Flumethrin
Adm.	External application
@	1 ml/L of water
Pres.	100 ml, 500 ml

Miscellaneous Ectoparasiticides

Benzyl Benzoate

It is an early ectoparasiticide consists of herbs inorganics aromatic petroleum derivatives and moieties. The mechanism of action is unknown. It is indicated in demodectic acariasis and control of sarcoptic form of scabies. These are safe for local application, when used in mild form. Scalding of skin can result when the agents are applied in high concentration. It is available in emulsion which is applied as spot treatment after cleansing. It should be washed off after 24 hours with soap and water. There can be irritation and hypersensitivity. Prevent contact with eyes.

Benzyl benzoate	Generic
Comp	25% Benzyl benzoate
Adm.	Local application
@	Apply as such on the spot
Pres.	100 ml, 200 ml, 400 ml, IL, 4 L

Miscellaneous

Megasunt powder	Bayer
Comp	Coumaphos+ Propoxyur + Sulfanilamide
Adm.	Locally sprayed in maggot wounds
@	As per need
Pres.	40 g

Maggacide liquid	**Cattle Remedies**
Indi: Scabies, psoriasis, Maggotwound, Estoparasitcide	
Comp: 100 mg contains Mallotus philippenis 3 g; Sulphursublimatum 3 g Oleum pinus rox burghii 65 ml; Oleum linum usitatissimum 95	
Adm: Local application	
@ : Local application or pack in maggot wound	
Pres: 100 ml, 450 ml	

Charmil gel	**Ayurvet**
Indi: ❖ Multiaction ensuring wide spectrum of protection against various skin infections mange, ring, worm, dermatomycosis, eczema, foot lesions in FMD etc. ❖ Active wound healer.	
Comp: Cedrus deidara Pongamia glabra	
Adm: Local application	
@ : Apply once or twice daily after cleaning the area, till complete recovery.	
Pres: 5 & 50 gm soft squeeze tube &100 ml aluminium can.	

Pestoban Liq.	**Indian Herbs**
Indi: Ectoparasiticide, Flyrepellent	
Comp: Not given	
Adm: Local application	
@ : Dilute10 times with water apply with swabor brushor spray daily for 3-4 days	
Pres: 100 ml, 1L	

Tickless Lotion	**Arosol Herbal**
Indi: Ectoparasiticide	
Comp: Not given	
Adm: Local application	
@ : Apply Locally	
Pres: 100 ml	

Flematic Oil/Ointment	**TTK Pharma**
Indi: Ectoparasiticide	
Comp: Extract of deodaroil and selected vegetable oils	
Adm: Local application	
@ : Apply on skin give bath after 60 minutes	
Pres: 100 ml	

Blaze	**Indian Herbs**
Indi: Body Coatshiner, grower	
Comp: Not given	
Adm: Local application	
@ : Apply Blaze all over body and rub to produce foam wash with water	
Pres: 100 ml bottle	

Dermocept Cream			**Concept Pharma**
Indi: Ectoparasiticide, Flyrepellant			
Comp:			
Kutaja	2.310%	Ratanjot	1%
Nimba	3.075%	Karanj oil	20%
Haridra	3.075%	Neem oil	5%
Daruharidra	1.540%		
Adm: Local application			
@ : Apply locally on affected part twice daily			
Pres: 2.5 g tube			

Supercure cure Plus Spray			**Venky's**
Indi: Antiseptic, Ectoparasiticide, Fly repellent			
Comp:			
Aloe vera	10%	Curcuma long	5%
Azadirachta indica	5%	Cedar wood oil	3%
Andrapogon citrates	3%		
Adm: Local application			
@ : Spray on affected part twice daily			
Pres: 100 ml Spray can			

Septiban spray	Phoenix
Comp	Devdarn 83% Neem 3% Haldi 4% Turpentine oil 10%
Adm.	Local spray
@	As per need
Pres.	75 ml, 100 ml, 200 ml

Endoparasiticides

Benzimidazoles

There are grouped according to their mechanism of action

These drugs interfere with energy production. Inhibit fumarate ruductase, block tubulin synthesis, inhibit glucose transport and kills the endo parasite via starvation of parasitis.

Different Chemical agents of this group are :

- Albendazole
- Cambendazole
- Fenbendazole
- Mebendazole
- Oxibendazole
- Oxygenbendazole
- Parbendazole
- Thiabendazole

Imidathiazoles: This group is ganglionic stimulant leading to spastic paralysis of parasite and death. These are:

- Tetramesole
- Levamesole

Macrolides: these are GABA potentiator causing fluecid paralysis of parasite

- Doramectin
- Ivermectin
- Milberrycine oxime

Organo phosphate: Those are cholinestrase inhibitor and kill the parsite via spastic paralysis

- Coumaphos

Pro Benzimedazole: Metabolised to Benzimidazoles in vivo and then kills parasite via starvation as the Benzimidazole

- Thiophanate
- Febantel

Salicylanides: causes uncoupled oxidative phosphorylation energy depletion of parasite and death

- Oxyclozanide
- Niclosamide
- Rafoxanide

Substituted phenols: Cause uncoupled oxidative phosphorylation and energy depletion of parasite

- Diclofolan
- Hexa chlorethane
- Hexa chlorphen

Tetrahydropyrimides:

- Morantel
- Pyrantel

Albendazole

Benzimidazole Chemical is effective against G.I round worms, lung worm, Tape worm, and adult liver fluke. It is larvicidal ovicidal, cysticidal in nature. It was developed by Smith Kline scientist in 1972. It is excreted in urine. Safety margin is 7.5 worm dose level and 5 fluke dose level. It is available in Tabs, Bolus, suspension and power form. These are administered oral @ 5mg/kg B.wt in SA, 7.5mg/kg B.wt in LA against worms. In fluke @ 7.5mg/kg B.wt in SA and 15mg/kg B.wt in LA. It is non toxic and safe for animals in field condition. No adverse effect at any stage of pregnancy is known on recommended dose. Milk should not be used for human for 72 hrs. Don't deworm cattle within 14 days and 10 days in sheep before slaughter.

Albidol Bolus/Susp	**Concept**
Comp	Albendazole Bol, 2.5% susp
Adm.	Oral
@	LA 7. 5 mg/kg B.wt SA 5 mg/kg B.wt
Pres.	150 mg, 1.5 g, 3 g 30 ml, 90 ml, IL, 5 L

Albidol Pow	**Concept**
Comp	15% Albendazole
Adm.	Oral
@	LA 7.5 mg/kg B.wt SA 5 mg/kg B.wt
Pres.	100 g

Albomar Bol	**Virbac**
Comp	Albendazole Bol, 2.5% susp
Adm.	Oral
@	LA 7.5 mg/kg B.wt SA 5 mg/kg B.wt
Pres.	150 mg, 3 g

Albomar Pow	**Virbac**
Comp	15% Albendazole
Adm.	Oral
@	LA 7.5 mg/kg B.wt SA 5 mg/kg B.wt
Pres.	100 g

Albomar Sus	**Virbac**
Comp	2.5% Albendazole
Adm.	Oral
@	LA 7.5 mg/ kg B.wt SA 5 mg/ kg B.wt
Pres.	30 ml, 60 ml, 90 ml, 500 ml

Almizole Bol/Sus.	**Alembic**
Comp	Albendezole Bol, 2.5% susp
Adm.	Oral
@	LA 7.5 mg/kg B.wt SA 5 mg/kg B.wt
Pres.	1.5 g, 3 g, 90 ml, 500 ml

Almizole Pow	**Alembic**
Comp	30% Albendazole
Adm.	Oral
@	LA 7.5 mg/kg B.wt SA 5 mg/kg B.wt
Pres.	100 g

Alzonex Bol	**Neospark**
Comp	5% Albendazole
Adm.	Oral
@	LA 7.5 mg/kg B.wt SA 5 mg/kg B.wt
Pres.	150 mg, 600 mg bol

Alzonex Pow	**Neospark**
Comp	30% Albendazole
Adm.	Oral
@	LA 7.5 mg/kg B.wt SA 5 mg/kg B.wt
Pres.	300 g

Alzonex Sus	**Neospark**
Comp	2.5% Albendazole
Adm.	Oral
@	LA 7.5 mg/ kg B.wt SA 5 mg/ kg
Pres.	IL, 5 L

Amzole Bol	**Pranav**
Comp	Albendazole 5%
Adm.	Oral
@	LA 7.5 mg/kg B.wt SA 5 mg/kg B.wt
Pres.	1.5 g, 3 g

Amzole Sus	**Pranav**
Comp	2.5% Albendazole
Adm.	Oral
@	LA 7.5 mg/kg B.wt SA 5 mg/kg B.wt
Pres.	IL, 5 L

Briben 1500 Bol.	Brihans
Comp	Albendazole 5%
Adm.	Oral
@	LA 7.5 mg/kg B.wt SA 5 mg/kg B.wt
Pres.	Strip of 4

Albacril Bol	Cattle Remedies
Comp	Albendazole 5%
Adm.	Oral
@	LA 7.5 mg/kg B.wt SA 5 mg/kg B.wt
Pres.	150 mg, 1.5 g(12), 3 g(6)

Albacril Sus	Cattle Remedies
Comp	2.5% Albendazole
Adm.	Oral
@	LA 7.5 mg/kg B.wt SA 5 mg/kg B.wt
Pres.	30 ml, 60 ml

Albendazole Sus	HAL/ Stallen
Comp	2.5% Albendazole
Adm.	Oral
@	LA 7.5 mg/kg B.wt SA 5 mg/kg B.wt
Pres.	60 ml, 120 ml, 500 ml, IL, 5 L

Albendos Sus	Satllen
Comp	2.5% Albendazole
Adm.	Oral
@	LA 7.5 mg/kg B.wt SA 5 mg/kg B.wt
Pres.	IL

Albenz Bol	Sterling Lab
Comp	Albendazole Bol, 2.5% susp
Adm.	Oral
@	LA 7.5 mg/kg B.wt SA 5 mg/kg B.wt
Pres.	150 mg x 2600 mg x 6

Albenz Sus	Sterling Lab
Comp	2.5% Albendazole
Adm.	Oral
@	LA 7.5 mg/kg B.wt SA 5 mg/kg B.wt
Pres.	90 ml, IL, 5 L

Albenz Pow	**Sterling Lab**
Comp	15% Albendazole
Adm.	Oral
@	LA 7.5 mg/kg B.wt SA 5 mg/kg B.wt
Pres.	30 g

Albendos Bol	**Merial (Dosch)**
Comp	Albendazole Bol
Adm.	Oral
@	LA 7.5 mg/kg B.wt SA 5 mg/kg B.wt
Pres.	3 g

Albendos Sus	**Merial (Dosch)**
Comp	2.5% Albendazole
Adm.	Oral
@	LA 7.5 mg/kg B.wt SA 5 mg/kg B.wt
Pres.	90 ml, IL, 5 L

Alzol Bol	**Vets Farma**
Comp	Albendazole Bol
Adm.	Oral
@	LA 7.5 mg/kg B.wt SA 5 mg/kg B.wt
Pres.	1.5 g x 2

Alzol Pow	**Vets Farma**
Comp	15% Albendazole
Adm.	Oral
@	LA 7.5 mg/kg B.wt SA 5 mg/kg B.wt
Pres.	30 g, 300 g

Alzol Sus	**Vets Farma**
Comp	2.5% Albendazole
Adm.	Oral
@	LA 7.5 mg/kg B.wt SA 5 mg/kg B.wt
Pres.	90 ml, IL

Analgon Bol	**Merial (Wockhardt)**
Comp	Albendazole
Adm.	Oral
@	LA 7.5 mg/kg B.wt SA 5 mg/kg B.wt
Pres.	1.5 g, 3 g

Analgon Sus	Merial (Wockhardt)
Comp	2.5% Albendazole
Adm.	Oral
@	LA 7.5 mg/kg B.wt SA 5 mg/kg B.wt
Pres.	60 ml, IL, 5L

Endoban Bol	TTK
Comp	Albendazole Bol
Adm.	Oral
@	LA 7.5 mg/kg B.wt SA 5 mg/kg B.wt
Pres.	750 mg x 4

Vetalben Sus.	Indian Immunology
Comp	Albendazole 2.5% susp
Adm.	Oral
@	LA 7.5 mg/kg B.wt SA 5mg/kg B.wt
Pres.	100 ml, 500 ml, IL, 5 L

Endoban Sus	TTK
Comp	2.5% Albendazole
Adm.	Oral
@	LA 7.5 mg/kg B.wt SA 5 mg/kg B.wt
Pres.	90 ml, IL

Eraworm Bol	Marc
Comp	Albendazole Bol
Adm.	Oral
@	LA 7.5 mg/kg B.wt SA 5 mg/kg B.wt
Pres.	600 mg x 20

Eraworm Sus	Marc
Comp	2.5% Albendazole
Adm.	Oral
@	LA 7.5 mg/kg B.wt SA 5 mg/kg B.wt
Pres.	60 ml, IL, 5 L

Helmigard Bol	Cargill (Unichem)
Comp	Albendazole Bol
Adm.	Oral
@	LA 7.5 mg/kg B.wt SA 5 mg/kg B.wt
Pres.	1.2 g

Helmigard Sus	**Cargill (Unichem)**
Comp	2.5% Albendazole
Adm.	Oral
@	LA 7.5 mg/kg B.wt SA 5 mg/kg B.wt
Pres.	30 ml, 60 ml, 450 ml, 5 L

Helmigard Granule	**Cargill (Unichem)**
Comp	15% Albendazole
Adm.	Oral
@	LA 7.5 mg/kg B.wt SA 5 mg/kg B.wt
Pres.	30 g

Kalbend Bol	**KAPL**
Comp	Albendazole Bol
Adm.	Oral
@	LA 7.5 mg/kg B.wt SA 5 mg/kg B.wt
Pres.	150 mg x 10, 600 mg x 4, 1.5 x 2

Kalbend Pow	**KAPL**
Comp	15% Albendazole
Adm.	Oral
@	LA 7.5 mg/kg B.wt SA 5 mg/kg B.wt
Pres.	500 g

Kalbend Sus	**KAPL**
Comp	2.5% Albendazole
Adm.	Oral
@	LA 7.5 mg/kg B.wt SA 5 mg/kg B.wt
Pres.	60 ml, 500 ml, IL, 5 L

Minthal Bol	**Alembic**
Comp	Albendazole Bol
Adm.	Oral
@	LA 7.5 mg/kg B.wt SA 5 mg/kg B.wt
Pres.	2000 mg, 600 mg

Minthal Sus	**Alembic**
Comp	2.5% Albendazole
Adm.	Oral
@	LA 7.5 mg/kg B.wt SA 5 mg/kg B.wt
Pres.	30 ml, IL

Minthal Pow	**Alembic**
Comp	15% Albendazole
Adm.	Oral
@	LA 7.5 mg/kg B.wt SA 5 mg/kg B.wt
Pres.	30 g, 300 g

Valbazen Bol	**Zydus (SKF)**
Comp	Albendazole Bol
Adm.	Oral
@	LA 7.5 mg/kg B.wt SA 5 mg/kg B.wt
Pres.	150 mg x 10, 600 mg x 6

Valbazen Sus	**Zydus (SKF)**
Comp	2.5% Albendazole
Adm.	Oral
@	LA 7.5 mg/kg B.wt SA 5 mg/kg B.wt
Pres.	60 ML, lL

Valbazen Pow	**Zydus (SKF)**
Comp	15% Albendazole
Adm.	Oral
@	LA 7.5 mg/kg B.wt SA 5 mg/kg B.wt
Pres.	30 g, 300 g

Woopar Bol/Tab.	**Carevet Pharma**
Comp	Albendazole Bol
Adm.	Oral
@	LA 7.5 mg/kg B.wt SA 5 mg/kg B.wt
Pres.	150 mg x 4, 1.5 g x 2, 3 g

Zomar Sus	**Cadila Pharma**
Comp	2.5% Albendazole
Adm.	Oral
@	LA 7.5 mg/kg B.wt SA 5 mg/kg B.wt
Pres.	60 ml, IL

Albex Pow	**Anmark**
Comp	15% Albendazole
Adm.	Oral
@	LA 7.5 mg/kg B.wt SA 5 mg/kg B.wt
Pres.	30 g, 300 g

Vibex Bol	**Cadila Health**
Comp	Albendazole Bol
Adm.	Oral
@	LA 7.5 mg/kg B.wt SA 5 mg/kg B.wt
Pres.	750 mg

Vibex Sus	**Cadila Health**
Comp	2.5% Albendazole
Adm.	Oral
@	LA 7.5 mg/kg B.wt SA 5 mg/kg B.wt
Pres.	30 ml, 60 ml, 500 ml

Vibex Pow	**Cadila Health**
Comp	15% Albendazole
Adm.	Oral
@	LA 7.5 mg/kg B.wt SA 5 mg/kg B.wt
Pres.	100 g, 250 g

Zerow Bol	**Sushima**
Comp	Albendazole Bol
Adm.	Oral
@	LA 7.5 mg/kg B.wt SA 5 mg/kg B.wt
Pres.	750 mg

Benvet Bol/Sus/Pow	**Cipla**
Comp	Albendazole Sus 2.5%, 10%, Bolus 250 mg, 500 mg, 1g, 2.5g , 3 g, Pow 10%
Adm.	Oral
@	LA 7.5 mg/kg B.wt SA 5 mg/kg B.wt
Pres.	150 mg, 1.5 g, 3 g 30 ml, 90 ml, IL, 5 L

Fenbendazole

It is a broad spectrum anthelmintic and is one of the benzimidazole compound for use in livestock with high margin of safety. It has efficacy against both mature and immature stages of nematodes, cestodes and trematodes. It has no adverse reaction on even at high dose or during pregnancy. No teratogenic effect. It is indicated in round worms, tapeworms and lung worm infestation. It is not effective against flukes. It has faster absorption. Due to longer half life it is wormicidal, larvicidal and ovicidal. Available in Tab, Liq, Bol, Powder form.

Curaminth Tab/Pow/Liq	**Zydus (Sarabhai)**			
Comp	Tablet	150 mg		
	Fenbendazole Bol	1.5 g		
	Liquid	2.5%	Powder	25%
Adm.	Oral			
@	5 mg/kg B.wt In heavy animals dose may be doubled			
Pres.	150 mg x 10, 1.5 g x 1, 60 ml, 120 g			

Fengard Tab/Bol/Pow	**Anmarks**
Comp	Tab, Bol, Powder Fenbendazole 25%
Adm.	Oral
@	5 mg/kg B.wt In heavy animals dose may be doubled
Pres.	Pow 60 gm, 120 g, 150 mg x 10, 1.5 g x 1

Fenomar Bol/Pow/Liq	**Virbac (Glaxo)**
Comp	25% Fenbendazole/Bol, Liq- 10%, 2.5%
Adm.	Oral
@	5 mg/kg B.wt In heavy animals dose may be doubled
Pres.	150 mg, 1.5 g, 10%, Sus 450 ml, 2.5%, 450 ml, IL, Pow 60 g, 120 g

Fentas Bol/Pow/Liq	**Intas**
Comp	Fenbendazole liq 10% Pow 25%
Adm.	Oral
@	5 mg/kg B.wt In heavy animals dose may be doubled
Pres.	1.5 g, Pow 6 g, 60 g, Liq 60 ml, IL

Fenorid Bol/Pow	**Sterling**
Comp	Pow 25% Fenbendazole, Bol.
Adm.	Oral
@	5 mg/kg B.wt In heavy animals dose may be doubled
Pres.	1.5 g, 120 g

Cipcur Bol/Pow	**Cipla**
Comp	Bol, Powder 25% Fenbendazole
Adm.	Oral
@	5 mg/kg B.wt In heavy animals dose may be doubled
Pres.	1.5 g, 6 g, 60 g, 120 g

Fenazol Bol/Pow	**Concept**
Comp	Bol, Pow 25% Fenbendazole
Adm.	Oral
@	5 mg/kg B.wt In heavy animals dose may be doubled
Pres.	1.5 g, 120 g

Helmicure Bol/Pow	**Centrury**
Comp	Bol, Powder 25% Fenbendazole
Adm.	Oral
@	5 mg/kg B.wt In heavy animals dose may be doubled
Pres.	1.5 g, 120 g

Panacure Tab/Bol/Pow/Liq	**Intervet (Hoechst)**
Comp	Tab, Bol, Powder 25%, Liq 2.5%, 10% Fenbendazole
Adm.	Oral
@	5 mg/kg B.wt In heavy animals dose may be doubled
Pres.	150 mg x 10, 1.5 g, 60 ml, 450 ml, IL(2.5%), 450 ml(10%), 60 g, 120 g

Panfugal Tab/Bol/Pow/Liq	**Merial (Wockhardt)**
Comp	Tab, Bol, Liq 2.5%, Pow 25%, Fenbendazole
Adm.	Oral
@	5 mg/kg B.wt In heavy animals dose may be doubled
Pres.	150 mg x 10, 1.5 g, 60 ml, 450 ml, 120 g

All clear Bolus	**Cargill**
Comp	Fenbendazole
Adm.	Oral
@	5 mg/kg B.wt In heavy animals dose may be doubled
Pres.	1.5g

Fenzole Tab/Bol/Liq/Pow	**KAPL**
Comp	Tab, Bol, Pow 25%, Liq 2.5% Fenbendazole
Adm.	Oral
@	5 mg/kg B.wt In heavy animals dose may be doubled
Pres.	150 mg x 10, 1.5 g, 60 ml, 450 ml, 6 g, 60 g, 120 g

Fenmax Bol	Animax Pharma
Comp	Fenbendazole
Adm.	Oral
@	5 mg/kg B.wt In heavy animals dose may be doubled
Pres.	3 g

Fendivet Bol	Vet Avenue
Comp	Fenbendazole
Adm.	Oral
@	5 mg/kg B.wt In heavy animals dose may be doubled
Pres.	3 g x 1

Vetfen Tab/Bol	Indian Immunology
Comp	Fenbendazole
Adm.	Oral
@	5 mg/kg B.wt In heavy animals dose may be doubled
Pres.	150 mg x 10, 1.5 g x 1, 2.5 g x 1

Fenbendazole Combination

Wesbo Plus Bolus	Wesfa Pharma
Comp	Fenbendazole 3 g Ivermectin 100 mg
Adm.	Oral
@	1 Bol for 300 kg B.wt
Pres.	1 Bolus

Fendymac Bol	Macnor
Comp	Bolus contains Fenbendazole 3 g Ivermectin 100 mg
Adm.	Oral
@.	One Bolus for 400 kg B.wt
Pres.	3 gm Bolus in pack of 15

Zomar IFS Bol/ Liq	Cadila Pharma
Comp	Each Bolus contains Fenbendazole 3 g Ivermectin 100 mg Silymarin 50 mg 1 ml Liquid contains F = 30 mg I = 1 mg S = 0.05 per ml
Adm.	Oral
@	1 Bol upto 500 kg B.wt 100 ml upto 500 kg B.wt
Pres.	Single Bol strip/100 ml

Mebendazole

It is broad spectrum anthelminitic introduced in 1972. It is one of the Benzimidazoles group anthelmintic and became very popular owing to its nontoxic effect over Thiabendazole. It gives 100% cure rate in Hook-worms infestation. Its action is by interfering with energy requirement of worms and does not effect the host in anyway. All type of nematodes, cestodes and lung worms are killed by it. With higher doses loss of hair, diarrhea and abdominal pain can be observed.

Animeb Pow/ Cap or Tab	**Novartis (Intercare)**
Comp	Cap 500 mg MBZ, Powder 10% MBZ
Adm.	Oral
@	LA 10 mg/kg B.wt In sheep 5 mg/kg B.wt
Pres.	4 Tab, 100 g

Helmin Tab, Pow	**Anmark**
Comp	Cap 500 mg MBZ, Powder 10% MBZ 50% MBZ
Adm.	Oral
@	LA 10 mg/kg B.wt In sheep 5 mg/kg B.wt
Pres.	500 mg x 4, 10%, 20 g, 100 g, 1 kg, Pow 50% 50 g, 100 g

Mebendal Tab/Pow	**Vets Farma**
Comp	Cap 500 mg MBZ, Powder 10% MBZ
Adm.	Oral
@	LA 10 mg/kg B.wt In sheep 5 mg/kg B.wt
Pres.	4 Tab, 100 g

Robendal Tab, Liq Granules	**TTK Pharma**
Comp	500 mg Tab, 2% Liq, 50% Granule MBZ
Adm.	Oral
@	LA 10 mg/kg B.wt In sheep 5 mg/kg B.wt
Pres.	10 Tab, 120 ml, 500 ml, 500 g

Zodex Bol/ Pow	**Concept**
Comp	1 g Bol, 50% Pow MBZ
Adm.	Oral
@	LA 10 mg/kg B.wt In sheep 5 mg/kg B.wt
Pres.	4 Bol, 100 g, 500 g

Banif Bol/ Pow	Brihans
Comp	10% and 50% Pow MBZ, Bol/g
Adm.	Oral
@	LA 10 mg/kg B.wt In sheep 5 mg/kg B.wt
Pres.	Bolus 4, Pow 10 g, 100 g, 500 g

Kalmeban Pow	KAPL
Comp	10% and 50% MBZ
Adm.	Oral
@	LA 10 mg/kg B.wt In sheep 5 mg/kg B.wt
Pres.	10%-20 g, 100 g, 500 g, 50%-50 g, 100 g

Wormin Tab/ Pow/ Liq	Cadila Pharma
Comp	100 mg, 600 mg, Pow 50%, Liq 2% MBZ
Adm.	Oral
@	LA 10 mg/kg B.wt In sheep 5 mg/kg B.wt
Pres.	100 x 10, 600 x 4, Pow 50 g, Liq 30 ml

Eshen Bol/Pow	Unjha
Comp	1 g Bol, 50% Pow MBZ
Adm.	Oral
@	LA 10 mg/kg B.wt In sheep 5 mg/kg B.wt
Pres.	4 Bol, 100 g, 500 g

Parbendazole

It is a broad spectrum anthelmintic indroduced in 1968 by Smith Klin Pharma scientists. Actions and activity is as per other membes of Benzimidazole as it is also one of Benzimidazole. Caution for slaughtered animal is to keep 6 days gap between dosing and slaughtering for human consumption.

Helatack Pow	Zydus (SKF)
Comp	30% Parbendazole
Adm.	Oral
@	30 g of Helatack per 40 kg B.wt
Pres.	480 g container

Oxibendazole

It is a broad spectrum anthelmintic of Benzimidazole group. Action is as good as Mebendazole.

Anthelmex Bol	Cipla
Comp	Oxibendazole 1g
Adm.	Oral
@	LA 1 Bol
Pres.	1 Bol

Thiabendazole

It is first compound of Benzimidazole group developed in 1960 by scientists. It is used for GI parasites of sheep, goat, cattle, camel, pigs, horses and birds. It is given orally in a single dose. For prophylaxis lower doses in feed for extended period is advised. It is larvicidal and ovicidal. Its action is similar to other group members of Benzimidazole group. It is not effective in several important swine helminths. It can be given in feed or water.

Thiabendole Bol/ Pow	Virbac (MSD)
Comp	Bol 2 g, Powder 50% Thiabendole
Adm.	Oral
@	66-110 mg/kg B.wt in cattle, 44-66 mg/kg B.wt in sheep and goat
Pres.	Bol 2 g, 3. 5 kg

Triclabendazole

It was developed in 1987 and a compound of Benzemidazole group. It is effective 98-100% in mature and immature infestation of liver fluke (Fascioliasis) in cattle, sheep and horses. It can be given with other antinematodes. It's plasma concentration is achieved within 12-36 hours. Excretion is via bile. It interferes with enzyme fumerate reductase and results diminished energy which leads to death. Its margin of safety is 17-20 times. Milk is not safe for human consumption upto 10 days. No claim for amphistomes

Fasinex Tab/Bol/Sus	Novartis
Comp	250 mg Tab, 900 mg Bol, 5% Triclabendazole
Adm.	Oral
@	12 mg/kg B.wt in cattle, 10 mg/kg B.wt in sheep and goat
Pres.	10 Tab, 2 Bol, 250 ml, 500 ml IL

Triclamar Tab/ Sus	Virbac (Glaxo)
Comp	900 mg, 5% Triclabenda zole
Adm.	Oral

@	12 mg/kg B.wt in cattle, 10 mg/kg B.wt in sheep and goat
Pres.	2 Bol 500 ml

Fluzic Sus	**Zydus (Ranbaxy)**
Comp	5% Triclabendazole
Adm.	Oral
@	12 mg/kg B.wt in cattle, 10 mg/kg B.wt in sheep and goat
Pres.	90 ml, 500 ml, IL

Triclasol Bol/Sus	**Merial (Dosch)**
Comp	900 mg, 5% Triclabendazole
Adm.	Oral
@	12 mg/kg B.wt in cattle, 10 mg/kg B.wt in sheep and goat
Pres.	2 Bol 500 ml

Piperazine

This antiparasitic compound was introduced in 1950. It is highly active against Ascaris and Enterobius achieving almost 100% cure rate. It blocks neuromuscular transmission of roundwords leading them paralised and then worms are expelled alive. It is used primarily for the treatment of Ascarids and Nodular worms in all species and animals including children. It can be given orally or mixed in drinking water. It is safe in all species. Diarrhea and abdominal pain can be seen in some animals. Piperazine has synergistic action with Phenothiazine compound.

Helmacid Liq	**Virbac**
Comp	Piperazine hydrate 45%
Adm.	Oral
@	44-66 mg/kg B.wt once for Pinworms, 75 mg/kg B.wt for others. in horses 110 mg/kg B.wt
Pres.	30 ml, 115 ml, 500 ml

Knock 45 Liq	**Zydus (Sarabhai)**
Comp	900 mg, 45% Piperazine hydrate
Adm.	Oral
@	44-66 mg/kg B.wt once for Pinworms, 75 mg/kg B.wt for others. in horses 110 mg/kg B.wt
Pres.	100 ml, 500 ml 5L

Piperazine Liq 45%	**HAL**
Comp	Piperazine hexachydrate 45%
Adm.	Oral
@	44-66 mg/kg B.wt once for Pinworms, 75 mg/kg B.wt for others. in horses 110 mg/kg B.wt
Pres.	500 ml 5L

Piperazine adipate oral/ Liq	**KAPL**
Comp	Piperazine adipate 45%
Adm.	Oral
@	44-66 mg/kg B.wt once for Pinworms, 75 mg/kg B.wt for others. in horses 110 mg/kg B.wt
Pres.	500 ml 5L

Piperazine adipate Pow	**Neospark**
Comp	Piperazine adipate 44.4%
Adm.	Oral
@	44-66 mg/kg B.wt once for Pinworms, 75 mg/kg B.wt for others. in horses 110 mg/kg B.wt
Pres.	15 g, 500 g, 1 kg

Vermex Liq	**Pfizer**
Comp	Piperazine hexachydrate 0.82 g in 5 L
Adm.	Oral
@	15-30 ml/30 kg B.wt
Pres.	100 ml, 500 ml

Piperol	**Indian Immunology**
Comp	Piperazine hydrate 45%
Adm.	Oral
@	44-66 mg/kg B.wt once for Pinworms, 75 mg/kg B.wt for others. in horses 110 mg/kg B.wt
Pres.	50 ml, 5 L

Piperaziine Hydrate Liq 61%	**Neospark**
Comp	Piperazine hydrate 61%
Adm.	Oral
@	44-66 mg/kg B.wt
Pres.	370 ml, I L, 5 L

Phenothiazine

It belongs to Heterocyclic compound. It was one of the early drug with fairly wide range of activity against GI nematodes. It was synthesized as early as 1885. It was extensively used in sheep, cattle and goats. With the advent of new products after 1960 and development of its resistance to some strain its use has been reduced. Discolouration of milk was its side effect. Anaemia can be seen.

Phenovis	**ICI**
Comp	Phenothiazine
Adm.	Oral
@	9-18 g in calves, S & G 4.5 g-13.5 g, cow 27-45 g Horses = 17g
Pres.	3.5 kg

Levamesole

It is an antiparasitic drug of Imidazothiazole class. It is a broad spectrum anthelmintic covering major GI nematodes including mature and immature worms. It is effective against lung worms also. Its action is to cause neuromuscular toxicity to the parasite. It has another quality. It provides immunostimulant action or known as Thymomimetic with host immunity and body resistance. It increases the antibody titre to vaccine thus relieves symptom of some diseases. Drug is excreted in urine. It is effective against mature and immature round worms of GI tract, lungworms, stomach worm, and improve the whipworm of pigs. It can be given to immunopotentiate in infections and improve the performance of animal. It can be given oral or injectable form in pregnants and lactating animals. It is non teratogemic and non embryotic. It acts longer and better due to immunostimulant action.

Almizol	**Alembic**
Comp	Levamesole 30%
Adm.	Add 5 g in 20ml
@	1 ml/kg B.wt
Pres.	5 g, 100 g

Curaminth L Pow	**Zydus**
Comp	Levamesole 30%
Adm.	Add 5 g in 20 ml
@	1 ml/kg B.wt
Pres.	10 g, 100 g

Helmisol Pow	**Sterling**
Comp	Levamesole 30%
Adm.	Add 5 g in 20ml
@	1 ml/k g B.wt
Pres.	50 g, 500 g

Levasole Pow	**Vets Farma**
Comp	Levamesole 30%
Adm.	Add 5 g in 20ml
@	1 ml/kg B.wt
Pres.	100 g

Nilverm Forte Pow	**Virbac**
Comp	Levamesole 30%
Adm.	Add 5 g in 20ml
@	1 ml/kg B.wt
Pres.	10 g, 100 g

Nematex L Pow	**Neospark**
Comp	Levamesole 30%
Adm.	Add 5 g in 20ml
@	1 ml/kg B.wt
Pres.	50 g, 100 g, 500 g

Levole Pow	**Merial (Wockhardt)**
Comp	Levamesole 30%
Adm.	Add 5 g in 20ml
@	1ml/kg B.wt
Pres.	10 g, 100 g

Kalmisole Pow/Tab/Bol	KAPL
Comp	Levamesole 30%, 150 mg Tab, 1500 mg Bol
Adm.	Add 5 g in 20 ml
@	1ml/kg B.wt or 75mg per or kg B.wt
Pres.	5 g, 50 g, 100 g, 250 g, Pow 150 mg, 1500 mg Bol

Kalmisole inj	KAPL
Comp	Levamesole 75 mg/ml
Adm.	IM/ SC
@	LA 15-20 ml
Pres.	30 ml

Lomox Plus Pow	Novartis
Comp	Levamesole 30%
Adm.	Add 5 g in 20 ml
@	1 ml/kg B.wt
Pres.	100 g, 1 kg

Lovam Forte Pow	Anmark
Comp	Levamesole 30%
Adm.	Add 5 g in 20ml
@	1ml/kg B.wt
Pres.	100 g, 500 g

L-Mezole Pow	Cargill (Vetcare)
Comp	Levamesole 30%
Adm.	Add 5 g in 20 ml
@	1ml/kg B.wt
Pres.	50 g, 250 g

Levole inj	Merial (Wockhardt)
Comp	Levamesole 150 mg/ ml
Adm.	IM/ SC
@	LA 10-15 ml
Pres.	10 ml, 30 ml

Ventrimisole Pow	Venky
Comp	Levamesole 30%

Adm.	Add 5 g in 20ml
@	1 g/4 kg B.wt
Pres.	100 g, 500 g

Levacip Bol	**Cipla**
Comp	400/ 600/ 1000 mg Levamesole
Adm.	Oral
@	kg B.wt
Pres.	400 mg x 10, 600 mg x 4, 1000 mg x 4

Levacip inj	**Cipla**
Comp	Levamesole 75 mg/ml
Adm.	IM/ SC
@	LA 15-20 ml
Pres.	30 ml

Lemasol inj	**Ranbaxy**
Comp	Levamesole 75 mg/ml
Adm.	IM/ SC
@	LA 15-20 ml
Pres.	30 ml

Tetramesole

It was developed late in 1960. It is active against many nematodes but use is restricted to ascariasis and ancyclostomiasis because action on other worms is poor. It kills strongyloides larvae. But adult worms are not sensitive. It stimulates ganglia in worms and cause paralysis which result in expulsion of live worms. It is indicated in Ascariasis, Hook worms and mixed infection with lung worms. Due to its activity, good tolerance and low dose it has been used in mass treatment of Round worms.

Curanminth Pow	**Zydus (Sarabhai)**
Comp	Tetramesole 30%
Adm.	Oral
@	LA 10 g in 300 ml or 100 g in 3L water LA 150 ml/ 100 kg B.wt SA 15-30 ml
Pres.	10 g, 100 g

Nilverm Pow	**Virbac**
Comp	Tetramesole 30%
Adm.	Oral

@	LA 10 g in 300 ml or 100 g in 3 L water LA 150 ml/ 100 kg B.wt SA 15-30 ml
Pres.	10 g, 100 g

Ranisol Pow	**Anmark**
Comp	Tetramesole 30%
Adm.	Oral
@	LA 10 g in 300 ml or 100 g in 3 L water LA 150 ml/ 100 kg B.wt SA 15-30 ml
Pres.	100 g

Tetracip Bol	**Cipla**
Comp	Tetramesole 300 mg, 600 mg, 1200 mg
Adm.	Oral
@	600 mg in animal of 200 kg or 1200 mg in 400 kg animal
Pres.	600 mg, 1200 mg

Thiophanate

It is a broad spectrum anthelmintic eliminating major GI nematodes in cattle, sheep, goat, pig, camels. It acts against adult and larval form of nematodes. It acts as benzimidazole when inside the body. It inhibits fumerate reductase system after absorption through cuticle of parasite. It is excreted within 72 hours through feces and urine. It has disadvantage of suspension. It has cross resistance with BZ family members. It is indicated in adult and larval form of GI worms, lung worms in sheep and goats, stomach worm, nodular worm and whip worm in pigs. It is active against ascarids when given as feed premix

Thiophanate	**Primavet**
Comp	70% thiophanate wettable powder
Adm.	Oral
@	50-100 mg/kg B.wt 100 g in 400 ml water which becomes 500 ml, 15 ml/40 kg or 3 g is dose. Sheep 50 ml or 10 g
Pres.	10 g, 100 g

Dichlorphene

It is substituted phenol anthelmintic. It blocks the channel of energy production and kill worms. It is similar to Niclosamide in certain properties. It is active against Tape worms like Taenia, Dipylidium in dogs and cats and Moniezia in sheep. It is also bactericidal and fungicidal. There can be vomiting, colic or diarrhea. It can be given only for Tape worms. It is safe with low toxicity.

Dichlorphen	**Anmark**
Comp	500 mg Tab
Adm.	Oral
@	50-100 mg/kg B.wt in sheep
Pres.	500 mg x 10

Niclosamide

It was developed in 1960 and used for tape worm infestation of domestic animals and dogs or cats. It is Salicylanilide anthelmintic. It is also effective against amphistomes. It is safe in all stage of pregnancy. Safety index is 40. It acts by energy depletion and accumulation of Lactic acid and with poor health. It is indicated in Tape worm, Amphistomes infestation of cattle and sheep. It is recommended to overnight fasting prior to treatment for better results.

Cestonex M Pow	**Neospark**
Comp	Niclosamide 750mg/g
Adm.	Oral
@	100-150 mg/kg B.wt LA 50 mg/kg B.wt SA 100 mg/kg B.wt
Pres.	50 g, 100 g

Niclomar Tab	**Virbac**
Comp	Niclosamide 500 mg
Adm.	Oral
@	50-100 mg/kg B.wt in sheep
Pres.	500 mg x 10 Tab

Oxyclozanide

It is practically effective against all flukes, few present in bile duct, amphistomes and paramphistomes in cattle, sheep, buffaloes and other live stock. It is effective against mature and immature flukes. It is also effective against Tapeworms Moniezia specie in sheep. Its exact mode of action is not known. It is excreted in bile tissue and body fluids. It is indicaited in Fascioliasis, amphistomiasis for treatment and control. It can be given with other treatments. It is safe for pregnants, lactating and sick animals. Animal may show loss of appetite for 1-2 days. Milk drops for 1-2 days cattle may pass softened feces. Safety index is 4.

Alzanide	**Alembic**
Comp	Sol 3.4%, Bol 1 g of Oxyclozanide
Adm.	Oral
@	LA 10 mg/kg B.wt SA 15 mg/kg B.wt
Pres.	1g Bol, 90 ml, IL

Banif Pow/ Bol	**Brihans**
Comp	20% in Pow, 1g Bol
Adm.	Oral
@	LA 10 mg/kg B.wt SA 15 mg/kg B.wt
Pres.	1 g Bol, 10 g, 100 g, 500 g

Distodin Bol/Sol	**Pfizer**
Comp	200 mg per g, 1 g, 3.4% solution
Adm.	Oral
@	LA 10 mg/kg B.wt SA 15 mg/kg B.wt
Pres.	200 mg x 10 Tab, 1 g x 4, 90 ml, IL

Neozide Bol/Sol	**Intas**
Comp	200 mg per g, 1 g, 3.4% solution
Adm.	Oral
@	LA 10 mg/kg B.wt SA 15 mg/kg B.wt
Pres.	1 g x 4, 90 ml, IL

Oxynide Bol/Sol	**Anmark**
Comp	200 mg per g, 1 g, 3.4% solution
Adm.	Oral
@	LA 10 mg/kg B.wt SA 15 mg/kg B.wt
Pres.	200 mg x 10, 1 g x 4, 90 ml, IL

Ocloz Bolus	**Cipla**
Comp	1 g
Adm.	Oral
@	LA 10 mg/kg B.wt SA 15 mg/kg B.wt
Pres.	Strip of 4

Zanil Susp Bol	**Virbac**
Comp	Sol 3.4%, Bol 1 g of Oxyclozanide
Adm.	Oral
@	LA 10 mg/kg B.wt SA 15 mg/kg B.wt
Pres.	100 ml, IL, Strip of 4

Zonax Tab/Bol/Sus	**Sterling**
Comp	Sol 3.4%, Bol 1 g of Oxyclozanide Tab 200 mg
Adm.	Oral
@	LA 10 mg/kg B.wt SA 15 mg/kg B.wt
Pres.	Tab 10, 1 g Bol, 90 ml, IL

Tolzan F Sus Tab/Bol	**Novartis (Hoechst)**
Comp	200 mg, 1 g, 3.4% solution, 1 g Bol
Adm.	Oral
@	LA 10 mg/kg B.wt SA 15 mg/kg B.wt
Pres.	200 mg x 10, 1 g x 4, 90 ml, IL, 5 L

Okazan Tab/Bol, Susp	**Merial (Wockhardt)**
Comp	200 mg, 1 g, 3.4% suspension, Bol 1 g
Adm.	Oral
@	LA 10 mg/kg B.wt SA 15 mg/kg B.wt
Pres.	Tab 10, 1 g x 4, 90 ml, IL

Hexanide Tab/Bol, Susp	**Zydus**
Comp	200 mg, 1g, 3.4% solution
Adm.	Oral
@	LA 10 mg/kg B.wt SA 15 mg/kg B.wt
Pres.	1 g x 4, 90 ml, IL

Distonex Tab/Bol	**Neospark**
Comp	200 mg, 1g,
Adm.	Oral
@	LA 10 mg/kg B.wt SA 15 mg/kg B.wt
Pres.	200 mg x 10, 1 g x 4,

Rafoxanide

It is an effective flukicide with wide range of activity against flukes and amphistomes in cattle buffaloes and sheep. It not only kills large adult fluke but also kills immature flukes. It is safe for pregnants and young. Its mode of action is energy depletion, The peak plasma level achieved in 12-24 hrs. It is indicated in fascioliasis and amphistomiasis. It has advantage over others. There is no need to treat the animal at intervals. It is effective against mature and immature severe infection. It is not recommended in milking animals. It is also effective against all stages of Haemonchus contortus and Oestrus ovis in sheep. Overdose may cause diarrhea and ocular dysfunctioning.

Amfanide Pow	**Merial**
Comp	Rofaxanide 200 mg/g
Adm.	Oral
@	7.5 mg of Rafoxanide/kg body weight. Dissolve 10 g in 80 ml of water. Give 3 ml/10 kg B.wt in sheep and 12.5 ml/20 kg in cattle
Pres.	15 g pouch

Fasinide Pow	**Neospark**
Comp	Rofaxanide 200 mg/g
Adm.	Oral
@	7.5 mg of Rafoxanide/kg body weight. Oissolve 10 g in 80 ml of water. Give 3 ml/10 kg B.wt in sheep and 12.5 ml/20 kg in cattle
Pres.	100 g

Rafox Pow/Tab/Bol	**Anmark**
Comp	2 g Bolus, 200 mg Tab, 200 mg/g Pow of Rafoxanide
Adm.	Oral
@	7.5 mg of Rafoxanide/kg body weight.
Pres.	200 mg x 10, 2 g x 1, 10 g, 100 g, 1 kg

Rafoxin Bol/Tab/ Pow	**Concept**
Comp	Rafoxin-200 mg/g, 2 g, 200 mg/g of Rafoxanide
Adm.	Oral

@	7.5 mg of Rafoxanide/kg body weight. Oissolve 10 g in 80 ml of water. Give 3 ml/10 kg B.wt in sheep and 12.5 ml/20 kg in cattle
Pres.	200 mg x 10, 2 g x 1 Bol, 10 g Pow

Raphomar Pow/Bol	**Virbac**
Comp	1.5 g, 200 mg/g
Adm.	Oral
@	7.5 mg of Rafoxanide/kg body weight. Oissolve 10 g in 80 ml of water. Give 3 ml/10 kg B.wt in sheep and 12.5 ml/20 kg in cattle
Pres.	1.5 g x 1, 10 g sachet

Rafocip Sus	**Cipla**
Comp	2.5%
Adm.	Oral
@	7.5 mg of Rafoxanide/kg body weight. Give 3 ml/10 kg B.wt in sheep and 12.5 ml/20 kg in cattle
Pres.	100 ml, IL

Rafoxin Tab	**Century**
Comp	200 mg Tab
Adm.	Oral
@	7.5 mg of Rafoxanide/kg body weight.
Pres.	Tab x 10

Carbon Tetrachloride

It was introduced in 1920. It is one of the halogenated hydrocarbons. Like hexachlerethane and strong flukicide effective against ruminal or immature flukes. This is considered to be toxic and should not be used in lactating cows and buffaloes. The drug taints milk for a few days. Drug should not be used within 3 weeks of calving. It is indicated in Fascioliasis in cattle and sheep. Due to toxicity the drug is not being used. Animals must be given calcium rich diet before treatment with it. It should be repeated after 4-5 weeks.

Carbon tetrachloride	**Generic**
Comp	Carbon tetrachloride
Adm.	Oral
@	LA 4 ml, SA ½ to 1ml
Pres.	100 ml, 500 ml

Hexachlorethane

It has very high efficacy in adult liver flukes, amphistomes and paramphistomes. Safety index is only 2. There is no claim for immature flukes. The full dose can not be given to weak, sick and heavily infected animals. The second dose is recommended after 3 weeks for high efficacy. For undersized poor conditioned animals dose should be divided in 2 equal parts and may be given after an interval of 48 hours. It is indicated in Fascioliasis, amphistomiasis and paramphistomiasis. Calcium deficient animals are sensitive.

Avlothane	**ICI**
Comp	Hexachlorethane
Adm.	Oral
@	10 g/kg B.wt
Pres.	500 g, 3 kg

Hexathane	**Zydus**
Comp	Hexachlorethane
Adm.	Oral
@	10 g/kg B.wt
Pres.	30 g, 500 g

Xethane	**Sarabhai**
Comp	Hexachlorethane
Adm.	Oral
@	10 g/kg B.wt
Pres.	30 g, 500 g

Hexachlorophene

It is substituted phenol anthelmintic. It is a flukicide which blocks the channels of energy products and consequently kills the parasites. In debilitated animals it should be given in divided doses. It is indicated in Fascioliasis and paramphistomiasis.

Flukaphene Pow	**Zydus**
Comp	20% Hexachlorophene
Adm.	Oral
@	10-20 mg/kg B.wt
Pres.	10 g, 250 g

Nitroxynil

It was developed in 1960. It is flukicide against mature and immature flukes. It is also effective in Haemonchas, Bunostomum and oesophagostomum sp. It is safe for pregnants. It has no claim on amphistomes. Milk is indicated in Fascioliasis (mature and immature). It is available in injectable dosage form and can be given S/C or IM. It can be given orally but parental is more effective. Maximum tolerated doses of 40mg/kg B.wt in sheep and calves. Higher dose cause increased heartbeat and respiration rate. It is slowly eliminated from body in urine and feces upto 60 days. It stains wool and hair. There is 2 months withdrawal before slaughter.

Nitronixing	**Cipla**
Comp	25% Nitroxynyl 250 mg/ml
Adm.	SC/ IM
@	10 ml/300 kg B.wt
Pres.	10 ml, 30 ml

Tetrahydropyrimidine

Morantel

It is a chemical compound of Tetrahydropyrimidine. It is a broad spectrum gastro intestinal roundworm anthelmintic. It kills both adult and immature roundworm. It kills by inhibition of Succinate dehydrogenase and also by depolarising neuro-muscular blocking action. There is no milk withdrawal period as the excretion is through feces and urine. It is safe even at 10-20 times the recommended dose. It is compatible with other treatments. It is indicated for control of immature and adult GI nematodes in cattle, buffaloes, sheep, goat, pig, horses and camels. It is safe with no side effects. It is effective even against Benzimidazole resistant worms.

Banminth Tab/Bol/ Sol/Pow	**Zydus (Pfizer)**
Comp	118.8 mg Tab, 594 mg Bol morantel tartrate 3% Sol of Morantel citrate, 9% Pow
Adm.	Oral
@	5.94 mg/kg B.wt in cattle, buffalo, sheep, goat, horses, camels, 1 g/15 kg. 2.97 mg/kg B.wt in pigs for ascariasis and 7.43 mg/kg B.wt in mature and immature round worms. 1 ml/ 5kg B.wt
Pres.	118.8 mg x 10 Tab, 594 mg x 4 Bol, 5 L 3% Sol, 20 g, 100 g Pow

Minthex M	Neospark
Comp	3% Sol
Adm.	Oral
@	1 ml/5 kg B.wt
Pres.	IL, 5 L

Vetminth Tab/Bol/ Sol/Pow	Anmark
Comp	118.8 mg Tab, 594 mg Bol morantel tartrate 3% Sol of Morantel citrate, 9% Pow
Adm.	Oral
@	5.94 mg/kg B.wt in cattle, buffalo, sheep, goat, horses, camels, 1 g/15 kg. 2.97 mg/kg B.wt in pigs for ascariasis and 7.43 mg/kg B.wt in mature and immature round worms. 1ml/5 kg B.wt
Pres.	118.8 mg x 10 Tab, 594 mg x 4 Bol, 5 L 3% Sol, 20 g, 100 g Pow

Exworm Tab/Bol	Cipla
Comp	150 mg, 750 mg Morantel tartrate
Adm.	Oral
@	5.94 mg/kg B.wt
Pres.	Tabx 10 Bol x 4

Combinations

Albendazole with Rafoxanide

Vetalben R Sus	Indian Immunology
Comp	ABZ 25 mg Rafoxanide 22.7 mg/ml
Adm.	Oral
@	LA 10 ml/30 kg SA 1 ml/3 kg
Pres.	100 ml, 500 ml

Tetramesole + Oxyclozonide

Flunil plus sus	Vets Farma
Comp	Tetramesole 3% Oxyclozonide 3%
Adm.	Oral

@	10 ml/30 kg B.wt
Pres.	IL

Nilzan Bol/Liq	**Virbac**
Comp	Tetramesole 1.5 g Oxyclozonide 1.5 g/3.4%, T 3.4% O
Adm.	Oral
@	LA 10 ml/30 kg 1 Bol for one adult
Pres.	1 Bol, IL

Levamisole Combination

Endex 8.75%	**Novartis**
Comp	Levamisole 3.75% + Triclabendazole 5%
Adm.	Oral
@	LA 1 ml/5 kg B.wt, SA 2 ml/5 kg B.wt
Pres.	60 ml, 250 ml

Endex 19.5	**Novartis**
Comp	L = 7.5%, T = 12%
Adm.	Oral
@	1 ml/10 kg B.wt
Pres.	30 ml, 60 ml, 250 ml

Fasnil Susp.	**Merial (Dosch)**
Comp	L = 1.5%, 3% Oxyclozanide
Adm.	Oral
@	La 5 ml/20 kg B.wt, SA 1 ml/4 kg B.wt
Pres.	90 ml, 500 ml, IL

Klozanide L Bol/Sus	**KAPL**
Comp	Bol oxycl 1 g L=0.5 g, Sus 3% oxy 1.5% L
Adm.	Oral
@	1 Bol or 90 ml for LA
Pres.	Bol x 4, 90 ml, IL

Anthelmect inj	**Cipla**
Comp	Levamesol 100 mg closantel 50 mg per ml
Adm.	SC/ IM
@	LA 10 ml
Pres.	10 ml, 30 ml

Levoxy H S Bol/Sus	Cipla
Comp	Bol L = 300 mg, O = 600 mg Sus. L = 15% O = 3%
Adm.	Oral
@	LA 4 Bolus
Pres.	Bol x 4

Trinex	Cipla
Comp	L = 7.5% Triclabendazole 12%
Adm.	Oral
@	1 ml/10 kg B.wt
Pres.	30 ml, 60 ml, 250 ml

Flukisyl Bol/Sus	Bovian
Comp	Bol Oxy 4000 mg + L 2000 mg + silymarin 300 mg Sus O = 60 mg L 30 mg, S 4 mg/ml
Adm.	Oral
@	LA 1 Bol or 90 ml
Pres.	Single Bol, 90 ml

Total out Bol/Sus	Avivet
Comp	Bol Oxy 4000 mg + L 2000 mg + silymarin 300 mg
Adm.	Oral
@	LA 1 Bol or 90ml
Pres.	Single Bolus

Devermax Bol	Animax Health
Comp	Bol Oxy 4000 mg + L 2000 mg + silymarin 300 mg
Adm.	Oral
@	LA 1 Bol or 90 ml
Pres.	Single Bol

MinflukeDS Sus	Animax Pharma
Comp	Bol Oxy 4000 mg + L 2000 mg + silymarin 300 mg Sus O = 60 mg L 30 mg, S 4 mg/ml
Adm.	Oral
@	LA 1 Bol or 90 ml
Pres.	Single Bol

Ozasol Bol/Sus	**Kepler**
Comp	Bol Oxy 4000 mg + L 2000 mg + silymarin 300 mg Sus O = 60 mg L 30 mg, S 4 mg/ml
Adm.	Oral
@	LA 1 Bol or 90 ml
Pres.	Single Bol, 90 ml

Helmicide DS Bol/ Sus	**Phoenix**
Comp	Bol Oxy 4000 mg + L 2000 mg + silymarin 300 mg Sus O = 60 mg L 30 mg, S 4 mg/ml
Adm.	Oral
@	LA 1 Bol or 90 ml
Pres.	Single Bol, 90 ml

Elzan Bol/Sus	**Anmarks**
Comp	Bol Oxy 4000 mg + L 2000 mg + silymarin 300 mg Sus O = 60 mg L 30 mg, S 4 mg/ml
Adm.	Oral
@	LA 1 Bol or 90 ml
Pres.	Single Bol, 90 ml

Macworm DS inj	**Macwell**	
Comp	Levamesole 75 mg	Oxyclozandie 150 mg
Adm.	SC	
@	1 ml/30 kg B.wt	
Pres.	30 ml vial	

Helino Sus	**Intas**
Comp	L = 37.5 mg Triclabendazole 50 mg/ml
Adm.	Oral
@	1 ml/10 kg B.wt
Pres.	250 ml, 500 ml

Macworm DS Bol/Sus	**Macwell**		
Comp	Oxyclozanide 4 g	Levamesole 2 g	Silymarine 300 mg in Bolus
	Oxyclozanide 6%	Levamesole 3%	Silymarine 0.3% in Susp

Adm.	Oral	
@	1 Bol for 400 kg animal	1 ml/4 kg B.wt

Antifluke Bol/ Sus	**Libra**		
Comp	Oxyclozanide 4 g	Levamesole 2 g	Silymarine 300 mg in Bolus
	Oxyclozanide 6%	Levamesole 3%	Silymarine 0.3% in Susp
Adm.	Oral		
@	1 Bol for 400 kg animal	1 ml/4 kg B.wt	

Macfluke Bol	**Macnor**		
Comp	Oxyclozanide 4 g	Levamesole 2 g	Silymarine 300 mg in Bolus
Adm.	Oral		
@	1 Bol for 400 kg animal		

Flukiban Bol/Susp	**Carevet Pharma**		
Comp	Oxyclozanide 4 g	Levamesole 2 g	Silymarine 300 mg in Bolus
	Oxyclozanide 6%	Levamesole 3%	Silymarine 0.3% in Susp
Adm.	Oral		
@	1 Bol for 400 kg animal	1 ml/4 kg B.wt	

Endwolf liq	**Agilis**	
Comp	Oxyclozandie 30 mg	levamesole 15 mg in each ml
Adm.	Oral	
@	10 ml/ 20 kg B.wt	
Pres.	100 ml, 1L	

Fasnil Bol/Sus	**Boehringer Ingelheim**	
Comp	Bolus	Sus
	Levamesol 2 g	Oxyclozandie 4 g
	Levamesol 1.5%	Oxyclozanide 3%
Adm.	Oral	
@	1 Bol/400 kg B.wt.	1 ml/2 kg B.wt
Pres.	6 g Bol, 90 ml, 1L, suspense	

Fastnot DS Bol	**Herstel**
Comp	Oxyclozanide 4 g Levamesole 2 g Silymarin 300 mg in one bolus
Adm.	Oral
@	1 Bol for 400 kg animal 1 ml/4 kg B.wt
Pres.	1 Bol strip, Susp 100ml

Wormivet — **Rakesh Pharma**

Indi: Endoparasiticide

Comp: 10 g contains

Bhrahamvriksha	2.6 g	Vatsak	1.0 g
Rochan	0.5 g	Ramath	0.250 g
Kitmari	0.5 g	Kuberakshya	1.5 g
Krimigna	1.2 g	Bhoomivalli	0.5 g
Bharhmdarbh	0.7 g	Keetari	0.7 g

Adm: Oral

@ : 60-75 g once daily for 2-3 days

Pres: 1 kg, 100 g

Wormkill — **Arosol Herbal**

Indi: Dewormer

Comp: Not given

Adm: Oral

@ : 100 g

Pres: 100 gm,1 kg

Wornil Pow. — **VetsFarma**

Indi: Rounduworm,Tapeworm infestation

Comp:

Ascaridia indica	10%	Mallotus philliplinesis	20%
Embeli aribes	20%	Hyoscyamas niger	5%
Areca catechu	5%	Azadirachta indica	3%
		Base	qs

Adm: Oral

@ : 100 g

Pres: 50 g, 1 kg

Wopell	Indian Herbs
Indi: Endoparasiticide	
Comp: Not given	
Adm: Oral	
@ : 50-75 g daily	
Pres: 100 g and 1 g	

Taenil Pow/Tab.	Indian Herbs
Indi: Against Taenia, cysts, worms	
Comp: Not given	
Adm: Oral	
@ :	
Pres: 500 g	

Endectoparasiticides

Avermectins

These are the compounds used to kill both internal and external parasites of liverstock.

Ivermectin

It is one of avermectins. It I used as endectocide of cattle, sheep, goat, camel and horses. Drug is neurotoxic to parasites by potentiating effect of inhibitory neurotransmitter GABA. It kills by flaccid paralysis. It is indicated in Gastro intestinal worms, lung worm, eyeworms, skin and muscle worm, ticks, grubs, mites, lice, nasal bots, cutaneous myiasis. It is used as injectable, powder for pour on and paste. Toxicity may occur with high doses. It is safe for pregnant and youngones, lactating or sick animals. Period of protection varies form 1-21 days.

Comectin	Concept
Comp	1% Ivermectin
Adm.	IM/ SC
@	1 ml/50 kg B.wt
Pres.	1 ml, 7 ml, 10 ml, 20 ml

Ectorid inj	Carevet Pharma
Comp	1% Ivermectin
Adm.	IM/ SC
@	1 ml/50 kg B.wt
Pres.	1 ml, 10 ml, 50 ml

Ivomac inj	**Virbac**
Comp	1% Ivermectin
Adm.	IM/ SC
@	1 ml/50 kg B.wt
Pres.	1 ml, 7 ml, 10 ml, 70 ml

Ivectin inj	**Indian Immunologicals**
Comp	1% Ivermectin
Adm.	IM/ SC
@	1 ml/50 kg B.wt
Pres.	1 ml, 7 ml, 10 ml, 50 ml

Mectin inj	**Alembic**
Comp	1% Ivermectin
Adm.	IM/ SC
@	1 ml/50 kg B.wt
Pres.	1 ml, 7 ml, 10 ml, 20 ml

Neomac	**Intas**
Comp	1% Ivermectin
Adm.	IM/ SC
@	1 ml/50 kg B.wt
Pres.	1 ml, 7 ml, 10 ml, 20 ml

Endact	**Merial (Wockhardt)**
Comp	1% Ivermectin
Adm.	IM/ SC
@	1 ml/50 kg B.wt
Pres.	1 ml, 7 ml

Ivomac oral Sol	**Virbac**
Comp	0.8% Ivermectin
Adm.	Oral
@	2.5 ml/kg B.wt
Pres.	IL

Parid	**Vets Farma**
Comp	1% Ivermectin
Adm.	IM/ SC
@	1 ml/50 kg B.wt
Pres.	1 ml, 7 ml, 30 ml

Trumectin	Zydus
Comp	1% Ivermectin
Adm.	IM/ SC
@	1 ml/50 kg B.wt
Pres.	1 ml, 10 ml

Clomectin LA inj	Macwell
Comp	Ivermectin 3.15%
Adm.	IM/ SC
@	1ml/50 kg B.wt
Pres.	10 ml, 50 ml

Ivera inj	Libra
Comp	Ivera 1% Ivera Gold 2% Iveraplatinum 3.15% of ivermectin
Adm.	IM
@.	1 ml or 10 mg/kg B.wt
Pres.	100 ml all

Ivera Tab/ Bol	Libra
Comp	15 mg, 30 mg, Tab 100 mg Bol, 150 mg Bol
Adm.	Oral
@.	10 mg/50 kg B.wt
Pres.	15 mg tab x5, 30 mg x 40, 100 mg x10 Bol, 150 mg x 10 Bol

Ivomec	Boehringer Ingelheim
Comp	Ivermectin 1%
Adm.	SC
@	1 ml/50 kg B.wt
Pres.	10 ml, 50 ml, 100 ml

Doramectin

It is one of avermectin. It is similar to ivermectin but it is little stronger and longer in action. It can be injected as well as used as pour on.

Dectomax inj	Pfizer
Comp	10 mg/ml of Doramectin
Adm.	IM/ SC
@	1ml/50 kg B.wt
Pres.	20 ml, 50 ml

Duromect inj	**Zydus**
Comp	Doramectin 10 mg/ml
Adm.	IM or SC
@	1 ml/50 kg B.wt
Pres.	10 ml, 50 ml

Closantel

It is a salicylanilide anthelmintic. Its action is like oxyclozanide or Rafoxanide. It is active against fasciola species and Haemonchus (in sheep) Drug can be used against Ancylostoma adult stage. It also acts as ectoparasitcide. It is indicated in mature, immature liver fluke, hematodes, cestodes and arthropods. It has no adverse effect even after high dosing. It has no action on amphistomes.

Exinot Liq	**Cadila Pharma**
Comp	15% closantel
Adm.	Oral
@	7.5-10 mg/kg B.wt or 1 ml/10-15 kg B.wt
Pres.	30 ml

Zenvet Sol/Bol	
Comp	Bol = 1000 mg, 150 mg/ml Sol
Adm.	Oral
@	7.5-10 mg/kg B.wt or 1 ml/10-15 kg B.wt
Pres.	Bolus x 4, 30 ml, 100 ml, 5 L

Zycloz Bol/Sol	**Zydus**
Comp	Bol = 1000 mg, 150 mg/ml Sol
Adm.	Oral
@	7.5-10 mg/kg B.wt or 1 ml/10-15 kg B.wt
Pres.	Bolus x 4, 30 ml, 100 ml, 5L

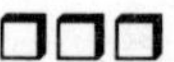

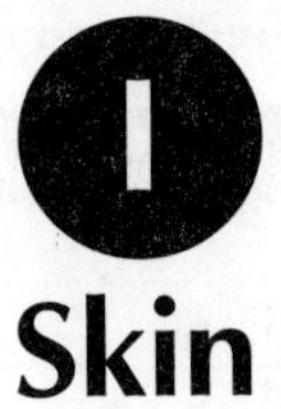

Skin

Diseases of Skin

Abcess: Local pouch of infection containing pus can be from injury to skin which gets complicated by entry of pus forming germ, swelling is there.

Abrasion: An injury in which breaking of integument and there is injury to underlying tissue.

Acne: It includes all infections of hair follicles caused by suppurative organism. Lesions begin as nodules on the base of hair.

Alopecia: Baldness or loss of hair or wool coat.

Anasarca: Accumulation of fluid in sub cutaneous tissue and extensive one.

Bruise: Injury by pressing the skin causing a sub-cutaneous haemorrhage.

Burns & Scalds: Former is caused by dry heat and later by moist heat with lesions on skin.

Carbuncle: Focal area of suppurative inflammation of skin in which there is discharge of pus into exterior.

Carcinoma: Cancer or uncontrolled cellular growth in any part of body.

Dandruff: Also called Pityriasis and is a condition characterised by the presence of bran like scales on the surface of skin.

Dermatitis: Inflammation of dermis and epidermis of skin.

Eczema: Inflammatory reaction of skin cells to substances to which cells are sensitized excessive wetting. Continuous scratching, continued soiling and accumulation of debris on skin.

Emphysema: Presence of free gas in subcutaneous tissue.

Folliculitis: Inflammation of hair follicle.

Gangrene: Death of tissue with sloughing of affected part.

Hyperkeratosis: Condition in which excessive keratinized cells accumulate on surface of skin.

Impetigo: Superficial eruption of thin walled small vesicles surrounded by a zone of erythema.

Melanoma: Cutaneous lesions on the back due to profuse haemorrhage.

Otitis: Suppurative, inflammatory condition of external ear. There is swelling at base, decrease in milk.

Pachydermia: Thickening of skin affecting all layers.

Papilla: A small nipple like or pimple like projection.

Papilloma: Abnormal growth arising from skin looks like wart. These vary in size and shape.

Papule: Circumscribed elevation of skin.

Parakeratosis: Condition of skin in which keratinization of skin cell is incomplete.

Petechia: Small spot on surface of organ or skin generally red or purple in colour.

Photosensitization: Disease caused by sensitization of superficial layers of lightly pigmented skin to light of certain wave lengths.

Pruritis: Itching sensation which gives rise to desire to scratch.

Purulent: Pertaining to pus.

Ringworm: Caused by invasion of keratinized epithelial cells and hair fibres by dermatophytes characterised by heavy, grey white crust raised above skin roughly circular in shape.

Scar: A mark remaining after the healing of a wound.

Seborrhoea: Excessive secretion of sebum on skin surface.

Tumor or Adenoma: Appearance and enlargement like papilloma can be Benign that is localized or malignant which means it has many branches.

Ulcer: Loss of entire epidermis and base of ulcer lies in subcutaneous tissue.

Urticaria: Allergic condition characterised by the appearance of wheals on skin surface.

Warts: Small solid growths arising upon surface of skin or mucous membrane.

Analgesics Topical

Irritants stimulate sensony nerve endings and induce inflammation at the site of application. Depending upon their nature, concentration and sensitiveness of the site these produce cooling sensation or warmth, numbness and vasodilation. These act as rubrefacients i.e. cause local hyperemia. Some irritants and counter-irritants produce a remote effect which tends to relieve pain and inflammation in deeper organs. Indicated for the relief of minor aches and pains of muscles and joints due to muscle strains, sprains and bruises as an adjunct in the management of minor stiffness. These are applied on the effected area and rubbed lightly until the cream vanishes. Neither massage nor bandage should be applied. Affected area should not be heated. It should not be applied on broken skin or wounds. These are applied externally so contact with eyes and mucous membrane should be avoided.

Iodine Methyl Salicylate

Iodex	**SKF**
Comp	Iodine 4%, Methyl Salicylate 5%
Adm.	Local application
@	As per need
Pres.	25 g

Iodyl oint	**Zydus**
Comp	Iodine 4.7%, Methyl Salicylate 5.9%
Adm.	Local application
@	As per need
Pres.	25 g

Briclofen Plus gel	**Brihans**
Comp	Diclofenae Sodium 1%, Methyl Salicylate 1%, Menthol 2%
Adm.	Local application
@	As per need
Pres.	30 g

Antifungal Topical

Clotrimazole

It is a synthetic imidazole derivative. It is used for skin infections due to yeasts and dermatophytes. In addition it has activity against certain Gram+ve bacterial and Trichomonas species used in fungal infections of skin and hair, for prevention of ringworm etc. Local irritation, itching and burning sensation can be there after its application

Myconil Powd	**Ranbaxy**
Comp	Clotrimazole 1% W/V
Adm.	Local application
@	As per need
Pres.	100 g

Canesten sol/cream	**Bayer**
Comp	Clotrimazole 1% W/V
Adm.	Local application
@	As per need
Pres.	100 g

Imidil Sol/ Cream/ Powder	Lyka
Comp	Clotrimazole 1% W/V
Adm.	Local application
@	As per need
Pres.	30 g Pow, 15 g Cream, 15 ml Sol

Antimicrobial Topical

Various topical ointments/ powders are available for the treatment of bacterial skin infections. These are applied or sprayed for primary and secondary skin infection. These are effective against various skin disorders. These are used locally after cleansing the effected part. These are also used in dressing of wounds, ulcers, cuts, yolk gall, foot rot, FMD lesions, burns and post operative lesions.

Gentim spray	Merial (Wockhardt)
Comp	Gentamicin sulphate 5 g/100 g
Adm.	Local application
@	As per need
Pres.	100 g

Gentamicine Sulphate	Lyka
Comp	Gentamicin sulphate 0.1%
Adm.	Local application
@	As per need
Pres.	50 g, 20 g

Oxytetracyclin

Oxytetracyclin Liq	Pfizer
Comp	Oxytetracyclin hydrochloride 50 mg/ml
Adm.	Local application
@	As per need
Pres.	60 ml

Oxy Liquid	Carevet Pharma
Comp	Oxytetracyclin hydrochloride 50mg/ml
Adm.	Local application
@	As per need
Pres.	60 ml, 100 ml

Ultrox Liq	Neospark
Comp	Oxytetracyclin hydrochloride 50mg/ml
Adm.	Local application
@	As per need
Pres.	60 ml, 100 ml

Miscellaneous combination

Spectrazole cream	Ranbaxy
Comp	Gentamicine sulphate 0.1% + clobetasol propionate 0.025% Miconazole nitrate 2%
Adm.	Local application
@	As per need
Pres.	20 g

Spectrocin oint	Zydus
Comp	Each g contains Neomycin sulphate 2.5 mg Gramicidine 0.25 mg Plastobase 9.5 mg
Adm.	Local application
@	As per need
Pres.	15 g tube

Vetbacin oint	Bayer
Comp	Each g contains Neomycin sulphate 5 mg Zinc bacitracin 500 IU
Adm.	Local application
@	As per need
Pres.	20 g tube

Micogel cream	Cipla
Comp	2% miconagale
Adm.	Local appllication
@	Aspect need
Pres.	15g

Kiskin Lotion	**Intas**
Comp	Miconazole nitrate 2%, clobetasol propionate 0.025% Gentamicin 0.1%
Adm.	Local
@	As per need
Pres.	30 ml, 100 ml

Furacin cream/Pow	**SKF**
Comp	Nitrofurazone 0.2%
Adm.	Local
@	As per need
Pres.	Cream 20 g, Pow 10 g

Canesten S cream	**Bayer**
Comp	Beclomethasone dispropionate 0.25 mg/10g
Adm.	Local application
@	As per need
Pres.	10 g tube

Coolmac oint	**Macnor** **126**
Comp	Boric acid 16% Zinc oxide 16% Cetrimide 0.8% Proflavin hemi sulphate 0.2% Iodoform 1.08%
Adm.	Local
@.	As per need
Pres.	50 g collapsible tube

Coolmac spray	**Macnor** **127**
Comp	Gamma benzene hexachloride 0.10% Proflavinhemi sulphate 0.10% Cetrimide 0.45%
Adm.	Local
@.	As per need
Pres.	100 ml bottle

Zymagout Wit liq	**Zydus** **262**
Comp	Turpentine oil 41.43% Neem oil 7.2% Camphor oil 6% Karanj oil 5.1% Turmeric oil 0.15%
Adm.	Spray local
As per nned	100-125 ml od
Pres.	40 ml, 100 ml

Wisporec cream/ Spray	**Boehringer Ingelheim**	**285**
Comp	Combination of Phytochemicals (1,8 Cineole, Eugonol, Menthrol and Ricinoleic acid)	
Adm.	Local	
@	As per need	
Pres.	100 ml, 200 ml aerosol spray, 25 g, 100 g tube	

Teeburb Cap.	**Indian Herbs**
Indi: Antibacteria in genital tract infection/mastitis	
Comp: Not given	
Adm: Local	
@ : 2 Cap. for 10 days or more	
Pres: 24 Cap. Pack	

Skinosole Cap.	**Arosol Herbal**
Indi: Skin in fections	
Comp: Not given	
Adm: Local	
@ : 2-3 Cap.2-3 times a day	
Pres: 20 Cap	

Septiban Spray			**Phoenix**
Indi: Wounds, FMD, Maggotwound, antiseptic			
Comp:			
Devdaru	83%	Neem	3%
Haldi	4%	T.T.oil	10%
Adm: Local			
@ : Spray on affected area 3-4 times a day.			
Pres: 75 ml, 100 ml, 200 ml			

Maggfite Spray	**Vet Avenue**
Indi: Ectoparasiticide, Kills maggots, heals wounds	
Comp: Seven oils of Indian Plants	
Adm: Local	
@ : Spray on affected area.	
Pres: 100 ml	

Povidone Iodine Preprations

Samodine spray	**Wockhardt**
Comp	Povidone Iodine 5.5% w/v
Adm.	Local
@	As per need
Pres.	80ml (60 g) spray can

Sterdine ointment	**Sterling Lab**
Comp	Povidone Iodine 5.5% w/v
Adm.	Local application
@	As per need
Pres.	100 ml, 500 ml

Wokadine Sol/ oint	**Wockhardt**
Comp	Povidone Iodine 5% w/v
Adm.	Local application
@	As per need
Pres.	100 ml, 500 ml, 30 g tube

Povisol sol.	**Vets Farma**
Comp	Povidone Iodine 5.5% w/v
Adm.	Local application
@	As per need
Pres.	100 ml, 500 ml, IL

Isopaint sol.	**Venkys**
Comp	Povidone Iodine 5% w/v
Adm.	Local application
@	As per need
Pres.	100 ml, 500 ml,

Pivodine sol.	**Vet Avenue**
Comp	Povidone Iodine 5.5% w/v
Adm.	Local application
@	As per need
Pres.	100 ml, 500 ml, IL

Betadin oint	Wockhardt
Comp	Povidone Iodine 5.5% w/v
Adm.	Local application
@	As per need
Pres.	30 g, 100 g

Cipladine Sol	Cipla
Comp	Povidone Iodine 5.5% w/v
Adm.	Local application
@	As per need
Pres.	100 ml, 500 ml

Indigenous

FM care Bolus	Rajshree
Comp	Not given
Adm.	Oral in FMD
@	LA 2 Bol bid for 5 day
Pres.	20's

Melabid tablet	Rajshree
Comp	Not given
Adm.	Oral
@	5-6 tab bid
Pres.	30's

Canisep cream	Himalya
Comp	Not given
Adm.	Local
@	As per need
Pres.	30 g

Charmil ointment	Ayurvet
Comp	Not given
Adm.	Local
@	As per need
Pres.	25 g, 50 g, 1 kg

Dermanol cream	**Indian Herbs**
Comp	Not given
Adm.	Local
@	As per need
Pres.	25 g

Dermocept cream	**Concept**
Comp	Not given
Adm.	Local
@	As per need
Pres.	25 g

Healup spray	**Century**
Comp	Not given
Adm.	Local
@	As per need
Pres.	250 ml

Dressol oint/ lotion	**Cattle Remedies**
Comp	Not given
Adm.	Local
@	As per need
Pres.	Ointment 50 g, 100 g, Lotion 450 ml

Ectosep ointment	**Zydus**
Comp	Not given
Adm.	Local (Antiseptic)
@	As per need
Pres.	50 g

Ectozee spray	**Venkys**
Comp	Not given
Adm.	Local (Antiseptic)
@	As per need
Pres.	200 ml

Himax oint/ Lotion	**Natural Remedies**
Comp	Not given
Adm.	Local (Antiseptic)
@	As per need
Pres.	Lotion 100 ml, Oint 10 g pouch 100 g tube 1 kg Jar

Himax D ointment	Indian Herbs
Comp	Not given
Adm.	Local (Antiseptic)
@	As per need
Pres.	25 g

HSD oint	Alembic
Comp	Not given
Adm.	Local Antibacterial, Antifungal
@	As per need
Pres.	50 g

Magout WH Liq	Zydus
Comp	Not given
Adm.	Local (Ectoparasite, Myasis)
@	As per need
Pres.	40 ml, 100 ml

Maggacite lotion	Cattle Remedies
Comp	Not given
Adm.	Local Myasis, Scabies
@	As per need
Pres.	100 ml, 450 ml

New Charm gel	Ayurvet
Comp	Not given
Adm.	Local Multiation
@	As per need
Pres.	25 g tube

Ostaderm ointment	Vets Farma
Comp	Not given
Adm.	Local Antibacterial, Antifungal
@	As per need
Pres.	50 g, 500 g

Scavon cream/ spray	Himalya
Comp	Not given
Adm.	Local Antibacterial, Antifungal application
@	As per need
Pres.	50 g cream, 120 ml spray

Wisprec oint	**Natural Remedies**
Comp	Not given
Adm.	Local Antibacterial, Antifungal application
@	As per need
Pres.	25 g tube

Vetomax omit	**Rakesh Pharma**
Comp	Not given
Adm.	Local Antibacterial, Antifungal application
@	As per need
Pres.	50 g tube, 1 kg tin

Topicure Spray/ Gel	**Natural Remedies**
Comp	Not given
Adm.	Local in wounds
@	Once/ twice a day
Pres.	Spray 75 ml, 250 ml, Gel 10 g, 50 g

Skinomen oitment	**Arosol Herbal**
Indi: Antiseptic dressing	
Comp: Not given	
Adm: Local	
@ : Apply locally	
Pres: 50 g, 1 kg	

Dermocept Cream			**Concept Pharma**
Indi: Ectoparasiticide, Fly repellant			
Comp:			
Kutaja	2.310%	Ratanjot	1%
Nimba	3.075%	Karanj oil	20%
Haridra	3.075%	Neem oil	5%
Daruharidra	1.540%		
Adm: Local			
@ : Apply locally on affected part twice daily			
Pres: 2.5 g tube			

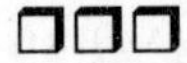

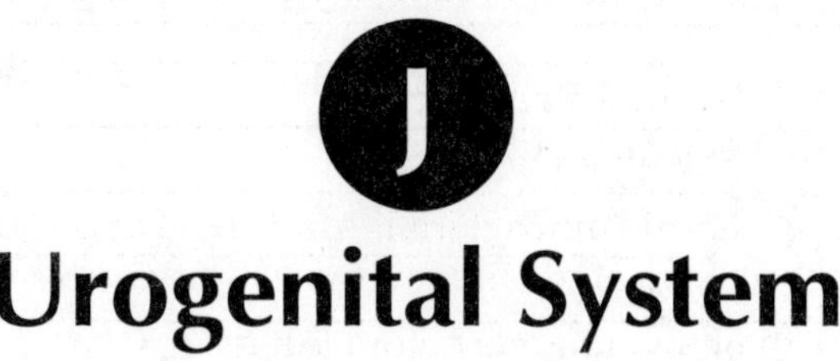

Urogenital System

Diseases/ Conditions of Urogenital System

Abortion: Foetus discharge from day 42 until normal day of parturition or prior to full gestation.

Anoestrus: Failure of oestrus cycle or heat.

Anuria: Complete absence of urine.

Cervicitis: Inflammation of cervix.

Congenital defects: Defects from the mother before birth.

Crystalluria: urine containing crystals of urea.

Cystitis: Inflammation of urinary bladder.

Dystokia: Difficult expulsion or birth of youngone or foetus even after full conception period.

Dysuria: Painful or difficult urination.

Early Enbryonic death: Death occurring from day of conception to day 42 of gestation.

Endometritis: Inflammation of inner wall of Uterus.

Glycosuria: Presence of glucose in urine.

Hematuria: Urine containing blood.

Hydrocele: collection of fluid present within outer coat of testicle.

Hydronephrosis: enlargement of kidney due to obstruction in ureter.

Infertility: Failure to breed.

Ketonuria: Presence of Ketone bodies in urine.

Mastitis: Inflammation of mammary gland, characterised by physical, chemical and usually bacteriological changes in milk and pathological changes in glandular tissues.

Metritis: Inflammation of uterus.

Miscarriage: Loss of products of conception from uterus before foetus is viable.

Mummification: Shrivelling of dead and retain foetus.

Myglobinuria: Presence of myoglobin in urine.

Neo-natal: Since birth or from mother's womb.

Nephritis: Inflammation of kidney.

Nephrosis: Degeneration with inflammatory lesion of renal tubules.

Oliguria: Reduction in daily output of urine.

Oophoritis: Inflammation of ovary.

Potency: Power gynaecologically ability of male to perform several act.

Premature birth: Birth of a youngone before full term.

Prolapse: Slipping down of some organ or structure. Usually applied to displacements of rectum & female generative organs.

Proteinuria: Urine containing small amounts of protein.

Pyelonephritis: Inflammation of kidney with pus in urine.

Pyometra: Inflammation of uterus with pus symptom of abnormal vaginal discharge.

Pyuria: Presence of pus in urine.

Repeat breeder: Animal does not conceive and there is regular oestrus after insemination

Retained Placente: ROP (Retention of Placenta) when placenta does not come out after parturition for 6-12 hrs.

Salpingitis: Inflammation of oviduct.

Silent Heat: Animal comes to heat with no apparent signs.

Still Birth: Expulsion of dead foetus at full term.

Summer Mastitis: Mastitis of non-lactating animals caused by Corynebacterium pyogenes.

Uraemia: Terminal stage of renal insufficiency with anuria and oliguria.

Urolithiasis: Urethral obstruction in urinary passage characterised by complete retention of urine unsuccessful efforts to urinate, distention of bladder. It is caused by deposition of carbonates, phosphates of Calcium and Magnesium.

Vaginitis: Inflammation of Vagina.

Vulvitis: Inflammation of Vulva.

Diuretics

These are the drugs which increase the rate of urine flow and induces natriuresis (Na-Sodium), Kaluresis (K-Potassium) and Chlorouresis (cl-chlorine) and modify renal handling of other ions and uric acids. Water is physiological diuretic.

There are various types of diuretics.

(A) Agents which increases glomerular filteration.

(B) Agents which increase renal solute excretion or osmotic diuretics.

(C) Agents which inhibit transport of sodium.

(D) Potassium sparing diuretics.

(E) Agents which depress Hydrogen for Na excretion.

Various diuretics are given to animals in acute pulmonary or cerebral oedema, Ascites and post-parturient oedema.

Frusemide

It is a loop of Henle diuretic. It is rapidly acting and high efficacious diuretic. Onset of action is prompt. Active absorption of sodium and chloride from the ultra filterate at the luminal phase of loop cells is reduced. The action is also associated with increased medullary blood flow and reduces intestinal hypertonocity and thus reduces the reabsorption efficiency of loop.

It is indicated in Odema of all type of forced diuresis in poisoning.

Lasix inj/ Tab	**Intervet – Novartis**
Comp	Frusemide 50 mg/ml 40 mg Tab
Adm.	Inj IM or IV Tablet orally
@	LA 5-10 ml SA 1ml/10 kg B.wt 6 hourly LA 0.5-1 mg/kg orally SA 1mg/kg B.wt
Pres.	10 ml, strip of 10

Ridema inj	**Wockhardt**
Comp	Frusemide 50 mg/ml
Adm.	IM/ IV
@	LA 5-10 ml SA 1 ml/10 kg B.wt 6 hourly
Pres.	10 ml

Urul	**Bhartiya Boote-Bhaven**
Comp	Not given
Adm.	Oral
@	LA 40-60 g bid SA 15-30 g bid
Pres.	100 g, 1 kg

Nephtone	**Indian Herbs**
Comp	Not given
Adm.	Oral
@	LA 40-60 g bid SA 15-30 g bid
Pres.	100 g, 1 kg

Urinary Antiseptics/ Antispasmodics

Due to Excretory function of urinary tract special antibiotics and antiseptics are used for the treatment of urinary tract infections. These are drugs which act on urinary tract before their elimination. These are indicated in acute and chronic genito-urinary infections.

Hexamine

It is hydrolysed to formaldehyde in the presence of acid and its action is due to this agent.

Hexamine inj	**Generic**
Comp	40% Sol. of Hexamine
Adm.	IM
@	LA 8-10 ml, SA 2-4 ml
Pres.	5 ml, 10 ml

Hexamine Powder	**Generic**
Comp	Hexamine powder
Adm.	Oral
@	LA 4-12 g
Pres.	100 g, 450 g

Cystone Tab/ Powder	**Generic**
Indi	Urinary calculi
Comp	Not given
Adm.	Oral
@	10 Tab tid 5 gm tid
Pres.	100 Tab, 50 g

Dicyclomine

It acts on G.I tract, biliary tract, ureter, uterus without producing any antisecretory effects. It acts directly on smooth muscles as muscle relaxant. It is indicated in renal colic & Spasmodic pain.

Picorex Bol	**Pranav**
Comp	Each Bol. Contains Dicyclomine hydrochloride 100 mg Diclofenac sod. 250 mg Paracetamol 1500 mg
Adm.	Oral
@	LA 1-2 Bol bid SA ½ -1 Bol bid
Pres.	Strip of 4

Jospas inj	**Animax Healthcare**
Indi	Uterine, GI tract, uterine smooth muscle
Comp	Dicyclomine hydrochloride 10 mg/ml
Adm.	IM
@	1 ml
Pres.	30 ml

Spas inj	**G.Loucotos**
Indi	Uterine, GI tract, uterine smooth muscle
Comp	Dicyclomine hydrochloride 10 mg/ml
Adm.	IM
@	1 ml
Pres.	30 ml

Spasmovet	**Wockhardt**
Indi	Uterine, GI tract, uterine smooth muscle
Comp	Dicyclomine hydrochloride 10 mg/ml
Adm.	IM
@	1 ml
Pres.	30 ml

Libragen Bol	**Libra**
Comp	Dicyclomine and Mefenamic acid
Adm.	Oral
@.	2-4 Bolus od
Pres.	4 Bol strip

Urolithiasis

Cystone Pow. — **Himalya**

Indi: Urinary Calculi, Haematuria

Comp: Each gm. contains

Onsoma bracteatum	72 mg	Didymocarpus pedicellata	291 mg
Saxifragaligulata	22 mg	Rubia cordifolia	72 mg
Cyperusscariosus	72 mg	Achryanthesaspera	72 mg
Croniacinerea	72 mg	Shilajit	58 mg
Hajroolyahood Bhasm	72 mg		

Adm: Oral
@ : 2-3½ g thrice daily for 4-6 days
Pres: 10 × 50 g pack

Stonil Pow.	**Indian Herbs**
Indications: Urinary Calculi, Diuretic	
Composition: Not given	
Dosage: 40-50 g daily	
Presentation: 100 g,1 kg	

Drugs Acting on Female Genital System (Ovaries)

Gonadotropin Releasing Hormone (GnRH)

(Buserelin)

It stimulates follicular development, ovulation and enhances release of Leutinising Hormone (LH) and /follicular stimulating hormone (FSH). This is GnRH analogue and is very potent as compared to others. Indicated in Anoestrus, silent heat, delayed ovulation, follicular cysts and for improving conception rete.

Receptal	**Intervet (Novartis)**
Comp	Each ml contains 0.0042 mg equivalent to 0.004 mg Buserelin
Adm.	IM/IV
@	For anoestrus LA 5 ml SA 1 ml Horse 10 ml For delayed Ovulation LA 2.5 ml SA 0.5 ml Horse 5 ml For cystic ovary LA 2.5ml SA 0.5ml Horse 5ml For conception rate after A1 and oestrous synchronization LA 2.5 ml SA 0.2 ml
Pres.	10 ml

Gynatone inj	**Libra**
Comp	Buserlin 0.004 mg/ml
Adm.	IM/ IV
@.	2.5 ml
Pres.	2.5 ml and 5 ml

Zydarelin inj	**Zydus**
Comp	Burserelin acetate 4.2 mcg/ml
Adm.	IM/IV/SC
@	5 ml for Synchronisation of heat 2.5 ml
Pres.	2.5 ml, 5 ml, 10 ml

Fertibin inj	**Alivira**
Comp	Buserelin 4 mcg/ml
Adm.	IM/ IV/ SC
@	Anoestrus 5 ml, Cyst 5 ml, Conception 2.5 ml
Pres.	2.5 ml, 5 ml with syringe and needle

Gonadorelin

It is a hypothalamic decapeptide that stimulates the secretion of both FSH and LH thus stimulates follicular development oestrous and ovulation. It is indicated in ovarian diseases, delayed ovulation, repeat breeder and improvement of fertility after post partum.

Fertagyl	**Intervet (Novartis)**
Comp	0.1 mg/ml of Gonadorelin
Adm.	IM or IV
@	For cystic ovaries 100 mcg. For ovulation or Repeaters 250 mcg
Pres.	1ml

Cystorelin	**BCAHP**
Comp	500 mcg/ml, 50 mcg/ml Gonadorelin
Adm.	IM/IV
@	For cystic ovaries 100 mcg. For ovulation or Repeaters 250 mcg
Pres.	1ml

Pituitary Gonadotropine

Follicular Stimulating Hormone (FSH)

It induces folliculogenesis in mature female ovaries. It is indicated for true oestrus in inactive ovaries for superovulation in embryotransfer technology in donor cows. It is contraindicated in swines.

Follitropin V	**Vets Farma**
Comp	FSH 400 mg/vial
Adm.	IM
@	LA 50 mg bid for 4 days
Pres.	400 mg vial with 20 ml diluent

Luteinizing Hormone (LH)

It is also a pituitary gonadotropin. It induces maturation and estrogen production which takes care of growth of corpus luteum and ovulation of Graffian follicles. It is indicated in delayed ovulation, anovulation, cystic ovaries and repeat breeders.

Lutropin V	**Vet Farma**
Comp	LH 25mg/ml
Adm.	IV
@	LA 2.5 mg SA 2.5 mg Swine 5 mg
Pres.	25 mg vial with 5ml diluent

Serum Gonadotropin

It stimulates growth of ovaries as well as its maturation. It influences ovulation rate. In males it stimulates development of testis and accessory sexual glands. It is useful in anoestrous and in active ovaries and impaired spermatogenesis.

Folligon inj	**Intervet**
Comp	Each ml contains 1000 or 5000 serum gonadotropin BVC
Adm.	SC/ IM
@	Anoestrous LA 1500-3000 IU In R.B after 10-14 days Miss first heat. Mares 3000-6000 IU
Pres.	1000 IU with 5 ml diluent

Non Pituitary Gonadotropins

Human Chorionic Gonadotropin

It is non pituitary Gonadotropin which acts as Pituitary Luteinizing hormone causing ovulation. It promotes the formation and maintenance of corpus luteum in females. It is indicated in Repeat Breeders, cystic ovaries, early abortion and delayed ovulation.

Chorulon Inj	**Intervet (Novortis)**
Comp	Each vial contains chorionic Gonadotropin (LH) 1500 IU
Adm.	IM / IU
@	LA 1500 IU- 3000 IU SA 100 IU-500 IU
Pres.	1500 IU vial

Corrogan	**BCAHP**
Comp	Each vial contains 250 IU/ml of chorionic Gonadotropin
Adm.	IM/ IV
@	LA 1500 IU- 3000 IU SA 100 IU-500 IU
Pres.	1000 IU, 2000 IU vials

Prolan inj	**Bayer**
Comp	Each ml contains 500 IU Human chorionic Gonodotropin
Adm.	IM/ IV
@	LA 1500 IU- 3000 IU SA 100 IU-500 IU
Pres.	2 ml vial

Gonadotropin Combination

Some formulations have both FSH and LH. These are indicated to improve the quality and yield of super ovulation in embryo transfer in bovines and ovines.

Apocrine inj Dry	**Bayer**
Comp	Each ampoule of 2 ml contains FSH = 500 IU LH = 1500 IU
Adm.	IM
@	LA 500-1000 IU SA 100-200 IU
Pres.	2 ml

Ovaset inj	**BCAHP**
Comp	FSH – 0.48 mg/9ml LH – 0.42 mg/ 3 ml
Adm.	IM
@	I day 6 ml bid II day 5 ml bid. III day 3 ml bid. IV day 2 ml bid
Pres.	9 ml FSH, 3 ml LH ampoules, 12 ml diluent

Menogen inj	**Associated Lab**
Comp	Each ml contains FSH activity 75 IU, LH activity 75 IU
Adm.	IM
@	1 ml in LA
Pres.	1 ml

Nymfalon	**Intervet**
Indi	Cystic ovary
Comp	Freeze dried Human chorionic Gonadotropin 3000 IU, Progestron 125 mg/ vial
Adm.	IV
@	1 vial slow
Pres.	1 vial

Pregnant Mare Serum Gonadotropin

It is used as Non pituitary gonadotropin. It effects FSH by inducing follicular growth in inactive ovaries of matured animals. It is indicated in anoestrus, inactive ovaries and to induce super ovulation for embryo transfer.

Folligon	**Intervet**
Comp	Each vial contains 1000 IU of PMSG
Adm.	IV/ SC
@	LA 1500-3000 IU Result in 2-5 days. Repeat 10-14 days SA 1000 IU Result in 24 hrs. if needed repeat after 72 hrs
Pres.	1000 IU vial with solvent

Synchro PMSG 400	**BCAHP**
Comp	400 IU PMSG in vial
Adm.	IV/ SC
@	LA 1500-3000 IU Result in 2-5 days. Repeat 10-14 days SA 1000 IU Result in 24 hrs. if needed repeat after 72 hrs
Pres.	400 IU vial + 2 diluent PSMG 500 IU vial + 2 ml diluent PSMG 700 IU + 2 ml diluent PSMG 600 IU vial + 2 ml diluent PSMG 6000 IU + 2 ml diluent

Trophovet	**Indian Immunology**
Comp	Each vial contains 1000 IU of PMSG
Adm.	IV/ SC
@	LA 1500-3000 IU Result in 2-5 days. Repeat 10-14 days SA 1000 IU Result in 24 hrs. if needed repeat after 72 hrs
Pres.	1000 IU vial with solvent

Ovarian Steroids

These are used to stimulate ovaries for inducing ovulation and strengthen the uterine wall and normal secretions and hormones.

Hydroxy Progestron

Its main function is prepration of uterus for nidation and maintenance of Pregnancy. It strengthens uterine wall and reduces its motility to maintain pregnancy. It inhibits immunological and rejection of foetus. It reduces T cell function and cell mediated immunity. It is indicated in habitual and threatened abortion, infertility due to corpus luteum insufficiency, prolapse of uterus and anoestrus due to delayed involution, early embryonic death, cystic ovarian disease as a supportive treatment.

Curaprogen	**Carevet Pharma**
Comp	Each ml contains 250 mg of 17 Hydroxyprogestrone caproate
Adm.	IM
@	LA 750 mg/ week of 3 weeks SA 125-250 mg/week
Pres.	3 ml

Duraprogen	**Cargill (Unichem)**
Comp	Each ml contains 250 mg of 17 Hydroxy progestrone caproate
Adm.	IM
@	LA 750 mg/ week of 3 weeks SA 125-250 mg/week
Pres.	2 ml

Hyprogen	**Vets Farma**
Comp	Each ml contains 250 mg of 17 Hydroxy progestrone caproate
Adm.	IM
@	LA 750 mg/ week of 3 weeks SA 125-250 mg/week
Pres.	2 ml, 3 ml

Nobort	**Vest**
Comp	Each ml contains 250 mg of 17 Hydroxy progestrone caproate
Adm.	IM
@	LA 750 mg/ week of 3 weeks SA 125-250 mg/week
Pres.	3 ml

Reset	Vet Pharma
Comp	Each ml contains 250 mg of 17 Hydroxy progestrone caproate
Adm.	IM
@	LA 750 mg/ week of 3 weeks SA 125-250 mg/week
Pres.	3 ml

Vetraprogen	Primavet Care
Comp	Each ml contains 250 mg of 17 Hydroxy progestrone caproate
Adm.	IM
@	LA 750 mg/ week of 3 weeks SA 125-250 mg/week
Pres.	2 ml

Fixo	Marc
Comp	Each ml contains 250 mg of 17 Hydroxy progestrone caproate
Adm.	IM
@	LA 750 mg/ week of 3 weeks SA 125-250 mg/week
Pres.	2 ml, 3 ml

P-Depot	Zydus
Comp	Each ml contains 250 mg of 17 Hydroxy progestrone caproate
Adm.	IM
@	LA 750 mg/ week of 3 weeks SA 125-250 mg/week
Pres.	3 ml

Progestagen Norgestomet

It is a synthetic Progestagen. Its effect increase LH activity resulting in oestrum and ovulation. It also acts as hypothalamic hypopyseal system preventing final growth and maturation of follicles. It can be used only in healthy animals. It is indicated to control or induce or synchronise ovulation in normal healthy animals.

Crester	Intervet
Comp	Norgestomet 3 mg (Oestradiol valerate 5 mg Norgestomet 3 mg/ml)
Adm.	SC implantation on ear. Or IM injection
@	3 mg implant or 2ml IM in LA 1.5 mg implant SC or 0.5 ml inj IM
Pres.	Implant +2 ml inj

Synchromate B	BCAHP		
Comp	Norgestomet 6 mg	Oestradiol valerate 5 mg	Norgestomet 3 mg/ml
Adm.	6 mg implant SC on ear or 2 ml IM inj in LA SA 3 mg implant SC on ear or 0.5 ml inj IM		
@	3 mg implant or 2 ml IM in LA 1.5 mg implant SC or 0.5 ml inj IM		
Pres.	Implant + 2 ml inj		

Nymfalon inj	Intervet
Comp	Freeze dried ovary Human chorionic gonadotrophin 3000 IU & Progestron 125 mg/ vial
Adm.	IV
@	1 vial
Pres.	Vial

Prostaglandin

Prostaglandin (PG) are members of endogenous fatty acid derivatives synthesized from cell membrane phospholipids. Naturally occurring PG is the derivative of fatty acid named Prostanoic acid. Classification is as a subscript to the letter e.g. PG1, PG2, PGE1, PGE3 etc. the involvement of PG in reproductive system is mainly associated with luteolysis, absorption and parturition. Mainly these cause regression of corpus luteum by their luteolytic action and induce fertile heat.

Cloprostenol Sodium

It is prostaglandin F2. It is indicated in subestrum, luteal cyst, synchronized breeding, removal of mummified foetus, treat chronic endometritis, pyometra and it induce parturition. It is contra-indicated in pregnancy except for termination of pregnancy. Drugs should be kept away from pregnant women & persons suffering with asthma or respiratory tract ailment.

Juramate inj	Vet Care
Comp	Cloprostenol sodium 263 mcg/ml provides 250 mcg/ml chloprostenol
Adm.	IM
@	LA 2 ml
Pres.	10 ml

Vetmate inj	**Vet Care**
Comp	Cloprostenol sodium 263 mcg/ml provides 250 mcg/ml chloprostenol
Adm.	IM
@	LA 2 ml
Pres.	2 ml

Synchromate inj	**Primavet Care**
Comp	Cloprostenol sodium 263 mcg/ml provides 250 mcg/ml chloprostenol
Adm.	IM
@	LA 2 ml
Pres.	4 ml

Metrum inj	**Macwell**
Comp	Cloprostenol sodium 263 mcg/ml provides 250 mcg/ml chloprostenol
Adm.	IM
@	LA 2 ml
Pres.	2 ml

Pragma	**Intas**
Comp	Cloprostenol sodium 263 mcg/ml provides 250 mcg/ml chloprostenol
Adm.	IM
@	LA 2 ml
Pres.	2 ml

Clostenol inj	**Zydus**	**228**
Comp	Cloprostenol 263 mcg provide 250 mcg	
Adm.	IM	
@	2 ml	
Pres.	2 ml with syringe	

Alpha 2 inj	**Boehringer Ingelheim**	**271**
Comp	Cloprostenol 263 mcg	Provides 250 mcg cloproslenol
Adm.	IM	
@	2 ml	
Pres.	2 ml vial	

PG X injection	Alivira 309
Comp	Cloprostenol inj 250 mcg/ml
Adm.	IM
@	2 ml
Pres.	2 ml

Dinoprost

PGF_2 is like all other PGF_2. Its action is also luteolytic. It also acts by constriction of uterovarian vessels. It also enhances cervical dilation. It is used as other PGF_2. All precautions indicated are same as other prostaglandin.

Dinofertin inj	Merial
Comp	Dinoprost 5 mg/ml
Adm.	IM
@	Bovine 5 ml, Equines 10 ml
Pres.	5 ml

Hermo P_2 Alpha	BCAHP
Comp	Dinoprost 5 mg/ml
Adm.	IM
@	Bovine 5 ml, Equines 10 ml
Pres.	5 ml

Lutalyse	Novartis
Comp	Dinoprost 5mg/ml
Adm.	IM
@	Bovine 5 ml, Equines 10 ml
Pres.	10 ml

Luprostiol

It is PGF_2 and also causes regression of corpus luteum followed by follicular growth, oestrus and ovulation in case of silent heaters or anoestrus cases. General precaution and contraindications are same as for other PG. site of injection must be cleaned and disinfected before injecting.

Prosolvin inj	Intervet
Comp	Luprostiol 7.5 mg/ml
Adm.	IM
@	LA 15 mg Heifers 7.5 mg
Pres.	2 ml, 10 ml, 20 ml

Tiaprost

It is also PGF_2. Its action indication, precaution and contraindications are same as for other PGF.

Iliren inj	Intervet
Comp	Tiaprost 0.196 mg/ml
Adm.	IM/ IV/SC
@	Bovines 5 ml IM or SC 2. 5 ml IV, Equines 3 ml IV Caprine 1-1.5 ml SC
Pres.	10 ml

Oxytocin

It is a nanopeptide hormone. It has very specific action on uterine smooth muscles as well as myoepithelial cells of mammary glands and myometrium. Due to their action oxytocin is used for the stimulation of uterine debris and helps in letting down of milk also. It can also be used in uterine prolapse, induction of parturition and expulsion of last offspring in polytochous animals.

Syntocinon	Novartis
Comp	Oxytocin 5 IU/ ml
Adm.	IM or IV
@	Mare 75-150 IU Cattle 75-100 IU, Sheep, goats 30-50 IU
Pres.	1 ml

Intertocine S inj	Intervet
Comp	Oxytocin 10 IU/ml
Adm.	IM or IV
@	LA 75-100 IU
Pres.	10 ml

Valethamate

It is a smooth muscle relaxant. It is useful in delayed dilation of cervix during parturition. It is indicated in spasm of smooth muscle and in normal labour to help easy expulsion of foetus in dystocia and hard cervix.

Epidosin inj	TTK
Comp	Valethamate bromide 10 mg/ml
Adm.	IM
@	LA 10-15 ml, SA 2.5-5 ml
Pres.	5 ml vial

Others

Oestrogen

These are steroidal oestrogens. These are natural estrogen like oestradiols, estrone and estriols. It is synthesized in the graffian follicle, corpus luteum & placenta. All are found in blood. Synthetic estrogens are also available which can be steroid or Non-Steroid. Natural oestrogen are inactive orally and have a short duration of action due to rapid metabolism in liver Estrogen bring about puberty. These can lead to polydipsia, polyuria, upsets G.I tract, suppresses Red blood cells production. Its chronic use may lead to impotency, feminization in males. These are used in Prostatic hypertrophy and excessive libido.

(No product available in veterinary)

Testosterone

This is androgen. Androgens are products of gonads and steroidal hormone. Their synthetic analogues have same properties. These cause development of secondary sex characters and growth of genitals. Testosterone is inactive orally. Duration of action after IM injection is also very short.

Testosterone propionate and esters of Testosterone have prolonged action. It may increase libido and have favourable effect on spermatogenesis. It is helpful in building body tissue, bones and in erythropoiesis. Thus effecting anabolic action. Indicated in Hypoganadism, infertility due to oligospermia, cryptorchidism, delayed puberty, premature sterility.

Durateston inj	**Intervet**
Comp	Combination 4 testosterone esters 30 mg T propionate 60 mg T phenylpropionate 60 mg T isocaprote 100 mg T decanoate
Adm.	IM/ SC
@	5 ml in adult LA
Pres.	Vial of 5 ml, 50 mg of easters/ ml

Drugs Acting on Uterus

Some of Drugs which act on ovaries also on uterus also cloprostenol, Dinoprost. Hydroxy Progesterone, Luprositol, oxytocin, Tiaprost, Valethamate are such products. Ergometrine is ergot alkaloid and used for action on uterus.

Methyl Ergometrin

It is ergot alkaloid and acts by stimulating Myometrium through alpha receptors and also constriction of vascular smooth muscles. It lacks vasoconstriction action. It is indicated to expel uterine debris and induce uterine involution.

Methergin inj	**Novartis**
Comp	Methyl ergotmetrine 0.5 mg/ml
Adm.	IM, IV
@	0.1 mg/10 kg B.wt
Pres.	1 ml ampoule

Ecobolics

These are the drugs or combination of ingredient which cleanse the uterus, expel uterine debris after parturition and helps in involution thus expedite timely ovulation. Mostly combination of herbs is used. These are also given as uterine tonic after parturition.

Bangshil	**Alarsin**
Comp	Not given
Adm.	Oral
@	LA 10 Tab od for 2 weeks SA 3 Tab bid for 2 weeks

CP Vet	**Rajshree**
Comp	Not given
Adm.	Oral
@	2 Bol bid x 10 days
Pres.	20

Metrigon liq	**Rajshree**
Comp	Not given
Adm.	Oral
@	30 ml
Pres.	60 ml

Metasil Bol	**Rajshree**
Comp	Not given
Adm.	Oral
@	2 Bol bid for 5-10 days
Pres.	20 Bol

Replanta Pow	Indian Herbs
Comp	Not given
Adm.	Oral
@	50 gm od x 5 days
Pres.	100 g

Exapar Liq/Bol	Ayurvet	
Comp	Plumbago zeylanical	Uraria picta
	Citrullus colocynthis	Leptadenia reticulate
	Tribulus terrestris	Leipidium sativum
	Rubia cordifolia	Saussurea lappa
	Gardenia gummifera	Aristolochia indica
	Taxus baccata	Gloriosa superba
	Gossypium herbaceum	Cyperus rotundus
	Caesalpinia crista	Aloe barbadensis
	Peganumhermala	Desmodium gangeticum
		Piper longum
Adm.	Oral	
@	4 Bol twice on first day followed by 50 ml or 2 Bol twice daily for 3 days	
Pres.	500 ml bottle 4 Bol strip	

Utronix Liq	Phoenix			
Comp	Chitkara	160 mg	Languli	120 mg
	Pippali	80 mg	Jivanti	160 mg
	Sthanuneya	120 mg	Rakt inravaruni	20 mg
	Candrasura	160 mg	Karpassa	160 mg
	Salaparni	60 mg	Harman	160 mg
	Latakranja	120 mg	Prsniparni	40 mg
	Manjishtha	160 mg	Kushtha	60 mg
	Kasis	120 mg	Nadihingu	80 mg
	Kumari	80 mg	Musta	120 mg
	Neela tootia	20 mg	ishvari	160 mg
	Zinc sulphate	20 mg	goksura	40 mg
Adm.	Oral			
@	100 ml daily for 10 days			
Pres.	500 ml, 1L			

Mactone Forte Liq/bol	**Macwell**			
Comp	5 ml contains		Bolus contains	
	Mai	25 mg	Vividang	50 mg
	Kamalpushpi	200 mg	Jeevanti	150 mg
	Lodhra	150 mg	Devdar	100 mg
	Harmal	400 mg	Mochras	100 mg
	Ashoka	400 mg	Arjunbark	150 mg
	Ashoka	1000 mg	Manjeeth	25 mg
	Ashvagandha	100 mg	Mochras	50 mg
	Amar beej	100 mg	Devidar	100 mg
	Shatawari	50 mg	Maju	50 mg
	Shatavari	500 mg	Lodhar	100 mg
	Amla	100 mg	Nagkesar	25 mg
	Dashmool	500 mg	Triphla	600 mg
	Bhringraj	50 mg	Jeevanti	50 mg
	Daruldi	500 mg	Balamood	100 mg
	Dashmool	50 mg	Kamalpushpi	150 mg
	Chandan	500 g	Jamhu seed	100 mg
	Chandan	25 mg	Sahera	200 mg
	Gokhru	100 mg	majeeth	50 mg
Adm.	Oral			
@	100 ml od for 5-10 days		4 Bol od for 5-10 days	
Pres.	1L, 4 Bol			

Utromaxx	**Vet Avenue**
Comp	Not given
Adm.	Oral
@	50 ml twice daily x 5 days
Pres.	500 ml

Avitone liq	**Avivet Pharma**
Comp	Not given
Adm.	Oral
@	100 ml bid
Pres.	1L

Utromac Pow/LIq	Macnor Life Science
Comp	Not given 12 herbs in Powder, 21 herbs in Liquid
Adm.	Oral
@	Liq 100 ml od x 10 days Pow 5 gm bid x 5 days
Pres.	1L, 5 gm x 4

Herboleen Liq	Rajshree
Comp	Not given
Adm.	Oral
@	100 ml od for 5-10 days
Pres.	500 ml, 1L

Utrilift Liq	Indian Herbs
Comp	Not given
Adm.	Oral
@	100 ml od x 5 days
Pres.	500 ml

Estrona Forte Bol	Rakesh Pharma
Comp	Not given
Adm.	Oral
@	100 ml od for 10 days
Pres.	10 Bol, 100 Bol

Endotrin liq	Cadila Pharma
Comp	Not given
Adm.	Oral
@	100 ml bid
Pres.	500 ml

Vetrotone Liq	Cattle Remedies			
Comp	10 ml contains			
	Desmodium gangetium	370 mg	Ginelina arborea	370 mg
	Uraria pica	370 mg	Tribulus terrestris	370 mg
	Saraca indica	370 mg	Caesalpinia bonduc	370 mg
	Solanum indicum	370 mg	Aloe barbadensis	74 mg
	Solanum xanthocarpum	370 mg	Sodium tetraboarte	74 mg

	Aegle marmelos	370 mg	Ferrous sulphate	74 mg
	Clerodendrum multiflorum	370 mg	Copper sulphate	37 mg
Adm.	Oral			
@	100 ml od x 5 days			
Pres.	225 ml, 450 ml, 900 ml			

Utrobolic	**Argano Organic**
Comp	Not given
Adm.	Oral
@	75 ml od x 5 days
Pres.	500 ml, 1L

Uklean	**Venky**			
Comp	100 ml provides extract of			
	Vasa	2.0 g	Copper	120 mg
	Karpasa	2.0 g	Cobalt	96 mg
	Candrika	1.5 g	Iron	240 mg
	Citraka	1.5 g	Zinc	48 mg
	Langeli	1.5 g	Harmale	0.9 g
Adm.	Oral			
@	200 ml day followed by 100 ml od x 3 days			
Pres.	500 ml, 1L			

Utroplanta Pow	**Arosol Herbal**
Comp	Not given
Adm.	Oral
@	50 g bid
Pres.	100 g, 500 g

Involon Bol	**Natural Remedies**
Comp	Not given
Adm.	Oral
@	1 Bol bid
Pres.	4 Bol

Utrasafe Liq	**Vetmankind**
Comp	Not given
Adm.	Oral
@	450 ml 6 hrs post parturition
Pres.	450 ml

Uclear Liq	Nicosia International		
Comp	21 herbs		
	Dashmoola	Vansmool	Ugragandha
	Vasaka	Mulethi	Ashoka
	Methi	Sonth	Bel
	Bahera	Safed jira	Brahmi
	Manjish	Harmol	Sonth
	Ishuwari	Kalimirch	Gajar seed
	Guggal	Gokhru	
Adm.	Oral		
@	100 ml od x 10 days		
Pres.	500 ml, 1L		

Gynatone Syp	Cattle Remedies			
Comp	200 ml contains			
	Ashoka	5g	Harmal	2g
	Kapas	1g	Ultakambal	3g
	Sonth	1g	Ghingwar	1g
	Methi	2g	Gudhal	1g
	Jeera	1g	Trikana	1g
	Raktshalmali	1g	Tapeswani	1g
	Agnishikha	1g	Shikhamulum	2g
	Nagarmothe	1g	Deepayaka	1g
	Pitohari	2g	Hapusha	1g
	Daru	1g	Isharman	1g
	Upkunchike	1g		
Adm.	Oral			
@	100 ml od x 5 days			
Pres.	225 ml, 450 ml, 900 ml			

Roptone Liq	Pranav
Comp	Not given
Adm.	Oral
@	100 ml od x 5
Pres.	450 ml

Garbhjali Liq	Patanjali
Comp	Not given
Adm.	Oral
@	100 ml od x10 days
Pres.	1L

Centroton Bol	**Century**
Comp	Each Bolus contains Rubia cordifolia 1g; Leptadania reticulata 1g Harmala 750 mg; Aristolochia bracteata 750 mg Myrrh 500 mg
Adm.	Oral
@	1-2 Bol
Pres.	Strip of 2 Bol

Centroton U Bol	**Century**
Comp	Herbs (Not given)
Adm.	Oral
@	1-2 Bolus bid
Pres.	Strip of 4

Clinosol Pow	**Bhartiya Boote Bhavan**
Comp	Herbs
Adm.	Oral
@	50-60 g daily
Pres.	100 g, 1 kg

Endotrin liq	**Cadila Pharma**
Comp	Not given
Adm.	Oral
@	100 ml od
Pres.	500 ml

Cleantone DS	**Wesfa Pharma**
Comp	Not given
Adm.	Oral
@	100 ml od, 100 ml bid in ROP
Pres.	500 ml, 1L

Uprotone liq	**Agilis**
Comp	100 ml contains Ashoka 2 g; Gokshure 1g; Lohbaan 500 mg Kantakari 2 g; Shatavari 1g; Jiwanti 500 mg Gamhari 1.5 g; Manjistha 800 mg

	Bael 1 g Ashwagandha 800 mg Shalparni 1 g Brihati 800 mg Kalonji 1 g Kalihari 800 mg
Adm.	Oral
@	200 ml od for 5 days
Pres.	1L

Utripulse	**Zydus**	**261**
Comp	Herbal ecobolic	
Adm.	Oral	
@	100-125 ml od	
Pres.	900 ml	

Utroclear O Pow/Liquid.			**Carevet Pharma**
Indi: Uterine tonic			
Comp: 150 gm contains			
Piper nigrum	20 g	Gossypium herbacum	10 g
Acorus calamus	20 g	Buteamono sperma	10 g
Rubia cordiofolio	20 g	Valeriana wallichi	10 g
Commiphora myrrha	20 g	Aristolochia indica	10 g
Saussurea lappa	10 g	Bosweilia glabra	10 g
Convolvulus pluricaulis	10 g		
Adm: Oral			
@ : 25 g powder 100 ml Liq. daily twice after calving for 3-6 days			
Pres: 150 gm, 500 ml, 1100 ml			

Uterotone Capsule			**Cattle Remedies**
Indi: Anoestrusovulatory			
Comp: Each Cap.			
Semicarpus anacardium	930 mg	Syzygium aromaticum	45 mg
Abrus precatorius	25 mg		
Adm: Oral			
@ : 4 Capsules daily for 4 days			
Pres: 8 Capsules pack			

Myrontab.	**Alarsin**
Indi: Antiseptic, antibacteria, Uterinetonic	
Comp: Not given	
Adm: Oral	
@ : 10 tabs. twice daily for 15-20 days	
Pres: Pack of 100, 1000 tablets	

Macbolic Liquid	**National Vet Pharma**
Indi: Ecobolic, Postpartum porblems	
Comp: 21 herbs	
Adm: Oral	
@ : 100 ml daily for 10 days	
Pres: 500 ml, 1L	

Gynatone Syp.			**Libra Biotech**
Indi: Ecobolic, Post parturient problems			
Comp: 200 ml contains			
Ashoka	5 g	Harmal	2 g
Kapas	1 g	Ultkambhal	3 g
Sonth	1 g	Ghingwar	1 g
Methi	2 g	Gudhal	1 g
Jeera	1 g	Trikana	1 g
Raktshalmali	1 g	Tapeswani	1 g
Agnishikha	1 g	Shikhamulm	2 g
Nagarmotha	1 g	Upakunchika	1 g
Pitohari	2 g	Hapusha	1 g
Deepayka	1 g	Darvi	1 g
Isharman	1 g		
Adm: Oral			
@ : 100 ml daily for 10 days			
Pres: 1 L, 5 L			

Intrauterine Preparations

In genital tract infections like Metritis, Endometritis, Pyometra, Vaginitis, Cervicitis, etc. topical use of some formulations is very common in veterinary field. Various preparations are deposited manually or infused with inseminating gun with the help of a syringe.

Antibiotics

Amikacin

Amikin Liq.	Vets Farma
Comp	Each ml contains Amikacin sulphate 250 mg/ml
Adm.	IU
@	2-4 ml in 40 ml D.W post-Insemination
Pres.	2 ml, 10, 30 ml

Ampicillin + Cloxacillin

Nepoclox Vet Inj	TTK
Comp	Ampicillin 1g Cloxacillin 1 g
Adm.	IU
@	Dissolve 2 g in 10 ml, then dilute in 20-25 ml water and infuse
Pres.	2 g vial

Ceftriaxone

Vetacef	Cargill (Unichem)
Comp	Ceftriaxone 1 g & ceftriaxone 2 g
Adm.	IU
@	LA 1 g diluted
Pres.	1 g, 2 g vial

Cephalexin

Ceflax Powd	Neospark
Comp	Cephalexin 20 g
Adm.	IU
@	20 g/50 ml distt water
Pres.	20 g sachet

Lixen Bol IU	Virbac
Comp	Each Bol contains Cephalexin 750 mg with urea 2.5 g
Adm.	IU
@	2 Bol IU
Pres.	Strip of 2

Lixen Susp (Dry) IU	**Virbac**
Comp	Cephalexin 1.5 g in 4.5 g Susp
Adm.	IU
@	Reconstitute to 60 ml
Pres.	4.5 g

Uteriguard IU Susp	**Zydus**
Comp	4 g contains Cephalexin 1.5 g Serratiopeptidase 10 mg
Adm.	IU
@	Reconstitute in 60 ml of water
Pres.	4 gm bottle with 60 ml water

Chloramphenicol

Kemicetine Bol	**Marc**
Comp	Chloramphenicol 500 mg/Bol
Adm.	IU
@	LA 2-4 Bol SA 1-2 Bol
Pres.	Strip of 3

Vetnicol	**Vets Pharma**
Comp	Chloramphenicol 500 mg/Bol
Adm.	IU
@	LA 2-4 Bol SA 1-2 Bol
Pres.	Strip of 4

Ciprofloxacin

C Flox TZ	**Intas**
Comp	Each 5 ml contains Ciprofloxacin 125 mg Tinidazole 150 mg
Adm.	IU
@	30-60 ml
Pres.	60 ml

Enrofloxacin

Enrocin Susp	Ranbaxy
Comp	Each ml contains Enrofloxacin 25 mg
Adm.	IU
@	Infuse 30-50 ml IU for 3-5 days
Pres.	50 ml

Gentamicin

Catlogena	Cattle Remedies
Comp	Each ml contains Gentamicin 40 mg/ml
Adm.	IU
@	5-10 ml in 20 ml of water
Pres.	30 ml

Genster Inj	Sterling
Comp	Each ml contains Gentamicin 40 mg/ml
Adm.	IU
@	5-10 ml in 20 ml of water
Pres.	30 ml

Gentamicin Inj	Vet Care
Comp	Each ml contains Gentamicin 40 mg/ml
Adm.	IU
@	5-10 ml in 20 ml of water
Pres.	30 ml, 100 ml

Gymcin inj	Carvet Pharma
Comp	Each ml contains Gentamicin 40 mg/ml
Adm.	IU
@	5-10 ml in 20 ml of water
Pres.	30 ml

Gentin inj	wockhardt
Comp	Each ml contains Gentamicin 40 mg/ml
Adm.	IU
@	5-10 ml in 20 ml of water
Pres.	30 ml

Kanamycin

Kancin Inj	Alembic
Comp	Kanamycin acid sulphate 1g
Adm.	IU
@	Dissolve the contents of vial in 40 ml of distt water and infuse IU before insemination or within 24 hrs after insemination
Pres.	1 g vial

Neomycin Sulphate

Unimycin Bol	Unichem
Comp	Each Bol contains Neomycin sulphate 350 mg
Adm.	IU
@	LA 1-2 Bol, Insert IU SA ½ -1 Bol
Pres.	Strip of 4

Nitrofurazone

Furacin Vet	Pfizer
Comp	Nitrofurazone 0.2%
Adm.	IU
@	30 ml Intrauterine
Pres.	30 ml

Furazone	Vets Pharma
Comp	Nitrofurazone 0.2%
Adm.	IU
@	30-90 ml Intrauterine
Pres.	30 ml, 120 ml

Oxytetracycline

Oxy Liquid	Carevet Pharma
Comp	Each ml contains Oxytetracycline HCl 50 mg/ml
Adm.	IU
@	20-30 ml of formulation diluted with equal quantity of sterile water for 3-5 days
Pres.	60 ml, 100 ml

Terramycine liq	**Pfizer**
Comp	Each ml contains Oxytetracycline HCl 50 mg/ml
Adm.	IU
@	20-30 ml of formulation diluted with equal quantity of sterile water for 3-5 days
Pres.	60 ml, 100 ml

Ultron Top liq	**Neospark**
Comp	Each ml contains Oxytetracycline HCl 50 mg/ml
Adm.	IU
@	20-30 ml of formulation diluted with equal quantity of sterile water for 3-5 days
Pres.	60 ml, 100 ml

Alycyclin O Bol	**Alembic**
Comp	Each Bolus contains 500 mg of oxytetracyclin hydrochloride
Adm.	IU
@	LA 2-4 Bol SA ½ -1 Bol
Pres.	Strip of 4

Amoly Bol	**Pranav**
Comp	Each Bolus contains 500 mg of oxytetracyclin hydrochloride
Adm.	IU
@	LA 2-4 Bol SA ½ -1 Bol
Pres.	Strip of 4

Oxytra Bol	**HAL**
Comp	Each Bolus contains 500 mg of oxytetracyclin hydrochloride
Adm.	IU
@	LA 2-4 Bol SA ½ -1 Bol
Pres.	Strip of 4

Neocyclin Bol	**Intas**
Comp	Each Bolus contains 500 mg of oxytetracyclin hydrochloride
Adm.	IU
@	LA 2-4 Bol SA ½ -1 Bol
Pres.	Strip of 4

Terramycin AF Tab	**Pfizer**
Comp	Each Bolus contains 500 mg of oxytetracyclin hydrochloride
Adm.	IU
@	LA 2-4 Bol SA ½ -1 Bol
Pres.	Strip of 4

Ultrox AF Tab	**Neospark**
Comp	Each Bolus contains 500 mg of oxytetracyclin hydrochloride
Adm.	IU
@	LA 2-4 Bol SA ½ -1 Bol
Pres.	Strip of 4

Vetoxy 500 Bol	**Vets Farma**
Comp	Each Bolus contains 500 mg of oxytetracyclin hydrochloride
Adm.	IU
@	LA 2-4 Bol SA ½ -1 Bol
Pres.	Strip of 4

Wolicyclin Bol	**Wockhardt**
Comp	Each Bolus contains 500 mg of oxytetracyclin hydrochloride
Adm.	IU
@	LA 2-4 Bol SA ½ -1 Bol
Pres.	Strip of 4

Tetracyclin

Steclin Bol	**Zydus Sarabhai**
Comp	Tetracycline hydrochloride 500 mg
Adm.	IU
@	LA 2-4 Bol SA ½ -1 Bol
Pres.	Strip of 4

Povidon Iodine

It is a complete broad spectrum microbiocidal which is also Trichomonocidal, fungicide and bactericidal to pathogens which commonly cause Genital Tract infection. It is inserted IU.

Povisol Sol	**Vets Farma**
Comp	Povidone iodine 5%
Adm.	IU
@	20-40 ml in LA
Pres.	100 ml, 500 ml, 1L

Sterdine Sol	**Sterling**
Comp	Povidone iodine 5%
Adm.	IU
@	20-40 ml in LA
Pres.	100 ml, 500 ml

Iodocure	**Anmark**
Comp	Povidone iodine 5%
Adm.	IU
@	20-40 ml in LA
Pres.	100 ml

Wokadin Sol	**Wockhardt**
Comp	Povidone iodine 5%
Adm.	IU
@	20-40 ml in LA
Pres.	100 ml, 500 ml

Metricure IU	**Zydus**
Comp	Povidone iodine 5%, Metronidazole 1%
Adm.	IU
@	20-40 ml in LA
Pres.	30 ml, 100 ml

Sulphonamide + Trimethoprim

Atrima Bol	**Primavet**	
Comp	Sulphadiazine 1g	Trimethoprim 200 mg
Adm.	IU	
@	LA 2-4 Bol SA ½ -1 Bol	
Pres.	Strip of 4	

Biotrim Bol	**Ranbaxy**	
Comp	Sulphadiazine 1g	Trimethoprim 200 mg
Adm.	IU	
@	LA 2-4 Bol SA ½ -1 Bol	
Pres.	Strip of 4	

Sparktrim Bol	Neospark	
Comp	Sulphadiazine 1 g	Trimethoprim 200 mg
Adm.	IU	
@	LA 2-4 Bol SA ½ -1 Bol	
Pres.	Strip of 4	

Sulcoprim Bol	Concept	
Comp	Sulphadiazine 1 g	Trimethoprim 200 mg
Adm.	IU	
@	LA 2-4 Bol SA ½ -1 Bol	
Pres.	Strip of 4	

Trisul Bol	Pranav	
Comp	Sulphadiazine 1 g	Trimethoprim 200 mg
Adm.	IU	
@	LA 2-4 Bol SA ½ -1 Bol	
Pres.	Strip of 4	

Vetran LA Bol	Vets Farma	
Comp	Sulphadiazine 1 g	Trimethoprim 200 mg
Adm.	IU	
@	LA 2-4 Bol SA ½ -1 Bol	
Pres.	Strip of 4	

Wocktrin Bol	Wockhardt	
Comp	Sulphadiazine 1 g	Trimethoprim 200 mg
Adm.	IU	
@	LA 2-4 Bol SA ½ -1 Bol	
Pres.	Strip of 4	

Sulphamethaxazole + Trimethoprim

Cotrimal Bol	Alembic
Comp	Sulphamethaxazole 1.25 g and Trimethoprim 250 mg
Adm.	IU
@	LA 2-4 Bol SA ½ -1 Bol
Pres.	Strip of 4

Duaprim Bol	Cargill	
Comp	Bol Sulphamaxazole 2 g	Trimethoprim 400 mg
Adm.	IU	
@	LA 2-3 Bol SA ½ -1 Bol	
Pres.	Strip of 4	

Intrim Bol	**Intas**
Comp	Sulphamethaxazole 1.25 g and Trimethoprim 250 mg
Adm.	IU
@	LA 2-4 Bol SA ½ -1 Bol
Pres.	Strip of 4

Orprim U Bol	**Sarabhai**
Comp	Sulphamethaxazole 1.25 g and Trimethoprim 250 mg
Adm.	IU
@	LA 2-4 Bol SA ½ -1 Bol
Pres.	Strip of 4

Robartan Bol	**TTK**
Comp	Sulphamethaxazole 1.25 g and Trimethoprim 250 mg
Adm.	IU
@	LA 2-4 Bol SA ½ -1 Bol
Pres.	Strip of 4

Sterbac Bol	**Sterling**
Comp	Sulphamethaxazole 1.25 g and Trimethoprim 250 mg
Adm.	IU
@	LA 2-4 Bol SA ½ -1 Bol
Pres.	Strip of 4

Sugaprim Bol	**Zydus**
Comp	Sulphamethaxazole 1.25 g and Trimethoprim 250 mg
Adm.	IU
@	LA 2-4 Bol SA ½ -1 Bol
Pres.	Strip of 4

Trepin Bol	**Cadila Pharma**
Comp	Sulphamethaxazole 1.25 g and Trimethoprim 250 mg
Adm.	IU
@	LA 2-4 Bol SA ½ -1 Bol
Pres.	Strip of 4

Other Combination

Furea Bol	**Pfizer**
Comp	Nitrofurazone 60 mg urea 6 g
Adm.	IU
@	LA 2-4 Bol daily
Pres.	Strip of 4

Furex Bol	**Vets Farma**		
Comp	Nitrofurazone 60 mg urea 6 g		
Adm.	IU		
@	LA 2-4 Bol daily		
Pres.	Strip of 4		

Orpisol Pessary	**Alved**		
Comp	Nitrofurazone 60 mg urea 6 g		
Adm.	IU		
@	LA 2-4 Bol daily		
Pres.	Strip of 4		

Uromet Bol	**Neospark**		
Comp	Nitrofurazone 60 mg urea 6 g		
Adm.	IU		
@	LA 2-4 Bol daily		
Pres.	Strip of 4		

Furex M	**Novartis**		
Comp	Nitrofurazone 60 mg	Metronidazole 1g	Urea 5 g
Adm.	IU		
@	LA 2-4 Bol SA 1-2 Bol		
Pres.	Strip of 4		

Uterofit	**Alembic**		
Comp	Nitrofurazone 60 mg	Metronidazole 1 g	Urea 5 g
Adm.	IU		
@	LA 2-4 Bol SA 1-2 Bol		
Pres.	Strip of 4		

Furazol M	**Century**		
Comp	Nitrofurazone 60 mg	Metronidazole 1 g	Urea 5 g
Adm.	IU		
@	LA 2-4 Bol SA 1-2 Bol		
Pres.	Strip of 4		

Utrox bol	**Vest**		
Comp	Nitrofurazone 60 mg	Metronidazole 1 g	Urea 5 g
Adm.	IU		
@	LA 2-4 Bol SA 1-2 Bol		
Pres.	Strip of 4		

Pesurea Bol	Indian Immunology
Comp	Nitrofurazone 60 mg Metronidazole 1 g Urea 5 g
Adm.	IU
@	LA 2-4 Bol SA 1-2 Bol
Pres.	Strip of 4

Cleanex Bol	Merial (Dosch)
Comp	Each Bol contains Nitrofurazone 60 mg Urea 6 g Metronidazole 100 mg
Adm.	IU
@	LA 2-4 Bol od
Pres.	Strip of 4

Ranvidon IU Liq	Ranbaxy
Comp	Povidone 10 days 5% Metronidazole 1%
Adm.	IU
@	LA 30-60 ml
Pres.	60 ml

Fazole Bol	Cargill (Unichem)
Comp	Each Bol contains Furazolidone 200 mg Metronidazole 1g
Adm.	IU
@	LA 2-4 Bol SA 1-2 Bol
Pres.	Strip of 4

Nildero Bol	Cargill (Unichem)
@	Each Bol contains Furazolidone 200 mg Metronidazole 1 g
Adm.	IU
@	LA 2-4 Bol SA 1-2 Bol
Pres.	Strip of 4

Metijet Sol	Intervet
Comp	Each Syringe contains Oxytetracycline hydrochloride 500 mg Furazolidone 500 mg Clioquinol 500 mg Ethinylestradiol 500 mg
Adm.	IU
@	1 syringe in mild cases in serious cases 1 syringe for 3 days
Pres.	19 g syringe

Uron Bol	**Pranav**
Comp	Nitrofurazone 60 mg Urea 6 g Povidon iodine 50 mg Metronidazole 100 mg
Adm.	IU
@	LA 2-4 Bol SA 1-2 Bol

Utroclear OZ	**Carevet Pharma**
Comp	5 ml contains Oflaxacin 50 mg Ornidazole 125 mg
Adm.	IU
@	60 ml
Pres.	60 ml

Utroclear U	**Carevet Pharma**
Comp	10 ml contains Ciprofloxacin 125 mg Tinidazole 150 mg Alfa tocopherol 5 mg
Adm.	IU
@	50 ml
Pres.	50 ml

Lenova Susp	**Intas**
Comp	Levofloxacin 20 mg, alpha tocopherol 5 mg in each ml
Adm.	IU
@	30-60 ml
Pres.	30 ml, 60 ml

Cleantone DSIU	**Wesfa Pharma 2**
Comp	5 ml contains Ofloxacin 50 mg Ornidazole 125 mg Urea 500 mg
Adm.	IU
@	30-60 ml
Pres.	60 ml, 100 ml, 500 ml

Clanex Bol	**Boehringer Ingelheim**
Comp	Bolus contains Metronidazole 100 mg Urea 6 g Nitrofurazone 60 mg Povidon iodine 60 mg
Adm.	IU
@	2-4 Bol for 3-5 days
Pres.	Strip of 4

Selvo IU XP liq	Alivira 302
Comp	Each ml has Levofloxacin 20 mg Ornidazole 25 mg Vit E 5 mg
Adm.	IU
@	30-60 ml
Pres.	60 ml

Metricare IU	Zydus 243
Comp	1 ml contains Povidone iodine 5% Metronidazole 1%
Adm.	IU
@	30-60 ml
Pres.	Both of 30 ml, 100 ml

Ovulation Inducing Drugs

These drugs induce luteolysis and smooth muscle contraction resulting in fertile heat in cows and buffaloes suffering from anestrous, persistent corpus luteum, Cystic corpus luteum.

Clomiphene

It is a non-steroidal agent. It is ovulation inducer. It inhibits the negative (feedback) mechanism of oestrogen on Gonadotrophin releasing hormone enabling the release of GnRH form hypothalamus. It does not interfere with any endocrinal gland function. In this way it induces ovulation.

Indications: Anoestrus, Repeat Breeding

Fertimed Tab	Cipla
Comp	Each tablet has clomiphene citrate 50 mg
Adm.	Oral
@	1 Tab daily for 5 days
Pres.	Pack of 5 Tab

Clomiphene and Copper Sulphate

Copper sulphate helps to retain clomiphene for long in body for activity. So it supports for better result.

Breed up	Phoenix
Comp	Clomiphene citrate 500 mg Copper sulphate 375 mg
	IU
Adm.	Oral
@	1 Tab of each in one day x 5 days
Pres.	Pack of 5 with 10 Tab

Fertibloom	**Macnor**	
Comp	Clomiphene citrate 500 mg	Copper sulphate 375 mg
Adm.	Oral	
@	1 Tab of each in one day x 5 days	
Pres.	Pack of 5 with 10 Tab	

Heat up	**Century**	
Comp	Clomiphene citrate 500 mg	Copper sulphate 375 mg
Adm.	Oral	
@	1 Tab of each in one day x 5 days	
Pres.	Pack of 5 with 10 Tab	

Fertizoom	**Vet Avenue**	
Comp	Clomiphene citrate 500 mg	Copper sulphate 375 mg
Adm.	Oral	
@	1 Tab of each in one day x 5 days	
Pres.	Pack of 5 with 10 Tab	

Fertigrow	**Vet Vision**	
Comp	Clomiphene citrate 500 mg	Copper sulphate 375 mg
Adm.	Oral	
@	1 Tab of each in one day x 5 days	
Pres.	Pack of 5 with 10 Tab	

Pashuvardhan Kit	**Macwell**	
Comp	Clomiphene citrate 300 mg	Copper sulphate 1500 mg
Adm.	Oral	
@	1 Tab of each in one day x 5 days	
Pres.	Pack of 5 with 10 Tab	

Vetykit	**Avivet**	
Comp	Clomiphene citrate 500 mg	Copper sulphate 375 mg
Adm.	Oral	
@	1 Tab of each in one day x 5 days	
Pres.	Pack of 5 with 10 Tab	

Heatfit Bol Heatfit Forte Bol	Libra
Comp	Bol clomifene 300 mg Copper sulphate 750 mg Forte bol clomifene 450 mg Copper sulphate 750 mg
Adm.	Oral
@.	1 Tab each in one day for 5 day
pres	Pack of 5 with 10 Tab

Heat kit Bol	Nicosia
Comp	Bolus contains Clomiphenecitrate 300 mg and copper sulphate 1500 mg
Adm.	Oral
@	One Bol od x 5 days
Pres.	Strip of 5

Miscellaneous

Heatsure Bol	Herstel 300
Comp	Saraca ashoka 2 mg Somecarpus anacardium 2 mg Tribuis terestris 3 mg Compiphora myroha 3 mg Asparagur racemosus 3 mg Valeriana wallichii 1 mg Abroma agusta 2 mg Copper sulphate, cobalt sulphate, ferrous sulphate
Adm.	Oral
@	1 Bol x 5-7 days
Pres.	1 Bol pack

Estrus Inducer

Janova Cap	Ayurvet
Comp	Citrullus colocynthis Zingiber officinalis Piper longum Piper nigrum
Adm.	Oral
@	3 Cap od for 2 days. Repeat after 10 days if heat is not observed
Pres.	6 Cap strip

Mintrus Caplet	**Ayurvet**
Comp	Not given
Adm.	Oral
@	1 Cap od for 20 days
Pres.	Strip of 10

Gyna Forte Bol	**Rajshree**
Comp	Not given
Adm.	Oral
@	2 Bol bid for 10-20 days
Pres.	20 Bol

Prajna HS Cap	**Indian Herbs**
Comp	Not given
Adm.	Oral
@	3 Cap for 3 days
Pres.	6 Cap

Heat up Cap	**Century**
Comp	Each cap contains Mrigakshi 600 mg, Pippali 60 mg Tiksina 60 mg, Sringaver 60 mg
Adm.	Oral
@	3 Cap for 2 days
Pres.	6 Cap

Estrona Cap	**Rakesh Pharma**
Comp	Loha bhasmi 50 mg, Nigella sativa 75 mg Myrsh 50 mg, Aloes indica 75 mg Harmula 50 mg, Rubia cordifolia 100 mg
Adm.	Oral
@	2 Cap daily for 5 days
Pres.	10 Tab

Gesta Forte Bol	**TTK Pharma**			
Comp	Each Bol contains			
	Andographis paniculata	660 mg	Piper longum	50 mg
	Phyllanthus niruri	300 mg	Zingiber officinalis	12.5 mg
	Pandanus odoratissmus	100 mg	Zinc sulphate	11.3 mg
	Mimusops elengi	100 mg	Copper sulpahte	31.0 mg
	Mimusops elengi	100 mg	Copper sulpahte	31.0 mg
	Dried yeast	150 mg	Cobalt choride	6.0 mg
	Iodine (KI)	19 mg	Ferrous sulphate	5.0 mg
	Selenium	0.9 mg	Phosphorous	25 mg
	Microcrystaline hydroxy apatite (ca)	55 mg		

Uterotone Cap	**Cattle Remedies**	
Comp	Each cap contains	
	Semicarpus anacardium	930 mg
	Abrus precatorious	25 mg
	Syzygium aromaticum	45 mg
Adm.	Oral	
@	4 Cap od x 4 days	
Pres.	8 Cap	

Sajan Cap	**Kepler**
Comp	Mrigkashi Pipalli Tikshna Shatavari Krishna
Adm.	Oral
@	2 Cap od x6 days
Pres.	6 Cap

Estrus care Cap	**Carevet Pharma**			
Comp	Alovera	100 mg	Rubia cordifoia	20 mg
	Strychnos nuxvomic	100 mg	Zingiber officinale	20 mg
	Gossypium herbaccum	100 mg	Piper longum	20 mg
	Sodi biborus	20 mg	Ferrous sulphate	20 mg
	Compiphora myrrh	100 mg		
Adm.	Oral			
@	4 Cap x 5 days			
Pres.	20 Cap			

Fertirich Pow	**Venky's**	
Comp	Packet I 20 g	Wavding, Mohari, Kamala, Palasbeej, Sonmukhi, Umber, Kalijiri, Kirmani, owa
	Packet II 20 g	Gokhu, Asvalkathi, Behda, Hirda, Daruhalad, Gorukhmundi, Ashawgandha, Indrayamool
	Packet III 20 g	Zinc, Copper, Cobalt, Manganese, Iron, Iodine, Calcium, Magnesium
	Packet IV 20 g	Ishwarmool, shatawari, Jatamansi, Ashok, Saal, Kalonji, Awalkathi, Manjistha
	Packet V 20 g	Balant shepa, Kavach beej, Gajar beej, Kalonji, Mohao
Adm.	Oral	
@	Daywise each packet for 5 days	
Pres.	Five packets of 20 g	

Heatsole Cap	**Arosol Herbal**
Comp	Not given
Adm.	Oral
@	3 Cap bid x 5
Pres.	20 Cap

Ovule Fort Bol	**Unjha Formulation**			
Comp	Each Bol contains			
	Mrigkashi	540 mg	Sringaver	60 mg
	Dhaturapatra	60 mg	Vadehi	60 mg
Adm.	Oral			
@	2 Bol bid x 3			
Pres.	Strip of 4			

Estrona Forte Bolus			**Rakesh Pharma**
Indications: Ecobolic, Estrogenic, Genitalproblems			
Comp: Each Bol. Contains			
Mandur Bhasma	2.50 mg	Aloes indica	197.50 mg
Abhrak Bhasma	50 mg	Sapindus trifoliatus	100 mg

Tuthya Bhasma	197 mg	Bambusa araudinacea	125 mg
Tir Bang Bhasma	75 mg	Foeniculum vulgarae	125 mg
Myrsh	125 mg	Citrullus colocynthis	125 mg
Commiphora mukul	150 mg	Raphanus sativus	50 mg
Tankan Khar	125 mg	Solanum xanth ocarpum	197.5 mg
Asfoetida compound	175 mg	Maringaoleifara	250 mg
Luffaechinata	125 mg	Daucuscarota	197 mg
Vitextrifolia	150 mg	Nigellasativa	250 mg
Harmala	175 mg	Rubiacordifolia	50 mg
Peristrophe bicaliculata	150 mg	Mimusops hexandra	125 mg
Adm: Oral			
@ : 1 Bol. daily for 10 days			
Pres: 10 Bol. 100 Bol. Pack			

Aloes Compound tab.	**Alarsin**
Indi: Ovulatory, Anoestrus	
Comp: Not given	
Adm: Oral	
@ : 5-10 tabs twice daily till animal conesin heat	
Pres: Pack of 100 tab.	

Stilbestrol

Stilbestrol injectable is used to induce estrous. It is non-steroidal synthetic estrogen. It brings about changes in the uterine growth, fallopian tubes and vagina. With estrogen only progesterone brings about secretory changes. These induce watery secretion from the cervix.

Indications: For the treatment of anoestrous in cows, retained placenta and mummified foetus, sterile pyometra. It prevents nidation if administration within 36 hrs of mating.

Stilbestrol inj	**Generic**
Comp	Each ml contains Stilbestrol dipropionate 10 mg
Adm.	IM
@	LA 20 mg for 3-3 Successive days SA 10 mg for 3-3 Successive days
Pres.	10 ml

Vetoestrol	Primavet Care
Comp	Each ml contains Stilbestrol dipropionate 10 mg
Adm.	IM
@	LA 20 mg for 3-3 Successive days SA 10 mg for 3-3 Successive days
Pres.	10 ml

Prolapse Cure-Prevention

Prolapse in Tab/ Pow	Cattle Remedies			
Comp	**Tablet contains**		**Pow contains**	
	Symplococos racemosa	3%	Brutea monosperms	4.5%
	Aluminium sulphate	0.5%	Quercus infectoria	2.0%
	Acacia nilotica indica	3.0%	Ficus glometra	2.0%
Adm.	Oral			
@	5 Tab od x 3 days with butter or ghee. Apply 20 g powder with glycerine on proplased organ and insert in			
Pres.	6 Tab, 20 gm Pow			

Lapsin Pow	Phoenix			
Comp	Bhasma nag	1.5 g	Symplocos racemosa	20 g
	Bhasma yashat	1.5 g	Tinospora cordifolia	55 g
	Bhasma bang	1.5 g	Asoka bark	15 g
	Rasinaflava	10 g	Acacia bark	15 g
	Soda vibros	10 g	Acacia ardica	10 g
	Quercus infectoria	10 g		
Adm.	Oral			
@	150 g bid followed by 100 g bid for 2 days			

Prolapsecure Pow	Rajshree
Comp	Not given
Adm.	Oral
@	150 gm od in 200 ml Sarson oil
Pres.	450 g

Proactive Bol	Rakesh Pharma			
Comp	Each Bol contains			
	Garbhphal ras	750 mg	Withania samnifera	200 mg
	Kumdudha ras	1580 mg	Rubia cordifolia	200 mg

	Kashish	100 mg	Curcuma aromatic	200 mg
	Glycerrhiza glabra	200 mg	Sympocos racemasa	170 mg
Adm.	Oral			
@	4-6 bolus od			
Pres.	20, 200 Pack			

Prolapgard	**Animax Healthcare**
Comp	Not given
Adm.	Oral
@	LA 100 g in 200 Mustard oil and 150 g of gram flour
Pres.	500 g

Proban Pow	**IHC (International Health Care)**
Comp	Herbal
Adm.	Oral
@	50 g 5 times daily
Pres.	1 kg

Prolapsyn Pow.			**Carevet Pharma**
Indi: Prepartum post part umprolap seuterus, vagina			
Comp: 150 g contains			
Extract umbesberis	234 g	Ferrous Sulphate	40.7 g
Tamarix gallica	13.9 g	Sodium Bi Carbonate	11.7 g
Procarpus santhalinus	13.9 g	Alum	9.3 g
Symplocos recemosa	13.9 g	Berberis aristata	9.3 g
Bombax pentadrum	13.9 g		
Adm: Oral			
@ : 75 g twice daily with gram flour for 3-7 days			
Pres: 150 g, 450 g			

Forlaps Pow.	**Avivet Pharma**
Indi: Uterine,Vaginal Prolapse	
Comp: 9 potent herbs	
Adm: Oral	
@ : 100 g in 200 ml of mustard oil with gram flour for five days	
Pres: 500 g pouch	

Prolapban	**Herstel**
Indi: Prolapse	
Comp: Not given	
Adm: Oral	
@ : 200 gm with 200 gm gram flour 200 ml Mustard oil	
Pres: 500 g	

Conceiver

Conceiver Bol	**Rajshree**
Comp	Not given
Adm.	Oral
@	1 Bol
Pres.	20 Bol

Cofe cu Tab/ Cofe cu plus	**Indian Herbs**
Comp	Not given
Adm.	Oral
@	1 Tab od x 20 days
Pres.	20 Tab

Utrovet	**Rakesh Pharma**
Comp	Rubia cordifolia 100 mg Myrsh 50 mg Harmala 75 mg Leptodaenia reticulata 100 mg Aristolochia bracteata 75 mg
Adm.	Oral
@	10-20 Tab bid
Pres.	100, 1000 Pack

Aisuse Liq	**Venky**
Comp	225 ml contains Herbal extract of Abroma angusta Cyperus rotundus Bacopa marinieri Rubia cordifolia Terminalia chebuls Cyndon dactylon
Adm.	Oral
@	225 ml after AI or NS
Pres.	900 ml

NRB Liq	Animax Healthcare			
Comp	Vit A	Vit D_3	Vit H	Selenium
	Cobalt	Zinc	Shatavari	Safedmusli
	Punarnava	Gokru	Dashmul	Satap
	Kale Til	Drum strick	Lodhra	Prepali
	Safed chandan			
Adm.	Oral			
@	LA 100 ml bid			
Pres.	1L			

Intra Mammary Preparations

Mastitis- It is inflammation of mammary glands. It leads to changes in physical and chemical properties of milk. It is caused by many infective agents including Gram+ve, -ve, fungus, mycoplasma. Disease can be initiated by any injury and through milking man. It is clinical/ subclinical/ acute/ subacute and chronic type. It can be in one quarter or more than one. In acute form it is associated with pain, abnormal milk (clumps of milk, blood or straw coloured liquid) sharp drop in milk flow with high body temperature. Chronic form show abnormal milk (lumpsy, off-coloured, flaky, stringy) and hard cheesy lumps may be felt in udder. Diagnosis depends upon clinical abnormality of milk. If not treated in time quarter or whole udder is lost.

Various antibiotics/ combinations/ formulations are used to treat mastitis. Apart from systematic therapy local intramammary preparations are used for early and higher cure rate. Intramammary formulations are infused in affected quarter after emptying it completely.

Alciclox Intramammary	Alembic
Comp	Ampicillin 75 mg, Cloxacillin 200 mg
Adm.	Intra- mammary
@	One syringe each quarter 12 hrly.
Pres.	7 g disposable syringe (Milk should not be consumed for 60 hrs)

Alincomycin Inj	Alved
Comp	Each ml contain Lincomycin HCL 20 mg/ml
Adm.	Intra- mammary
@	10-20 ml
Pres.	30 ml

Amilox I	**Pranav**
Comp	Each syringe contains Cloxacillin 200 mg Colistin sulphate 5000000 IU
Adm.	Intra- mammary infusion
@	One syringe each quarter 12 hrly.
Pres.	Single use syringe

Campidex	**Cadila**
Comp	Ampicillin 75 mg Cloxacillin 200mg
Adm.	Intra- mammary
@	1 syringe/quarter 12 hrly
Pres.	10 ml syringe

Chlorectin Intrammary	**Dosch – Merial**
Comp	Tube of 10 gm contains Cephacetrile sodium 235 mg/tube
Adm.	Intramammary
@	1 tube/ quarter 24 or 48 hourly
Pres.	10 g tube

Megaclox Infusion	**Cipla**
Comp	5 gm tube contains Ampicillin 75 mg Cloxacillin 200 mg in tube
Adm.	Intramammary
@	1 tube/ quarter 12 hourly
Pres.	5 g tube

Cobactan LC Im	**Intervet**
Comp	Each syringe contains Cefquinome 75 mg
Adm.	Intra mammary
@	1 syringe/ quarter 12 hrly
Pres.	8 g syringe

Floclox D Infusion	**Ranbaxy**
Comp	Each syringe contains Cloxacillin 500 mg
Adm.	Intra mammary
@	1 syringe/ quarter 12 hrly
Pres.	3 g syringe

Mammitel Im	Intas Pharma
Comp	Each syringe contains Colistin sulphate 500000 IU
Adm.	Intra mammary Cloxacillin 200 mg
@	1 syringe/ quarter 12 hrly
Pres.	10 g syringe

Masticure Im	Pranav
Comp	Each tube contains Ampicillin 75 mg Cloxacillin 200 mg
Adm.	Intra mammary
@	1 tube/ quarter 12 hrly
Pres.	5 g tube

Maxomast Im	Sterling Lab
Comp	Each tube contains Ampicillin 75 mg Cloxacillin 200 mg
Adm.	Intra mammary
@	1 tube/ quarter 12 hrly
Pres.	5 g syringe

Nefuran	Pfizer
Comp	Each tube contains Nitrofurazone 150 mg
Adm.	Intra mammary
@	1 tube/ quarter 12 hrly
Pres.	3 g syringe

Pendistrin Oint	Sarabhai Zydus
Comp	Each tube contains Penicillin G potassium 1 lac IU Streptomycin sulphate 75 mg
Adm.	Intra mammary
@	1 tube/ quarter 12 hrly
Pres.	7.5 ml tube

Pendistrin SH oint	**Sarabhai Zydus**
Comp	Each tube contains Procaine penicillin 100000 IU Streptomycin sulphate100 mg Subfamerazine 500 mg Hydrocortisone acetate 20 mg in Plastobase
Adm.	Intra mammary
@	1 tube every 12 hrly in each quarter
Pres.	6 ml tube

Penicure D Syringe	**Marc**
Comp	Each tube contains Ampicillin 100 mg Cloxacillin 200 mg Dexamethasone 0.5 mg
Adm.	Intramammary
@	1 tubc/ quarter 12 hrly
Pres.	5 g syringe

Rifijet	**Intervet**
Comp	8 g syringe with Rifamycin 50 mg
Adm.	Intramammary
@	1 syringe/ quarter 12 hrly
Pres.	8 g syringe

Tilox Intramammary	**wockhardt**
Comp	Each tube contains Ampicillin 75 mg Cloxacillin 200 mg
Adm.	Intra mammary
@	1 tube/quarter 12 hrly
Pres.	5 g tube

Timutin 10% inj	**Novartis**
Comp	Each ml contains Tiamutin 100 mg
Adm.	Intra mammary
@	5 ml in each quarter
Pres.	20 ml vial

Vetclox Intramammary	**Sarabhai Zydus**	
Comp	Each tube contains Cloxacilliin 200 mg	
Adm.	Intra mammary	
@	1 tube/quarter 12 hrly	
Pres.	10 ml tube	

Vetclox Plus	**Sarabhai Zydus**	
Comp	Each tube contains Ampicillin 75 mg	Cloxacillin 200 mg
Adm.	Intramammary	
@	1 tube/ quarter 12 hrly	
Pres.	10 ml tube	

Vetimast Sus	**Novartis**
Comp	Each tube contains Cephacetrile sodium 235 mg/tube
Adm.	Intra mammary
@	1 tube/quarter every 24 hrly or 48 hrly
Pres.	10 ml tube

Ubrolexin	**Boehringer**	
Comp	10 gm syringe contain Cephalexin 200 mg	Kanamycin 100000 IU
Adm.	Intra mammary	
@	1 syringe in each QR	
Pres.	10 gm syringe	

Cefaject Infusion	**Cipla**	
Comp	7 gm tube contain Cefaperazone Procaine penicillin	 250 mg 150000 IU
Adm.	Intra mammary	
@	1 tube in each oR	
Pres.	7g tube	

Cefamast Infusion	**Cipla**
Comp	8 gm tube contain Cefquinone 750 mg/8g
Adm.	Intra mammary
@	1 tube each oR
	10 g syringe
Pres.	8 g tube

Clavet LC Infusion	**Cipla**
Comp	Tube of Amoxicillin 200 mg Clavulanic acid 50 mg
Adm.	Intra mammary
@	1 tube each or
Pres.	Tube

Multibact Infusion	**Cipla**
Comp	5 gm tube contains Procaine penicillin 100000 IU Speptomycin sulphate 100 mg Neomycin sulphate 100 mg Prednisolone 10 mg
Adm.	Intra mammary
@	1 tube in each or
Pres.	5 g tube

Cefasafe	**Intervet**
Comp	Each syringe has 300 mg Cefaprin
Adm.	Intra mammary
@	1 syringe each or
Pres.	Syringe

Mastijet Forte	**Intervet**
Comp	Each syringe contains Tetracyclin hydrochloride 200 mg Neomycin sulphate 250 mg Bacitracin 2000 IU Prednisolone 10 mg
Adm.	Intra mammary
@	1 syringe
Pres.	Syringe

Neo Mastitar	**Intervet**
Comp	Each syringe contains Procaine penicillin 500 mg (500000 IU) Neomycin 300 mg
Adm.	Intra mammary
@	1 syringe
Pres.	Syringe

Uddercef	**Zydus**	
Comp	3.5 g syrine contains	Cefuroxime 250 mg
Adm.	Intra mammary	
@	1 syringe each qr bid	
Pres.	3.5 g pre filled syringe	

Masticare tube	**Carevet Pharma**
Comp	Herbal extract
Adm.	Intra mammary
@	Infuse in each oR
Pres.	Intube with nozzle

Pendizyd	**Zydus**	
Comp	6 ml syringe	
	Procaine penicillin	100000 IU
	Streptomycin sulphate	100 mg
	Suephadimidine	500 mg
	Hydrocortisone	20 mg
Adm.	1 Mammary	
@	1 syringe each qr bid	
Pres.	6 ml syringe	

Mastitis Supportive

Uniselit Pow	**Ayurvet**
Comp	Not given
Adm.	Oral
@	10g Od for 15 days
Pres.	10 gm sachet

Lactilet M	**Rajshree**
Comp	Not given
Adm.	Oral
@	2 Bol bid
Pres.	20 Bol pack

Teatkit	**PAIL**
Comp	12 g contains Vit A 300000 IU Lactobacillus sporogenes 60 million CFO Amino nitrogen 100 mg Vit E 30 mg Trisodium citrate 60 g Vit K 30 mg Leptadaenia reticulata 6 g Selenium 30 mg Potassium iodine 120 mg Vit D_3 600 IU
Adm.	Oral
@	1st day I pouch 2nd day 2 pouch, 3rd day 3 pouch
Pres.	3 Pouches

Wisprec Pow	**Natural Remedies**
Comp	Not given
Adm.	Oral
@	To be applied on teat/ udder/ twice a day
Pres.	25 g

Mammidium Pow	**Intas**
Comp	50 g contains Trisodium citrate 25 g Vit A 70000 IU D_3 20000 IU E 100 mg Niacin 2000 mg $B_1$200 mg B_2 200 mg Pantothenic acid 50 mg Biotin 25 mg Methionine Manganese sulphate 10 g
Adm.	Oral
@	50 g od in jaggery for 4 day
Pres.	50g sachet

Mastilep oint	**Ayurvet**	
Comp	Cedrus deodar Curcuma longea Glycerrhiza glabra	Euclyptus glabulus Paedara fetida Sulphur
Adm.	Apply Twice daily after each milking for 5 days	
@	As per need	
Pres.	50 g	

Mammiflam cream	**Indian Herbs**
Comp	Not given
Adm.	Apply on teats after milking
@	As per need
Pres.	50 g

Inflamin	**Indian Herbs**
Comp	Not given
Adm.	Apply on affected part
@	As per need
Pres.	50 g, 125 g tube

Fibrokit MRF Pow	**Wesfa pharma**	
Comp	Each 60 g contains	
	Trisodium citrate	35 g
	Vit A	4000 IU
	Lactobacillus	200 million
	Amino nitrogen	100 mg
	Vit E	1500 IU
	Serratiopeptidose	120 mg
	Potassium iodide	7 g
	Vit K	400 IU
	Live yeast culture	7500 million
	Zinc sulphate	150 mg
	Bromelian	320 mg

	Ocimum sanctum	1000 mg
	Sodium selenite	10 mg
	Aloevira	100 mg
	Azadirachta indica	4000 mg
Adm.	Oral	
@	30 gm bid	
Pres.	60 g	

Mastahelp Plus Pow	**Macwell**		
Comp	Tri sodium citrate	Vit A	Sea weeds
	Magnesium sulphate	Vita D_3	Neem extract
	Zinc sulphate	Vit E	Glucose
	Potassium iodide	Vit B_1	Enzymes
	Ammonium chloride	Vit B_2	Lactobacillus
	Potassium alum	Vit B_6	Bhasma
	Fatty acid	Vit K	Herbs
	Chelated mineral	Vit C	Serratiopeptidase
Adm.	Oral		
@	50 g od x 5 days		
Pres.	250 g		

Mastikit Pow	**Nicosia**
Comp	Not given
Adm.	Oral
@	50 g od with Jaggary
Pres.	50 g pouch in 3's pack

Mastisol	**Alivira**
Comp	Trisodiumcitrate 25 mg Lactobacillus acidophilus 60 millions Vit A 3000 IU E 1000 IU Amino nitrogen 100 mg
Adm.	30 g
@	30 g bid
Pres.	60 g sachet

Qatercare Spray	**Nicosia International**
Indi: Ectopasasiticide, wound healing, FMD, Fly repellant	
Comp: Not given	
Adm: Spray on body	
@ : As per need	
Pres: 100 ml	

Mastigo Cap.			**Libra Biotech.**
Indi: Galactagogue, Utdommilk			
Comp: Each Contains			
Bhasam Parad	14%	Kachnar	7%
Bhasam Tamra	7%	Lahsoon	14%
Bhasam Shubhra	14%	Chiniakapoor	2%
Bhasam Godanti	7%	Sendha Lavan	14%
Bhasam Kashish	7%	Naushadar	7%
Bhasam Yarad	7%		
Adm: Oral			
@ : 1-2 Cap. twice a day in banana.			
Pres: 6 Cap.			

Drugs acting on Male Genital System

Certain drugs are used to enhance the growth of genital organs and their function. Some are used to increase libido or fertility by helping better sperm production. Some help to produce sperms fertile motile and more in number.

Gonadotropins

These are used in genital hypoplasia and crytorchidisin in males also. These are used to increase sex desire and libido.

Human Chorionic Gonadotropin

A non pituitary Gonadotropin

(Refer Female genital organ drugs)

Chorulon	**Intervet**
Comp	HCG 1500 IU in a vial
Adm.	IM
@	Stallion 1500 IU twice in a week for 4-6 weeks Boar/ Ram 500 IU twice in a week for 4-6 weeks
Pres.	1500 IU vial

Pregnant Mare Serum Gonadotropin

(Refer Drugs acting on Female Genital organs)

Folligon	**Intervet**
Indi	Used in impaired spermatogenesis
Comp	1000 IU vial
Adm.	IM
@	Bull 1000-3000 IU twice a week for 4-6 weeks Ram /Boar 500-750 IU twice a week for 4-6 weeks
Pres.	1000 IU vial with solvent

Miscellaneous

Fortege Tab	**Alarsin**
Comp	Not given
Adm.	Oral
@	10 tab bid x 15 days
Pres.	100 Tab, 1000 Tab

Speman Pow/Tab	**Himalya**
Comp	Not given
Adm.	Oral
@	12 g od for 2-6 weeks. Tablet for SA
Pres.	50 g, 100 Tab

Tentex Forte Pow/Bol	**Himalya**
Comp	Not given
Adm.	Oral
@	4 ½ g od x 7-10 days for impotent for 30 days 2 tab for SA
Pres.	10 gm, strip of 10

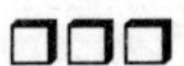

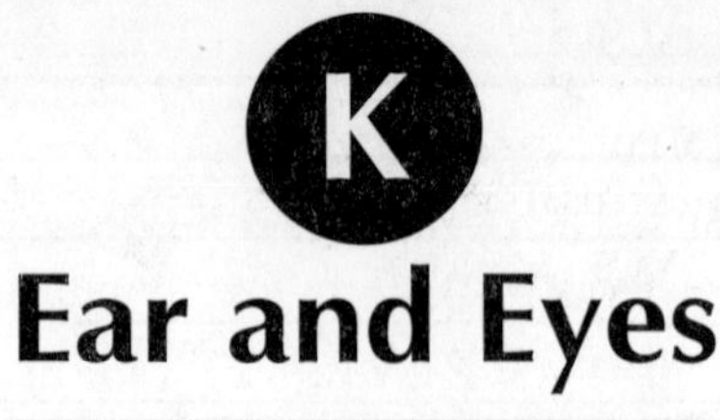

Ear and Eyes

Eye & Ear Diseases

Asteroid hyalosis: Degenerative condition of eye involving small white opacities in vitreous humor.

Canine glaucoma: Increase of pressure within eye caused by abnormal development of drainage angle of eye.

Cataract: Opacity of the lens

Chalazion: Granuloma that forms in the eyelid due to blocked secretions from meibomian gland. It may result inflammation of eyelid

Cherry eye: The gland of third eyelid prolapses and becomes visible

Chronic superficial Keratitis: Inflammation of cornea

Conjunctivitis: Inflammation of conjunctiva caused by mechanical irritation, allergies or bacterial infection.

Corneal dystrophy: A condition characterised by bilateral non-inflammatory opacity of cornea. It appears as grayish white lines, circles or clouding of cornea.

Corneal ulcer or Ulcerative Keratitis: It is an inflammatory condition of cornea involving loss of its outer layer. It is caused by trauma, detergent, burns and infection

Distichia: An eyelash that arises form an abnormal spot on eyelash. These can irritate the eye causing tearing, squinting and inflammation and corneal ulcers.

Ear otitis media: Inflammation of middle ear canal

Ectropion: Eyelid folding outwards

Entropion: Eyelid folding inward

Eye proptosis: A condition resulting in forward displacement and entrapment of eye from behind by the eyelids.

Florida Keratopathy: Presence of multiple spots within both corneas

Fly strike dermatitis: Caused by bites of stable fly. It occurs at the tip and folds of ear

Horner's Syndrome: It results from damage to sympathetic innervation of the eye. Signs include sunken eye, small pupil elevated third eyelid and dropping of upper eyelid.

Iris cysts: Small hollow structures attached to the iris of eye or flouting free in anterior chamber

Kerato conjunctivitis sicca: There is eye redness, a yellow or greenish discharge, ulceration of cornea, pigmented cornea

Lens luxation: Displacement of lens from its normal position

Nuclear sclerosis: It appears as a bilateral bluish grey haziness at the centre of lens

Optic neuritis: Inflammation of optic nerve caused by granulomatous meningoencephelitis or infection.

Otitis media: Inflammation of middle ear canal

Retinal dysplasia: It is caused by viral infection, drugs or vitamin A deficiency. It is characterised by folds or rosettes (round clumps) of retinal tissue

SARD: Sudden acquired Retinal degeneration: It is caused by toxin, or cushing's disease or unknown reason. Symptoms include permanent blindness, dilated pupils and loss of pupillary light reflex

Trichiasis: It is from the eyelid growing in wrong direction and rubbing on eye, causing irritation. Usually occurs at lateral upper eyelid

Uveitis: Inflammation within eye caused by trauma, cataract, infectious hepatitis, leptospirosis or fungal infections

Betnesol N Eye/Ear oint	**Intas**
Comp	Betamethasone sod Phos 0.1% Neomycin sulphate 0.5%
Adm.	Ear drop, Eye drop locally
@	1-2 drops in each eye/ear
Pres.	5 ml

Betnesol N Eye/Ear drops	**Glaxo**
Comp	Betamethasone sod Phos 0.1% Neomycin sulphate 0.5%
Adm.	Ear drop, Eye drop locally
@	1-2 drops in each eye/ ear
Pres.	5 ml

Ciplox Eye Drop	**Cipla**
Comp	Ciprofloxacin hydrochloride 0.3% Benzalkonium chloride 0.0225%
Adm.	Eyes locally
@	1-2 drops in each eye qid
Pres.	5 ml

Dexona Eye/Ear Sol	**Cadila Healthcare**
Comp	Dexamettsone sodium phosphate 0.1% Neomycin sulphate 0.5% Benzal- kornium chloride 0.02%
Adm.	Eye – Ears locally
@	1-2 drops qid
Pres.	3 ml

Neosperin H Ear drop	Glaxo
Comp	Polymyxin B sulph 10000 IU Neomycin sulphate 3400 IU Hydrocortisone 10 mg per ml
Adm.	Ear locally
@	1-3 drops tid
Pres.	5 ml

Otirel Ear drop	Ranbaxy
Comp	Gentamycin sulphate 0.3% Clotrimazole 1% Betamethasone dipropionate 0.025% Liqnocain hydrochloride 2%
Adm.	Ear locally
@	1-3 drops tid
Pres.	15 ml

Kittu eye drop	Macnor
Comp	Each ml contains Potassium iodide 3.3% Sodium chloride 0.83% Calcium chloride 1.0% Propylparaben 0.011% Methylparaben 0.023%
Adm.	Local in eyes
@.	2-4 drop bid
Pres.	15 ml vial

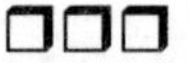

Endocrine System/ Hormones

Terms associated with Endocrines

Adrenal gland: These are two in number. Each one is situated close to the kidney. In ruminants left is C shaped and right is V shaped

Anterior pituitary: It is one lobe of pituitary gland. It secretes Adrenocorticotropic hormone (ACTH) Follicle stimulating hormone (FSH), Growth hormones (GH), Luteinizing hormone (LH), Prolactin and thyroid stimulating hormone (TSH).

Estrogen: It produces all manifestation of estrus. It prepares genitalia for reception of fertlised ova and responsible for secondary sex characters. Hormone of females, is secreted by ovary.

Endocrine glands: These are specialized glands that synthesise, store and release their secretions directly into blood stream. They respond to changes in internal and external environment to coordinate and maintain homeostasis. These are ductless.

Epinephirme: It causes Vasoconstriction and increases heart rate and blood pressures. It increases sweating and helps in regulation of body temperature. It is a hormone of fight and flight.

Epinephrine: It is a hormone released by adrenal medulla. It is also known as adrenaline. This responds to stress by increase heart rate and rushing blood to brain and muscles. Its spikes blood sugar level.

Glucocorticoids: It is a group of hormones secreted by Adrenal cortex. These are Hydrocortisone and Corticosterone hormones.

Hormones: These are chemical messengers secreted directly into the blood which carries them to organs and tissues of the body to exert their functions. There are many types of hormones. Hormones are secreted from endocrine glands.

Mineral corticoides: It is a group of hormones secreted by Adrenal cortex. Aldosterone is major hormone which maintain the right balance of salt and water while helping blood pressure control.

Insulin: It is secreted by pancreas. The hormone regulates carbohydrate metabolism and protein synthesis.

Luteinizing hormone (LH): It Stimulates development of corpus luteum in females and production of progesterone from ovary. It also synergises the action of Follicular stimulating hormones. In males its stimulates testes to produce testosterone.

Norepinephrine: this hormone is known as noradrenaline and secreted by adrenal medulla. It works with epinephrine in respond to stress. It can cause vasoconstriction and result is high blood pressure.

Oxytocin: Secreted by pituitary, the hormone causes letdown of milk and acts upon oestrogen smooth muscles of uterus causing contraction.

Parathormone: It regulates the calcium Phosphorus and vitamin D metabolism in the body.

Parathyroid gland: These are four reddish yellow coloured small bodies situated at variable positions close to thyroid glands.

Pituitary gland: This is an oval reddish grey colored body about the size of a large pea situated at the base of brain. It consists of two lobes. Anterior and Posterior. Both secrete hormones. It is master gland.

Posterior Pituitary: It is posterior lobe of pituitary and secretes Antidiuretic hormone (ADH) and oxytocin.

Pancreas: It is endocrine gland that maintains the body's blood sugar balance. It secretes insulin and glucagon hormones. These both regulate blood glucose.

Sex hormones: These are hormones released by adrenal cortex known as sex steroids or sex hormones. Small amount of male and female sex hormones are released by adrenal cortex.

Testosterone: It helps in the development of secondary sexual characters in male. It is essential for the maintenance of normal male genital trait. It acts as anabolic agent in retaining Nitrogen. It is secreted by testes.

Thyroxine: It is secreted by Thyroid. It helps in normal functioning of sex glands. It controls growth maturation and tissue differentiation. It regulates metabolism of carbohydrate and fat.

Thyroid gland: These are two triangular dark brown coloured glands situated at ventrolateral junction of larynx and trachea. It secretes Thyroxin hormones, calcitonin.

Antithyroid Drugs

Carbimazole

Ind. Hyper Thyrodisim

Ifer H Iodine Prepration

(Refer Minerals in Metabolism)

Corticosteroids

- **Glucocorticoids**
- **Hydrocortisone**

- **Betamethasone**
- **Dexamethasone**
- **Prednisolone**
- **Triamcinolone**
- **Isoflupredone**

Refer SAID in Musculo - skeleton system

Anabolic Steroids

These are synthetic derivatives of testosterone. These are indicated to promote nitrogen retention in animals. These stimulate appetite, increase muscle mass, increase skin thickness, increase skeletal mass and production of erythrocytes.

Nandrolone Refer Metabolism

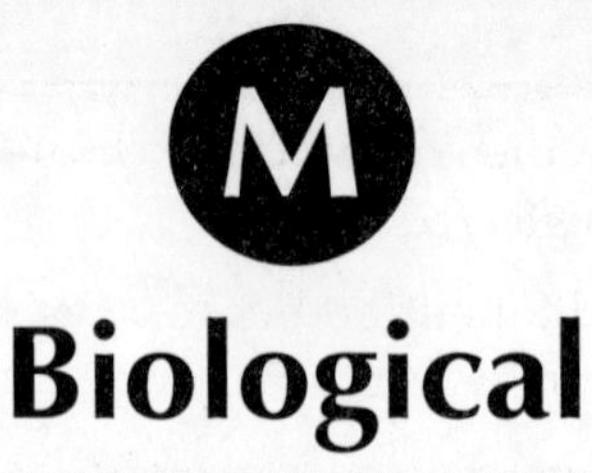

Biological

Veterinary Biologicals of India

In India, the production of veterinary biological was initiated in 1898 at Indian Veterinary Research Institute. The major activity of Institute was the production of various antisera against Rinderpest, Hemorrhagic septicaemia, Anthrax, Teanus, black quarter at Mukteswar in 1910. A new laboratory was established at Izat Nagar in 1913 to produce biological in large scale. The Veterinary Biological Products came under the purview of Drugs and cosmetic Acts 1940, in 1969.

The biologicals produced at present fall into two major groups viz. antibacterial and antiviral. There have been important changes and advances in the production and processing biological. Regular training programme in the technique of manufacture and standardization of veterinary biologicals to the state Vets were carried out here. With the passage of time, more and more states developed their own Biological Product Sections. After 1970, private manufacturers also entered this field.

Vaccines & Immunotherapy

The immunologic defenses of the body respond to antigen stimulation by production of antibodies or by activation of cell modulated immunity or both. Administration of specific antigen (as in a vaccine) may result in the development of a specific immune response to the inducing antigen only. A nonspecific antigen stimulates the immune system as a whole or increases disease resistance in general. Vaccines provoke effective, specific and long term immunity.

Immunologial Terms

Active Acquired Immunity: Animal produces in his own body, as a result of disease followed by recovery or vaccination.

Active Immunisation: Involves administration of antigen derived from an infectious agent so that animals mount a specific immune response and achieves resistance to that agent. It should not cause adverse side effects.

Adjuvant: Material used to increase the antigencity of a substance added in vaccine.

Antibody: product of those cells of the animal body which synthesise globulins in response to the presence of specific antigen.

Antigen: It is the substance introduced in the animal body, stimulate the formation of a specific antibody.

Antisera: Readymade antibodies (produced by any other animal who has been actively immunized) are transferred.

Antitoxins: Is the name used for antibodies to a toxin. It is produced by body cells in response to a stimulus by toxins. Antitoxins are stable on low temperature 3-50C.

Attenuation: Killed organisms are commonly less immunogenic than living ones. Virulence of an organism can be reduced to the point that it replicate but not pathogenic. This is attenuation. It also enables organisms to adapt unusual conditions.

Bivalent Vaccine: Combination of antigens made in which 2 strains of same species or organisms are combined to make the vaccine.

Hyperimmunisation: Repeated injection of large amount of an antigen which produce maximum antibodies is called hyper-immunisation. Also called Booster Dose.

Immunization: Introduction of vaccine to produce immunity is known as Immunisation.

Immunity: An attack of a disease gives certain protection against subsequent attack of same disease. Such resistance is called immunity.

Immunopotentiating or Immunomodulator: Agent that enhances immune system.

Immunosuppressant: Agents that suppress the immune system.

Inactivated Vaccine: Composed of killed inactivated bacteria or virus mixed and emulsified. These are safe with respect to residual virulence and contamination. It is easy to store but may be weaker immunogens.

Live Vaccine: Vaccines composed of live virulent virus or reduced virulence virus or live bacterial of reduced virulence or live bacterial spore. These stimulate good response but pose risks of residual virulence and contamination with unwanted organisms even to spread to unvaccinated animals.

Mixed Vaccine: Vaccine containing more than one organisms. These save time and effort. Commonly used in Dogs and Cats.

Monovalent Vaccine: A vaccine with single specific antigen of particular disease.

Passive Immunity: it involves transfer of animal body from individual by natural transfer or by infection. It is short lived.

Polyvalent Vaccine: More than two vaccines.

Serum: Pathogenic bacteria grown more abundantly when medium is enriched with blood serum. Blood serum is aspirated from blood taken under aseptic conditions.

Toxin: A bacterial substance which is capable of producing disease in a susceptible animal.

Toxoids: These are immunostimulants to induce a short term non-antigenic specific enhancement of immune system. Generally these are detoxified bacterial toxins but antigencity is retained.

Trivalent Vaccine: Combination of antigens made in which 3 several strains of same species or organisms or more than 2 combined to make the vaccine.

Vaccine: Composed of live or killed bacterial or viral antigens prepared commercially for the purpose of active immunisation against disease.

Types of Vaccines

Vaccines are of 3 types-

(a) Inactivated vaccine or killed

(b) Live attenuated vaccines

(c) Toxoids

Route of Biological Administration

Vaccination is done differently in different animals

Livestock

- Mostly subcutaneous injection: Neck region is preferred
- Intramuscular (rarely used)

Canines

- Subcutaneous or Intramuscularly

Poultry

- **Intraocular or (Eye drop method) :** Bird is held with one eye turned up. Vaccine or dropper bottle is used for instilling one drop in eye.
- **Intranasal (IN):** Instead of eye vaccine drop is instilled in one of nostrils. By momentarily pressing of beak expedite inhalation of vaccine by the chick. Handler should ensure that nasal drop is inhaled by the bird.
- **Drinking water method:** Birds at the age of 5-6 week and above can be vaccinated through drinking water. Cool clean water should be used which is free from iron and chlorine.
- **Intramuscular (IM):** Injected on lower neck region or breast muscle or thigh.
- **Subcutaneous injection (SC):** Injected on the back of neck or brisket region.
- **Wingweb:** Needle should be inserted through wingweb from beneath taking care to avoid feather of the wingweb.
- **Spray Method:** Cool clean water free from iron and chlorine is used to prepare vaccine for spraying. Vaccine is spread by spraying apparatus which should be free from sediments, corrosion and traces of disinfectant.

Precautions to keep in mind while vaccinating

- Vaccinate with asceptic precautions.
- Do not vaccinate sick or convalescent animals
- Do not apply any antiseptic at the site of vaccination
- Always check the shelf life of vaccine
- Store vaccine as per instruction of manufacturer (4-100C) and avoid freezing
- Equipment should be clean, sterile and free for traces of disinfectants used

To Remember on Post vaccination

- Slight swelling at the site of injection can occur which subside subsequently
- Slightly body temperature may elevate after vaccination
- Reduced intake of water and feed
- Production is lowered

Ideal Vaccine

An ideal vaccine should-

- Confer prolonged and strong immunity in the vaccinated animal
- Not cause adverse effect
- Be stable
- Be adaptable to mass vaccination
- Stimulate immune response distinguishable from that due to natural infection
- Be easy to administer
- Be inexpensive
- Initiate onset of immunity rapidly
- Develop uniform level of immunity

Abbreviations Used

Anti Rabic Vaccine	ARV
Black Quarter	BQ
Enterotoxaemia	ET
Foot and Mouth Disease	FMD
Freezed dried	FD
Haemorrhagic Septicaemia	HS
Infectious Bovine Rhino tracheitis	IBRT
Intra Ocular	IO
Intra Nasal	IN

Intra Muscular	IM
Rinderpest	RP
Sheep Pox	SP
Strain	Str
Subcutaneous	SC
Tissue Culture	TC

Vaccine Producing Institutes

Full Name	Abbreviation
Andhra Pradesh Veterinary Biological & Research Institute Hyderabad (A.P)	APVBRI
Animal Vaccine Institute, Gandhi Nagar (Gujart)	AVI
Bayer India Ltd. B.E. Animal Health Bayer House Central Avenue Hiranandani Gardens, Sec-12, Powai Mumbai 400 076	Bayer
Biological Product Centre, Jammu & Kashmir (J & K)	BPC
Biological Product Division Indian Vety. Research Institute Izat Nagar	BPDIVRI
Biological Products Section, Calcutta (W.B)	BPS
Biomed Private Ltd. C-96, Site No.1, Buland Shahar, Ghaziabad 201 001	Biomed
Brilliant India Ltd. Gr. Floor, K.S. Complex, 4/304, Bhagya Nagar, Kurnool 518 004	Brilliant
Haffekine Bio Pharmaceuticals Corp. Ltd. Parel, Mumbai 400 012	HBPC
Haryana Vety. Vaccine Institute, Hisar	HVVI
Hester Pharmaceuticals Ltd. 16/10, Devendra Society, Naranpura, Ahmedabad 380 013 (Guj.)	Hester
Indian Immunology Road No. 44, Jubilee Hills, Hyderabad 500 033	Ind.Imm.
Indian Veterinary Research Institute Regional Station, Hebbal, Bangalore (Karnataka)	IVRI
Indovax Pvt. Ltd. Corporate Heights, Sco-24, Sector-14, Gurgoan 122 001	Indovax

Institute of Animal Health & Production, Patna (Bihar)	IAHP
Institute of Animal Health And Vety. Biological Products Bangalore (Karnataka)	IAHVBP
Institute of Animal Health Veterinary Biological Products Mhow (M.P)	IAHVBP
Institute of Veterinary Biological, Khanapara, Guwahati 781 022 (Assam)	IVB
Institute of Veterinary Preventive Medicine Ranipet, Tamil Nadu 632 402	IVPM
Institute of Vety. Biological Products (Animal Husbandry Deptt. U.P.) Lucknow	BPI
Intervet (India) Ltd. No.5, Istmani Road, Cit Colony, Mylapore, Chennai 600 004	Intervet
Orissa Biological Product Institute, Bhubneshwar (Orissa)	OBPI
Panjab Vety. Vaccine Institute, Ludhiana	PVVI
Pfizer Ltd. Animal Health Division 5, Patel Estate, Sv Road, Jogeshwari West, Mumbai 400 102	Pfizer
Ranbaxy Animal Health A-3 Okhla Industrial Area, Phase-I, New Delhi	Ranbaxy
Regiona Vety. Biological Institute, Jaipur (Rajasthan)	RVBI
Sarabhai Zydus Animal Health Ltd. Administration Building, Gorwa Road, Baroda 390 023	Sarabhia Zydus
Serum Institute Of India Vety. Division 212/2, Hadapsar, Pune 411 028 (Behind Akashvani)	SII
Solvay B.E. Animal Health Ltd. Durgabhai Deshmukh Colony, Adikmet, Hyderabad 500 007	Solvay
Stallen South Asia Pvt. Ltd. 101, Shyam Kamal 'D' Building, Vile Parle East, Mumbai 400 057	Satllen
Ventri Biological Division Of Venkateshware Hatcheries Ltd. Pune Panshet Road, Giri Nagar, Pune 411 025	Ventri
Veterinary Biological Institute, Palode Pocha (Kerala)	VBI
Veterinary Biological Product, Pune	VBP

Infectious Diseases of Livestock

Bacterial

Anthrax

Disease can occur in cattle, sheep and horses. A bacterial disease caused by Bacillus anthracis. Symptoms are blood tinged foamy discharge from mouth, nostrils, and anus. Sudden death after high temperature with pain. Treatment is not possible. Anti anthrax serum are available. Prophylaxis- vaccines are also there. Hygiene is the biggest single factor in prevention of spread of disease.

Black Quarter

It is caused by Bacteria Clostridrium chauvoei or Clostridium septicum. Symptoms are high fever, hot and painful swelling in one of the legs commonly hindlegs, may be in neck region also. Swelling becomes cold, painless, crepitates on pressure due to pressure of gas with putrefied smell of rancid butter. Control by serum and antibiotic therapy. Prophylaxis- Vaccines

Botulism

A bacterial disease caused by Clostridium botulinum. It causes paralysis of muscles of throat and tongue by the toxins. Spread through stored dry fodder where carcase of rats are mixed. Muscular weakness and salivation has been observed. Symptoms appear 3-7 days after infection depending upon amount of toxins. Paralysis of chest muscles result in abdominal type respiration. Stiffness in walking can be seen.

Bovine Lymphangitis

It is a contagious disease caused by Corynebacterium pseudotuberculosis. Infection occurs through abrasions and unhygienic quarters. Nodules develop in sub/cut tissue around fetlock. These rupture to discharge green creamy pus.

Brucellosis or Bang's Disease or Contagions Bovine Abortion

Bacterial disease caused by Brucella abortus. In females it causes catarrhal metritis which leads to abortion in 5th or 8th month. Opaque discharge from vagina. In males orchitis and epididymitis occur occasionally. Retention of placenta is very common. Prophylaxis vaccines are used.

Enterotoxaemia Sheep

A bacterial diseases caused by different strains of Clostridium (welchii, perfringens, Clos. oedematiens) also known as Pulpy kidney disease. Kidney is damaged so heavily that it decomposes soon after the death. Toxins are liberated in intestine, which cause the death in 3-4 hours after onset of disease. Adult sheep can survive for 24 hours. Dullness, depression, yawning and loss of interest in food. In severe cases pasty diarrhea, staggering and convulsions are seen. Antitoxins and vaccines are used.

Haemorrhagic septicaemia (HS)

It is caused by bacteria. Pasteurella multocida. Symptoms are – very high temperature, swelling below jaw, throat, dewlap, brisket. Sometimes bloody diarrhea (intestinal form), sign of bronchopeneumonia and labored breathing. Unable to respire due to inflammation and the animal dies. Can be treated with antibiotics. For prophylaxis there are vaccines.

Johne's Disease or Para-Tuberculosis

Bacterial disease caused by Mycobacterium paratuberculosis. Animal passes loose diarrhoeic faeces intermittently, a number of times with general unthriftness with oedematous swelling under jaw. Faeces are frothy and with mucus. Disease is transmitted by ingestion of contaminated food and water.

Salmonella Abortive equine

Abortion in female caused by Salmonella abortive equina. Mostly pathogensis is not clear but involve effects of stern and systemic endotoxaemia of foetus. Infection is due to ingestion of foodstuff contaminated with uterine discharge from carrier or mares. Abortion occurs in 7-8 months. Retention of placenta and metritis are common. Can be in male and showing fever, oedematous swelling of prepuce, scrotum and arthritis.

Tetanus

Highly fatal infectious disease of all species of domestic animals caused by Clostridium tetani. It is characterised by hyperaesthesia, tetany and convulsions. Entry or organism is through deep puncture wounds. Increase in muscle stiffness with tremors, prolapse of third eyelid, stiffness of hindlegs dilatation of nostrils. There is constipation, retention of urine and bloat. Fatal illness in 5-10 days in cattle and horses. But in dogs and sheep 2-3 days.

Tuberculosis

Caused by Mycobacterium bovis. All species and age group are susceptible. Infected animal is the main source of transmission. Organisms are in exhaled air, in sputum and faeces, milk, urine, uterine discharges and enteres through inhalation or ingestion. Fluctuating temp. with rough hair coat and cough are noticed. It lead to dyspnea and involvement of lymph nodes. Tuberculous mastitis, vaginitis are also seen.

Viral

African Horse Sickness (Arbonons)

Caused by viserotropic arbovirus present in all body fluids and tissues of affected animals form the onset of fever till recovery. Disease is spread by biting insects. Incubation period is 5-7 days. It is a disease of horse, mule and donkeys. Initially there is fever followed by laboured breathing and severe coughing. There is profuse nasal discharge of yellow serous fluid and froth, profuse sweating and weakness.

Death follows within 4-5 days. A few can recover. In subacute cases oedema in head region especially eyelids, lips and has been noticed even to chest. It can also be fatal.

Foot and Mouth Disease

A viral caused by strain O, A, C and Asia-1. Incubation period is 2-5 days. Virus enters through injury of membrane of mouth, tongue and intestine, cleft of hooves. There is formation of vesicles on foot and mouth. These rupture into raw, red ulcers and blisters. Animals loose weight and appetite. Secondary complications are pus formation, maggot wound, shedding of hooves or permanent deformity, lameness, panting conditions. Disease can be in cattle, buffalo, sheep and goats.

Infectious bovine Rhino Tracheitis (IBRT)

Cause is herpes virus.

It is a disease of cattle, buffalo, sheep and goat. It causes placentitis, then infects the foetus and kills it in 24 hours. Abortion can occur any time but usually is from 4 month to end of pregnancy. Foetus is autolyzed with excess fluid in body cavities. Prophylaixs vaccines available.

Pox Disease

Also called sheep pox, goat pox, cow or buffalo pox, horse and camel pox. Caused by virus with incubation period of 2-5 days. Symptoms are rise in body temperature with pinpoint red spots and papules of mustard size on teat and udder. These can be felt by hand and becomes vesicles. In males lesions are on thigh and scrotum. Lesions heal in 15-20 days. Transmission is through milker's hands. For propxylaxis vaccines are available.

Rabies

Caused by virus and is of 2 forms (a) Furious form- behavior changes, restless, excited, develops hoarse voice as a result of paralysis of muscles of throat and larynx. Desires to bite and runs aimlessly. If survives paralysis of lower jaw, tongue, throat etc and dies (b) Dumb rabies- animal is inattentive, paralysis soon extends to muscles of throat. Animal is unable to bark or bite. If in late stage, killing of animal is advised. Virus may be present in saliva for 4-5 days before signs are evident. It is transmitted through dog mainly but cat, fox, wolves, monkey, squirrel and bats also are carriers. Incubation period is 3 weeks can be 5-6 months. Drooling of saliva is most constant sign.

Rinderpest

Cause- myxovirus. A viral disease of cattle, sheep and goats with 3-7 days incubation period. Symptoms are congested conjunctiva, lachrymation and dryness of muzzle. Arching of back with diarrhea of foeted smell. Lesions on buccal mucous membrane inside lips and gums also develop in the intestine, so mucus comes in faeces. Reduced to skeleton and animal dies in 7-10 days form onset of symptoms. Vaccines are used for prophylaxis and Serum are used for treatment.

Swine Fever or Hog cholera

Caused by virus, with high temperature and showing loss of appetite, extreme weakness, inflamed eyes, vomiting and convulsions resulting in death, may be complicated with pneumonia and enteritis. It is highly infectious viral septicaemia. All ages of pigs are effected. It is transmitted through inert-material and uncooked meat. Birds and humans can also spread. Signs appear 5-10 days after infection. Incubation period is 35 or more days. Even young pigs may die in the beginning of outbreak. High temperature of 40.5-41.5 °C is usual. Nervous sign also appear showing convulsions of tetanic or clonic type.

Protozoan

Theileriasis

It is a protozoan disease of cattle and sheep caused by Theileria. Important species are T. annulata and T.parva in sheep. The infective sporozoite stage of parasite is transmitted through saliva of infected ticks. These invade lymphocytes and within a few days develop to schizonts. With this, the multiplication of parasites starts and spreads throughout the lymphoid system. a portion of schizonts form merozoites, infect RBC and cause piroplasmosis. Symptoms are high fever, loss of appetite, anaemia, jaundice, swelling lymphnodes, spleen, liver, gums and mouth. Instestines are inflamed causing diarrhea. High dose of oxytetracycline and special antitheileria drugs are used for treatment. Prophylactive vaccines are available.

Bacterial Diseases Vaccines

Anthrax Vaccine

Anthrax Spore Vaccine (Live)	**Intervet**
Comp	Live spores of highly antigenic non capsulated avirulant strain of Bacillus anthracis in glyceine saline
Adm.	SC
@	1 ml in L and S animal (annual)
Pres.	100 ml

Anthrax Spore Vaccine (Live)	**Ranipet (IVPM)**
Comp	Live spores of highly antigenic non capsulated avirulant strain of Bacillus anthracis in glyceine saliva
Adm.	SC
@	1 ml in L and S animal (annual)
Pres.	100 ml

Anti Anthrax Serum	**IAHVB Delhi**
Comp	Serum of Anthrax activated animal
Adm.	SC
@	LA 50 ml SA 20 ml
Pres.	10 ml, 30 ml, 50 ml, 100 ml,

Anthrax Spore Vaccine (Live)	**IAHVBP Banglore**
Comp	Live spores of highly antigenic non capsulated avirulant strain of Bacillus anthracis in glyceine saline
Adm.	SC
@	1 ml in L and S animal (annual)
Pres.	100 ml

Anthrax Spore Vaccine (Live)	**VBI Palode**
Comp	Live spores of highly antigenic non capsulated avirulant strain of Bacillus anthracis in glyceine saline
Adm.	SC
@	1 ml in L and S animal (annual)
Pres.	100 ml

Anthrax Spore Vaccine (Live)	**RVBI Jaipur**
Comp	Live spores of highly antigenic non capsulated avirulant strain of Bacillus anthracis in glyceine saline
Adm.	SC
@	1 ml in L and S animal (annual)
Pres.	100 ml

Anthrax Spore Vaccine (Live)	**IAHVB Delhi**
Comp	Live spores of highly antigenic non capsulated avirulant strain of Bacillus anthracis in glyceine saline
Adm.	SC
@	1 ml in L and S animal (annual)
Pres.	100 ml

Anthrax Spore Vaccine (Live)	**BPI Lucknow**
Comp	Live spores of highly antigenic non capsulated avirulant strain of Bacillus anthracis in glyceine saline
Adm.	SC
@	1 ml in L and S animal (annual)
Pres.	100 ml

Anthrax Spore Vaccine (Live)	**BPS Calcutta**
Comp	Live spores of highly antigenic non capsulated avirulant strain of Bacillus anthracis in glyceine saline
Adm.	SC
@	1 ml in L and S animal (annual)
Pres.	100 ml

Anthrax Spore Vaccine (Live)	**IVBI Guwahati**
Comp	Live spores of highly antigenic non capsulated avirulant strain of Bacillus anthracis in glyceine saline
Adm.	SC
@	1 ml in L and S animal (annual)
Pres.	100 ml

Anthrax Spore Vaccine (Live)	**IAHD Patna**
Comp	Live spores of highly antigenic non capsulated avirulant strain of Bacillus anthracis in glyceine saline
Adm.	SC
@	1 ml in L and S animal (annual)
Pres.	100 ml

Anthrax Spore Vaccine (Live)	**BVDIVRI Izat Nagar**
Comp	Live spores of highly antigenic non capsulated avirulant strain of Bacillus anthracis in glyceine saline
Adm.	SC
@	1 ml in L and S animal (annual)
Pres.	100 ml

Anthrax Spore Vaccine (Live)	**IVBP Puna**
Comp	Live spores of highly antigenic non capsulated avirulant strain of Bacillus anthracis in glyceine saline
Adm.	SC
@	1 ml in L and S animal (annual)
Pres.	100 ml

Anthrax Spore Vaccine (Live)	**IAHVBP Mhow**
Comp	Live spores of highly antigenic non capsulated avirulant strain of Bacillus anthracis in glyceine saline
Adm.	SC
@	1 ml in L and S animal (annual)
Pres.	100 ml

Anthrax Spore Vaccine (Live)	**APVBRI Hyderabad**
Comp	Live spores of highly antigenic non capsulated avirulant strain of Bacillus anthracis in glyceine saline
Adm.	SC
@	1 ml in L and S animal (annual)
Pres.	100 ml

Anthrax Spore Vaccine (Live)	**OBPI Bhubneshwar**
Comp	Live spores of highly antigenic non capsulated avirulant strain of Bacillus anthracis in glyceine saline
Adm.	SC
@	1 ml in L and S animal (annual)
Pres.	100 ml

Black Quarter Vaccine

Black Quarter Vaccine	**Biomed**
Comp	Formalin inactivated Alumunium hydroxide gel adjuvant
Adm.	SC
@	2 ml Primary 6 months Revaccination annually
Pres.	100 ml or 50 doses

Black Quarter Vaccine	Brilliant
Comp	Inactivated Clostridum chauvei antigens adsorbed in aluminium hydroxide gel
Adm.	SC
@	2 ml Primary 6 months Revaccination annually
Pres.	100 ml or 50 doses

Black Quarter Vaccine	Intervet
Comp	Formalin inactivated Alumunium hydroxide gel adjuvant
Adm.	SC
@	2 ml Primary 5 months Revaccination annually
Pres.	100 ml or 50 doses

Black Quarter Vaccine	HVVI Hisar
Comp	Formalin inactivated Alumunium hydroxide gel adjuvant
Adm.	SC
@	LA 5 ml SA 2-3 ml Immunity for year
Pres.	250 ml

Black Quarter Vaccine	IAHVBP Mhow
Comp	Formalin inactivated Alumunium hydroxide gel adjuvant
Adm.	SC
@	LA 5 ml SA 2-3 ml Immunity for year
Pres.	250 ml

Black Quarter Vaccine	APVBRI Hyderabad
Comp	Formalin inactivated Alumunium hydroxide gel adjuvant
Adm.	SC
@	LA 5 ml SA 2-3 ml Immunity for year
Pres.	250 ml

Black Quarter Vaccine	IVB Guwahati
Comp	Formalin inactivated Alumunium hydroxide gel adjuvant
Adm.	SC
@	LA 5 ml SA 2-3 ml Immunity for year
Pres.	250 ml

Black Quarter Vaccine	**IAHP Patna**
Comp	Formalin inactivated Alumunium hydroxide gel adjuvant
Adm.	SC
@	LA 5 ml SA 2-3 ml Immunity for year
Pres.	250 ml

Black Quarter Vaccine	**AVI Gadhi Nagar**
Comp	Formalin inactivated Alumunium hydroxide gel adjuvant
Adm.	SC
@	LA 5 ml SA 2-3 ml Immunity for year
Pres.	250 ml

Black Quarter Vaccine	**BPC Jammu**
Comp	Formalin inactivated Alumunium hydroxide gel adjuvant
Adm.	SC
@	LA 5 ml SA 2-3ml Immunity for year
Pres.	250 ml

Black Quarter Vaccine	**VBI Palode**
Comp	Formalin inactivated Alumunium hydroxide gel adjuvant
Adm.	SC
@	LA 5 ml SA 2-3 ml Immunity for year
Pres.	250 ml

Black Quarter Vaccine	**OBPI Bhubaneshwar**
Comp	Formalin inactivated Alumunium hydroxide gel adjuvant
Adm.	SC
@	LA 5 ml SA 2-3 ml Immunity for year
Pres.	250 ml

Black Quarter Vaccine	**PVVI Lundhiana**
Comp	Formalin inactivated Alumunium hydroxide gel adjuvant
Adm.	SC
@	LA 5 ml SA 2-3 ml Immunity for year
Pres.	250 ml

Black Quarter Vaccine	BPDIVRI Izat Nagar
Comp	Formalin inactivated Alumunium hydroxide gel adjuvant
Adm.	SC
@	LA 5 ml SA 2-3 ml Immunity for year
Pres.	250 ml

Black Quarter Vaccine	BPI Lucknow
Comp	Formalin inactivated Alumunium hydroxide gel adjuvant
Adm.	SC
@	LA 5 ml SA 2-3 ml Immunity for year
Pres.	250 ml

Black Quarter Vaccine	IAHVBP Bangalore
Comp	Formalin inactivated Alumunium hydroxide gel adjuvant
Adm.	SC
@	LA 5 ml SA 2-3 ml Immunity for year
Pres.	250 ml

Black Quarter Vaccine	IVPM Ranipet
Comp	Formalin inactivated Alumunium hydroxide gel adjuvant
Adm.	SC
@	LA 5 ml SA 2-3 ml Immunity for year
Pres.	250 ml

Black Quarter Vaccine	IVBP Pune
Comp	Formalin inactivated Alumunium hydroxide gel adjuvant
Adm.	SC
@	LA 5 ml SA 2-3 ml Immunity for year
Pres.	250 ml

Black Quarter Vaccine	RVBI Jaipur
Comp	Formalin inactivated Alumunium hydroxide gel adjuvant
Adm.	SC
@	LA 5 ml SA 2-3 ml Immunity for year
Pres.	250 ml

Black Quarter Vaccine	**IAHVB Delhi**
Comp	Formalin inactivated Alumunium hydroxide gel adjuvant
Adm.	SC
@	LA 5 ml SA 2-3 ml Immunity for year
Pres.	250 ml

Black Quarter Vaccine	**Indian Immunology**
Comp	Inactivated antigen
Adm.	SC
@	2 ml
Pres.	100 ml

Anti BQ	**IAHVB Delhi**
Comp	Serum of BQ activated animal
Adm.	SC
@	LA 15 ml SA 10 ml
Pres.	300 ml

Botulism Vaccine

Multi Component Clostridial vaccine	**BVDIVRI Izat Nagar**
Comp	Multi clostridium antigen
Adm.	SC
@	2 ml
Pres.	50 ml

Botulism vaccine	**IVBP Pune**
Comp	Multi clostridium antigen
Adm.	SC
@	2 ml
Pres.	50 ml

Brucellosis Vaccine

Brucella abortus Vaccine (S-19)	**IVPM Ranipet**
Comp	Suspension of pure smooth (living) culture of Brucella abortus of Low virulence
Adm.	SC
@	LA 5 ml Primary at 8 month in females once
Pres.	50 ml

Brucella abortus Vaccine (S-19)	**BPDIVRI Izat Nagar**
Comp	Suspension of pure smooth (living) culture of Brucella abortus of Low virulence
Adm.	SC
@	LA 5 ml Primary at 8 month in females once
Pres.	50 ml

Brucella abortus Vaccine (S-19)	**PVVI Ludhinana**
Comp	Suspension of pure smooth (living) culture of Brucella abortus of Low virulence
Adm.	SC
@	LA 5 ml Primary at 8 month in females once
Pres.	50 ml

Brucella abortus Vaccine (S-19)	**VBP Pune**
Comp	Suspension of pure smooth (living) culture of Brucella abortus of Low virulence
Adm.	SC
@	LA 5 ml Primary at 8 month in females once
Pres.	50 ml

Brucella abortus Vaccine (S-19)	**Intervet**
Comp	Suspension of pure smooth (living) culture of Brucella abortus of Low virulence
Adm.	SC
@	LA 5 ml Primary at 8 month in females once
Pres.	50 ml

Brucella Vaccine Freeze dried	**Intervet**
Comp	Suspension of pure smooth living culture of Brucella abortus of low virulence but freeze dried
Adm.	SC
@	LA 5 ml Primary at 8 month in females once
Pres.	50 ml

Brucella Vaccine Strain 10	**Intervet**
Comp	Suspension of pure smooth living culture of Brucella abortus of low virulence but freeze dried
Adm.	SC
@	LA 5 ml Primary at 8 month in females once
Pres.	25 ml

Enterotoxemia Vaccine

Enterotoxemia Vaccine	**Biomed**
Comp	Clostridium welchi (Type D) toxoid and Bacterium formalin inactivated Aluminium hydroxide gel adjuvanted
Adm.	SC
@	Sheep & Goat 1ml vaccine in 1st week Booster in 4-6 weeks
Pres.	40 ml

Enterotoxemia Vaccine	**HVVI Hisar**
Comp	Clostridium welchi (Type D) toxoid and Bacterium formalin inactivated Aluminium hydroxide gel adjuvanted
Adm.	SC
@	2.5 ML Repeat after 2 weeks. Then annually
Pres.	250 ml

Enterotoxemia Vaccine	**IVPM Ranipet**
Comp	Clostridium welchi (Type D) toxoid and Bacterium formalin inactivated Aluminium hydroxide gel adjuvanted
Adm.	SC
@	2.5 ML Repeat after 2 weeks. Then annually
Pres.	250 ml

Enterotoxemia Vaccine	**AVI Gandhi Nagar**
Comp	Clostridium welchi (Type D) toxoid and Bacterium formalin inactivated Aluminium hydroxide gel adjuvanted

Adm.	SC
@	2.5 ML Repeat after 2 weeks. Then annually
Pres.	250 ml

Enterotoxemia Vaccine	**OBPI Bhubneshwar**
Comp	Clostridium welchi (Type D) toxoid and Bacterium formalin inactivated Aluminium hydroxide gel adjuvanted
Adm.	SC
@	2.5 ML Repeat after 2 weeks. Then annually
Pres.	250 ml

Enterotoxemia Vaccine	**RVBI Jaipur**
Comp	Clostridium welchi (Type D) toxoid and Bacterium formalin inactivated Aluminium hydroxide gel adjuvanted
Adm.	SC
@	2.5 ML Repeat after 2 weeks. Then annually
Pres.	250 ml

Enterotoxemia Vaccine	**BVDIVRI Izat Nagar**
Comp	Clostridium welchi (Type D) toxoid and Bacterium formalin inactivated Aluminium hydroxide gel adjuvanted
Adm.	SC
@	2.5 ML Repeat after 2 weeks. Then annually
Pres.	250 ml

Enterotoxemia Vaccine	**IAHVBP Bangalore**
Comp	Clostridium welchi (Type D) toxoid and Bacterium formalin inactivated Aluminium hydroxide gel adjuvanted
Adm.	SC
@	2.5 ML Repeat after 2 weeks. Then annually
Pres.	250 ml

Enterotoxemia Vaccine	IVPP Pune
Comp	Clostridium welchi (Type D) toxoid and Bacterium formalin inactivated Aluminium hydroxide gel adjuvanted
Adm.	SC
@	2.5 ML Repeat after 2 weeks. Then annually
Pres.	250 ml

Enterotoxemia Vaccine	IAHVBP Mhow
Comp	Clostridium welchi (Type D) toxoid and Bacterium formalin inactivated Aluminium hydroxide gel adjuvanted
Adm.	SC
@	2.5 ML Repeat after 2 weeks. Then annually
Pres.	250 ml

Enterotoxemia Vaccine	APVBRI Hyderabad
Comp	Clostridium welchi (Type D) toxoid and Bacterium formalin inactivated Aluminium hydroxide gel adjuvanted
Adm.	SC
@	2.5 ML Repeat after 2 weeks. Then annually
Pres.	250 ml

Enterotoxemia Vaccine	BPI Lucknow
Comp	Clostridium welchi (Type D) toxoid and Bacterium formalin inactivated Aluminium hydroxide gel adjuvanted
Adm.	SC
@	2.5 ML Repeat after 2 weeks. Then annually
Pres.	250 ml

Enterotoxemia Vaccine	PVVI Ludhiana
Comp	Clostridium welchi (Type D) toxoid and Bacterium formalin inactivated Aluminium hydroxide gel adjuvanted
Adm.	SC
@	2.5 ML Repeat after 2 weeks. Then annually
Pres.	250 ml

Enterotoxemia Vaccine	**IVB Guwahati**
Comp	Clostridium welchi (Type D) toxoid and Bacterium formalin inactivated Aluminium hydroxide gel adjuvanted
Adm.	SC
@	2.5 ML Repeat after 2 weeks. Then annually
Pres.	250 ml

Enterotoxemia Vaccine (Type D)	**Intervet**
Comp	Clostridium welchi (Type D) toxoid and Bacterium formalin inactivated Aluminium hydroxide gel adjuvanted
Adm.	SC
@	Primary 4-6 week age Booster 3-6 week after. Then every 6 months
Pres.	100 ml

Enterotoxemia Vaccine	**IAHVB Delhi**
Comp	Clostridium welchi (Type D) toxoid and Bacterium formalin inactivated Aluminium hydroxide gel adjuvanted
Adm.	SC
@	2.5-3 ml
Pres.	300 ml

Multi component Enterotoxemia Vaccine (C and D Type)	**Inervet**
Comp	Clostridium welchi (Type C, D) toxoid and Bacterium formalin inactivated Aluminium hydroxide gel adjuvanted
Adm.	SC
@	5 ml Primary 4-6 weeks. Repeat every 6 months
Pres.	100 ml

Raksha ET (Type D)	**Indian Immunology**
Comp	Clostridium welchi (Type D) toxoid and Bacterium formalin inactivated Aluminium hydroxide gel adjuvanted
Adm.	SC
@	5 ml Primary 4-6 weeks. Repeat every 6 months
Pres.	100 ml

Raksha ET (Type D)	**HVVI Hisar**
Comp	Clostridium welchi (Type D) toxoid and Bacterium formalin inactivated Aluminium hydroxide gel adjuvanted
Adm.	SC
@	2 ml Primary 4 month age repeat annually
Pres.	100 ml

ET Vaccine	**Brilliant**
Comp	Clostridium welchi (Type D) toxoid and Bacterium formalin inactivated Aluminium hydroxide gel adjuvanted
Adm.	SC
@	5 ml Primary 4-6 weeks age repeat every 6 months
Pres.	100 ml

H.S Vaccine

(A) Oil Adjuvant

H.S (OA) Vaccine	**HVVI Hisar**
Comp	It is killed bacteria of Pasteurella multocids with oil as adjuvant
Adm.	SC
@	3 ml Immunity for 1 year
Pres.	100 ml

H.S (OA) Vaccine	**IVPM Pune**
Comp	It is killed bacteria of Pasteurella multocids with oil as adjuvant
Adm.	SC
@	3 ml Immunity for 1 year
Pres.	100 ml

H.S (OA) Vaccine	**IAHVBP Mhow**
Comp	It is killed bacteria of Pasteurella multocids with oil as adjuvant
Adm.	SC
@	3 ml Immunity for 1 year
Pres.	100 ml

H.S (OA) Vaccine	ADVBRI Hyderabad
Comp	It is killed bacteria of Pasteurella multocids with oil as adjuvant
Adm.	SC
@	3 ml Immunity for 1 year
Pres.	100 ml

H.S (OA) Vaccine	VBI Palode
Comp	It is killed bacteria of Pasteurella multocids with oil as adjuvant
Adm.	SC
@	3 ml Immunity for 1 year
Pres.	100 ml

H.S (OA) Vaccine	Brilliant
Comp	It is killed bacteria of Pasteurella multocids with oil as adjuvant
Adm.	SC
@	3 ml Immunity for 1 year
Pres.	100 ml

H.S (OA) Vaccine	IAHVB Delhi
Comp	It is killed bacteria of Pasteurella multocids with oil as adjuvant
Adm.	SC
@	3 ml Immunity for 1 year
Pres.	100 ml

H.S (OA) Vaccine	BPDIVRI Izat Nagar
Comp	It is killed bacteria of Pasteurella multocids with oil as adjuvant
Adm.	SC
@	3 ml Immunity for 1 year
Pres.	100 ml

H.S (OA) Vaccine	BPI Lucknow
Comp	It is killed bacteria of Pasteurella multocids with oil as adjuvant
Adm.	SC
@	3 ml Immunity for 1 year
Pres.	100 ml

H.S (OA) Vaccine	**IAHVBP Bangalore**
Comp	It is killed bacteria of Pasteurella multocids with oil as adjuvant
Adm.	SC
@	3 ml Immunity for 1 year
Pres.	100 ml

H.S (OA) Vaccine	**IVPM Ranipet**
Comp	It is killed bacteria of Pasteurella multocids with oil as adjuvant
Adm.	SC
@	3 ml Immunity for 1 year
Pres.	100 ml

HSOA Vaccine	**PVVI Ludhiana**
Comp	It is killed bacteria of Pasteurella multocids with oil as adjuvant
Adm.	IM
@	2 ml for 150 kg B.wt 3 ml above 150 kg B.wt
Pres.	300 ml

HSUA Vaccine	**OBPI Bhubneshwar**
Comp	It is killed bacteria of Pasteurella multocids with oil as adjuvant
Adm.	IM
@	2 ml upto 137 kg, 3 ml above 137 kg B.wt
Pres.	300 ml

HS Vaccine	**Intervet**
Comp	It is killed bacteria of Pasteurella multocids with oil as adjuvant
Adm.	SC
@	2 ml primary at 6 month of age. Repeat every year but 6 monthly in endemic area
Pres.	100 ml

HS Vaccine (OA)	**Biomed**
Comp	It is killed bacteria of Pasteurella multocids with oil as adjuvant
Adm.	SC or IM
@	2.5 ml 6 monthly
Pres.	50 dose

B. Alum Precipitated

HS (AP) Vaccine	HVVI Hisar
Comp	Inactivated Pasteurella multocida organisms absorbed in Aluminium hydroxide as an adjuvant
Adm.	SC
@	5 ml To repeated 6 monthly
Pres.	250 ml or 50 dose

HS (AP) Vaccine	PVVI Ludhainana
Comp	Inactivated Pasteurella multocida organisms absorbed in Aluminium hydroxide as an adjuvant
Adm.	SC
@	5 ml To repeated 6 monthly
Pres.	250 ml or 50 dose

HS (AP) Vaccine	IVPM Ranipet
Comp	Inactivated Pasteurella multocida organisms absorbed in Aluminium hydroxide as an adjuvant
Adm.	SC
@	5 ml To repeated 6 monthly
Pres.	250 ml or 50 dose

HS (AP) Vaccine	IVBP Pune
Comp	Inactivated Pasteurella multocida organisms absorbed in Aluminium hydroxide as an adjuvant
Adm.	SC
@	5 ml To repeated 6 monthly
Pres.	250 ml or 50 dose

HS (AP) Vaccine	IAHVPB Mhow
Comp	Inactivated Pasteurella multocida organisms absorbed in Aluminium hydroxide as an adjuvant
Adm.	SC
@	5 ml To repeated 6 monthly
Pres.	250 ml or 50 dose

HS (AP) Vaccine	**BPI Lucknow**
Comp	Inactivated Pasteurella multocida organisms absorbed in Aluminium hydroxide as an adjuvant
Adm.	SC
@	5 ml To repeated 6 monthly
Pres.	250 ml or 50 dose

HS (AP) Vaccine	**BPS Calcutta**
Comp	Inactivated Pasteurella multocida organisms absorbed in Aluminium hydroxide as an adjuvant
Adm.	SC
@	5 ml To repeated 6 monthly
Pres.	250 ml or 50 dose

HS (AP) Vaccine	**RVBI Jaipur**
Comp	Inactivated Pasteurella multocida organisms absorbed in Aluminium hydroxide as an adjuvant
Adm.	SC
@	5 ml To repeated 6 monthly
Pres.	250 ml or 50 dose

HS (AP) Vaccine	**IVB Guwahati**
Comp	Inactivated Pasteurella multocida organisms absorbed in Aluminium hydroxide as an adjuvant
Adm.	SC
@	5 ml To repeated 6 monthly
Pres.	250 ml or 50 dose

HS (AP) Vaccine	**AVI Ghandhi Nagar**
Comp	Inactivated Pasteurella multocida organisms absorbed in Aluminium hydroxide as an adjuvant
Adm.	SC
@	5 ml To repeated 6 monthly
Pres.	250 ml or 50 dose

HS (AP) Vaccine	BP Central Jammu
Comp	Inactivated Pasteurella multocida organisms absorbed in Aluminium hydroxide as an adjuvant
Adm.	SC
@	5 ml To repeated 6 monthly
Pres.	250 ml or 50 dose

HS Vaccine	Brilliant
Comp	Inactivated Pasteurella multocida organisms absorbed in Aluminium hydroxide as an adjuvant
Adm.	SC
@	2 ml To be repeated annually
Pres.	100 ml

Raksha HS	Indian Immunology
Comp	Inactivated Pasteurella multocida organisms absorbed in Aluminium hydroxide as an adjuvant
Adm.	SC
@	2 ml to be repeated annually
Pres.	250 ml or 50 dose

HS Vaccine	IAHVB Delhi
Comp	Inactivated Pasteurella multocida organisms absorbed in Aluminium hydroxide as an adjuvant
Adm.	SC
@	5 ml to be repeated 6 monthly
Pres.	300 ml

HS Vaccine	OBPI Bhubneshwar
Comp	Inactivated Pasteurella multocida organisms absorbed in Aluminium hydroxide as an adjuvant
Adm.	SC
@	5 ml upto 273 kg 10ml above 273 kg B.wt
Pres.	250 ml

Tetanus

(i) Toxoid

Tetanus Toxoid	Glaxo
Comp	It is adsorbed toxoid of Clostridium tetani in purified form used for Prophylaxis

Adm.	IM
@	LA 2 ml SA 0.5-1 ml
Pres.	1 ml, 2 ml

Tetanus Toxoid	**Serum Institute Pune**
Comp	It is adsorbed toxoid of Clostridium tetani in purified form used for Prophylaxis
Adm.	IM
@	LA 2 ml SA 0.5-1 ml
Pres.	0.5 ml, 10 ml

(ii) Antitoxin

Tetanus Antitoxin inj	**Bengal immunity**
Comp	It is antitoxin of Clostridium tetani used for Prophylactic and therapeutic use against tetanus
Adm.	IM
@	LA Prophylactic -3000 IU Therapeutic 150000 – 200000 IU SA Prophylactic -500-1500 IU Therapeutic 25000-50000 IU
Pres.	1500 IU, 10000 IU, 20000 IU

Tetanus Antitoxin (Enzyme Refined)	**Serum Institute India Pune**
Comp	It is antitoxin of Clostridium tetani used for Prophylactic and therapeutic use against tetanus
Adm.	IM
@	LA Prophylactic -1500 IU Therapeutic 10000 IU
Pres.	2000 IU, 50000 IU

Vaccines – Viral Diseases

African Horse Sickness Disease

Horse Sickness Vaccine	**BVDIVRI Izat Nager**
Comp	Not given
Adm.	Not given
@	Not given
Pres.	Not available now.

Foot and Mouth Diseases

Clovax	Intervet
Comp	Trivalent oil adjuvant vaccine containing FMD virus O, A, C Asia I Monovalent, bivalent, Trivalent vaccines with different virus types
Adm.	SC/ IM
@	LA 1 ml Mono 1.5 ml Bivalent 2 ml Trivalent 3 ml Tetravalent SA 1ml Mono 1 ml Bivalent 1.5 ml Trivalent 2ml Tetravalent Primary 3 weeks I Booster 12-14 week, II Booster after 6 months Revaccination annual
Pres.	All types 30 ml, 90 ml

FMD Vaccine	Brilliant
Comp	Contains O, C, Asia and A22 strain inactivated concentrated oil adjuvanted
Adm.	IM/ SC
@	1 ml
Pres.	50 ml, 100 ml

FMD Vaccine	Brilliant
Comp	In Aluminium gel
Adm.	IM/ SC
@	1 ml
Pres.	100 ml

Foot and Mouth Disease Vaccine	Intervet
Comp	Concentrated monovalent vaccine containing FMD virus type either One of Asia I, O, A_{22}, C or A_{10}
Adm.	SC
@	2.5 ml
Pres.	50 ml, 100 ml

Foot and Mouth Disease Vaccine	Intervet
Comp	Concentrated Trivalent vaccine containing FMD virus types A, O_{22}, C or Asia I,
Adm.	SC
@	LA 10 ml, SA 5 ml Primary 6-8 weeks or 3 month Booster 45 days after Revaccination every 6 months
Pres.	100 ml

Foot and Mouth Disease Vaccine	**Intervet**
Comp	Super concentrated tetravalent vaccine containing FMD virus types O, A_{22}, C and Asia I
Adm.	SC
@	LA 5 ml SA 2.5 ml
Pres.	50 ml, 100 ml

Raksha FMD	**Indian Immunology**
Comp	Tissue culture inactivated FMD virus antigens O, A, C and Asia I adosorbed into Aluminium hydroxide and saponin added as an adjuvant
Adm.	SC
@	LA 3 ml SA 1 ml, Primary at 4 months. Booster 2-4 weeks later Revaccination every 6 month
Pres.	30 ml, 90 ml, 300 ml

Raksha OVAC	**Indian Immunology**
Comp	Inactivated tissue culture FMD virus antigens O, A, C and Asia I adjuvanated into mineral oil
Adm.	IM
@	LA 2ml SA 1ml Primary at 4 months Revaccination after every 9 months
Pres.	20 ml (10D) 30 ml (15D) 50 ml (25D)

Foot and Mouth Disease Vaccine	**BDDIVRI Izat Nagar**
Comp	Concentrated monovalent vaccine containing FMD virus either one of Asia I, O, A_{22}, C or A_{10}
Adm.	IM
@	2.5 ml
Pres.	50 ml, 100 ml

FMD vaccine	**IVRI Herbal Bangalore**
Comp	Concentrated monovalent vaccine containing FMD virus either one of Asia I, O, A_{22}, C or A_{10}
Adm.	IM
@	2.5 ml
Pres.	50 ml, 100 ml

FMD vaccine (IVRI Vaccine)	**IAHVB Delhi**
Comp	Concentrated monovalent vaccine containing FMD virus either one of Asia I, O, A_{22}, C or A_{10}
Adm.	IM
@	2.5 ml
Pres.	50 ml, 100 ml

Infectious Bovine Rhiotracheitis Vaccine

IBRIVAX	**Intervet**
Comp	Bovine Herpes virus grown in cell culture chemically inactivated and emulsified with fortified special oil adjuvant
Adm.	SC/ IM
@	2 ml Primary vaccine 4-6 weeks. Booster 3 months later. Then annually
Pres.	20 ml

Pox Vaccines

Sheep Pox Vaccine

Raksha SP	**Indian Immunology**
Comp	Live attenuated sheep pox virus grown on lambs testicle cells
Adm.	IM
@	1 ml
Pres.	25 ml, 50 ml, 100 ml + Diluent

Sheep Pox Vaccine	**Intervet**
Comp	Live attenuated sheep pox virus grown on lambs testicle cells
Adm.	IM
@	1 ml
Pres.	25 ml, 50 ml

Goat Pox Vaccine	**Biomed**
Comp	Virus TCID 50 per dose live attenuated freeze dried
Adm.	SC or intradermal
@	0.2 ml annual
Pres.	50 doses or 25 doses with diluent

Goat Pox Vaccine	**IAHVB Delhi**
Comp	Virus TCID 50 per dose live attenuated freeze dried
Adm.	SC or intradermal
@	0.2 ml annual
Pres.	50 doses or 25 doses with diluent

Sheep Pox Vaccine	**IAHVB Delhi**
Comp	Virus TCID 50 per dose live attenuated freeze dried
Adm.	SC or intradermal
@	1ml annually
Pres.	50 doses or 25 doses with diluent

Sheep Pox Vaccine	**IAHBP Mhow**
Comp	Live attenuated sheep pox virus grown on lambs testicle cells
Adm.	IM
@	1ml
Pres.	25 ml, 50 ml, 100 ml + Diluent

Sheep Pox Vaccine	**IVBP Pune**
Comp	Live attenuated sheep pox virus grown on lambs testicle cells
Adm.	IM
@	1 ml
Pres.	25 ml, 50 ml, 100 ml + Diluent

Sheep Pox Vaccine	**IVPM Ranipet**
Comp	Live attenuated sheep pox virus grown on lambs testicle cells
Adm.	IM
@	1ml
Pres.	25 ml, 50 ml, 100 ml + Diluent

Sheep Pox Vaccine	**IAHVBP Bangalore**
Comp	Live attenuated sheep pox virus grown on lambs testicle cells
Adm.	IM
@	1ml
Pres.	25 ml, 50 ml, 100 ml + Diluent

Sheep Pox Vaccine	**BPDIVRI Izat Nagar**
Comp	Live attenuated sheep pox virus grown on lambs testicle cells
Adm.	IM
@	1ml
Pres.	25 ml, 50 ml, 100 ml + Diluent

Sheep Pox Vaccine	**RVBI Jaipur**
Comp	Live attenuated sheep pox virus grown on lambs testicle cells
Adm.	IM
@	1 ml
Pres.	25 ml, 50 ml, 100 ml + Diluent

Sheep Pox Vaccine	**BIP Lucknow**
Comp	Live attenuated sheep pox virus grown on lambs testicle cells
Adm.	IM
@	1 ml
Pres.	25 ml, 50 ml, 100 ml + Diluent

Sheep Pox Vaccine	**APVBRI Hyderabad**
Comp	Live attenuated sheep pox virus grown on lambs testicle cells
Adm.	IM
@	1ml
Pres.	25 ml, 50 ml, 100 ml + Diluent

Sheep Pox Vaccine	**HVVI Hisar**
Comp	Tissue culture inactivated Pox virus adsorbed into Aluminium hydroxide gel as adjuvant
Adm.	SC
@	0.5 ml
Pres.	50 doses (25ml)

Sheep Pox Vaccine	**IVBP Pune**
Comp	Live attenuated strain Russian of sheep pox virus grown is secondary sheep thyroid cell culture
Adm.	SC
@	0.5 ml
Pres.	50 doses (25)

Sheep Pox Vaccine	**IAHBP Mhow**
Comp	Live attenuated strain Russian of sheep pox virus grown is secondary sheep thyroid cell culture
Adm.	SC
@	0.5 ml
Pres.	50 doses (25)

Sheep Pox Vaccine	**BPI Lucknow**
Comp	Live attenuated strain Russian of sheep pox virus grown is secondary sheep thyroid cell culture
Adm.	SC
@	0.5 ml
Pres.	50 doses (25)

Sheep Pox Vaccine	**IAHVB Delhi**
Comp	Tissue culture inactivated Pox virus adsorbed into Aluminium hydroxide gel as adjuvant
Adm.	SC
@	0.5 ml
Pres.	50 doses (25 ml)

Rabies

ARV (inactivated) 5%	**HVVI Hisar**
Comp	Inactivated and stablised rabies virus vaccine
Adm.	SC/ IM
@	7 injections are needed, LA 30 ml SA 10ml Animal weighing less than 50 kg 5 ml daily
Pres.	70 ml, 210 ml, 420 ml

ARV 20%	HVVI Hisar
Comp	Inactivated and stablised rabies virus vaccine
Adm.	SC/ IM
@	One dose
Pres.	Single dose

ARV (inactivated) 5%	APVBRI Hyderabad
Comp	Inactivated and stablised rabies virus vaccine
Adm.	SC/ IM
@	7 injections are needed, LA 30 ml SA 10 ml Animal weighing less than 50 kg 5 ml daily
Pres.	70 ml, 210 ml, 420 ml

ARV (inactivated) 5%	IVBP Pune
Comp	Inactivated and stablised rabies virus vaccine
Adm.	SC/ IM
@	7 injections are needed, LA 30 ml SA 10 ml Animal weighing less than 50 kg 5 ml daily
Pres.	70 ml, 210 ml, 420 ml

ARV (inactivated) 5%	OBVI Bhubneshwar
Comp	Inactivated and stablised rabies virus vaccine
Adm.	SC/ IM
@	7 injections are needed, LA 30 ml SA 10 ml Animal weighing less than 50 kg 5 ml daily
Pres.	70 ml, 210 ml, 420 ml

ARV (inactivated) 5%	PVVI Ludhiana
Comp	Inactivated and stablised rabies virus vaccine
Adm.	SC/ IM
@	7 injections are needed, LA 30 ml SA 10 ml Animal weighing less than 50 kg 5 ml daily
Pres.	70 ml, 210 ml, 420 ml

ARV (inactivated) 5%	**IVB Guwahati**
Comp	Inactivated and stablised rabies virus vaccine
Adm.	SC/ IM
@	7 injections are needed, LA 30 ml SA 10 ml Animal weighing less than 50 kg 5 ml daily
Pres.	70 ml, 210 ml, 420 ml

ARV (inactivated) 5%	**BPDIVIR Izat nagar**
Comp	Inactivated and stablised rabies virus vaccine
Adm.	SC/ IM
@	7 injections are needed, LA 30 ml SA 10 ml Animal weighing less than 50 kg 5 ml daily
Pres.	70 ml, 210 ml, 420 ml

ARV (inactivated) 5%	**IAHVBP Bangalore**
Comp	Inactivated and stablised rabies virus vaccine
Adm.	SC/ IM
@	7 injections are needed, LA 30 ml SA 10 ml Animal weighing less than 50 kg 5 ml daily
Pres.	70 ml, 210 ml, 420 ml

Candor R	**Intervet**
Comp	Inactivated Rabies virus grown in purified chicken (rabies virus/ IU) embryo cell culture
Adm.	SC/ IM
@	Prophylactic 7 weeks of age. Booster 4-6 weeks later. Revaccination annually Postexposure on 0,3,7,14, 28, 90th days
Pres.	1ml vial, 10 ml multi dose

Megavac -R	**Indian Immunology**
Comp	Tissue culture rabies virus CNS strain produced on BHK 21 cell line and inactivated with aziridine compound
Adm.	SC/ IM

@	1ml Prophylactic at 3 month Booster 2-4 weeks. Revaccination annually
Pres.	1 ml, 10 ml

Rabdomun	**Zydus**
Comp	Flurry egg passage strain of rabies grown in BHK 21 cell culture inactivated with Aziridine compound and adsorbed on to Aluminium hydroxide. Single dose contains antigenic value not less than 5 IU
Adm.	SC/ IM
@	1 ml post exposure on 0, 3, 7, 14, 28, 90 th day
Pres.	1ml

Rabies Vaccine	**Biomed**
Comp	HEP Flurry strain virus $10^{45}MLD_{50}$ per dose. Attenated live freeze dried
Adm.	SC/ IM
@	Day 1 2nd – 2nd, 3rd 3 day and on 5th day
Pres.	4 dose

Raksharab	**Indian Immunology**
Comp	Inactivated tissue culture rabies virus CVBS strain produced on BHK21 cell line adjuvanted with Aluminium hydroxide
Adm.	SC/ IM
@	1ml dose on 0 day or within 24 hrs of dog bite followed by vaccination 3rd, 7th, 14th, 28th & 90th day
Pres.	1 ml, 5 ml, 10 ml

Rinderpest

Raksha RP	**Indian Immunology**
Comp	Live attenuated Rinderpest virus grown in bovine kidney cells
Adm.	SC
@	1ml 1st at age of 4 months. Repeat annually
Pres.	25 ml + diluent, 100 ml+ diluent

Rinderpest GAT Vaccine	**PVVI Ludhiana**
Comp	Freezed dried Tissue cell cultured goat adopted tissue live
Adm.	SC
@	2ml Dissolve 200ml water in 100 dose. Repeat annually
Pres.	100 dose

Rinderpest GAT Vaccine	**BPS Calcutta**
Comp	Freezed dried Tissue cell cultured goat adopted tissue live
Adm.	SC
@	2ml Dissolve 200ml water in 100 dose. Repeat annually
Pres.	100 dose

Rinderpest GAT Vaccine	**IVB Guwahati**
Comp	Freezed dried Tissue cell cultured goat adopted tissue live
Adm.	SC
@	2ml Dissolve 200ml water in 100 dose. Repeat annually
Pres.	100 dose

Rinderpest GAT Vaccine	**IAHP Patna**
Comp	Freezed dried Tissue cell cultured goat adopted tissue live
Adm.	SC
@	2ml Dissolve 200ml water in 100 dose. Repeat annually
Pres.	100 dose

Rinderpest GAT Vaccine	**OBPI Bhubneshwar**
Comp	Freezed dried Tissue cell cultured goat adopted tissue live
Adm.	SC
@	2ml Dissolve 200ml water in 100 dose. Repeat annually
Pres.	100 dose

Rinderpest GAT Vaccine	**HVVI Hisar**
Comp	Freezed dried Tissue cell cultured goat adopted tissue live
Adm.	SC
@	2ml Dissolve 200ml water in 100 dose. Repeat annually
Pres.	100 dose

Rinderpest GAT Vaccine	IVPM Ranipat
Comp	Freezed dried Tissue cell cultured goat adopted tissue live
Adm.	SC
@	2ml Dissolve 200ml water in 100 dose. Repeat annually
Pres.	100 dose

Rinderpest GAT Vaccine	IVBP Pune
Comp	Freezed dried Tissue cell cultured goat adopted tissue live
Adm.	SC
@	2ml Dissolve 200ml water in 100 dose. Repeat annually
Pres.	100 dose

Rinderpest GAT Vaccine	IAHVBP Mhow
Comp	Freezed dried Tissue cell cultured goat adopted tissue live
Adm.	SC
@	2ml Dissolve 200ml water in 100 dose. Repeat annually
Pres.	100 dose

Rinderpest GAT Vaccine	BPL Lucknow
Comp	Freezed dried Tissue cell cultured goat adopted tissue live
Adm.	SC
@	2ml Dissolve 200ml water in 100 dose. Repeat annually
Pres.	100 dose

Rinderpest GAT Vaccine	IAHVB Delhi
Comp	Freezed dried Tissue cell cultured goat adopted tissue live
Adm.	SC
@	1 ml Immunity 5 years
Pres.	10 ml

RP Vaccine Tissue culture	IAHVB Delhi
Comp	Freezed dried Tissue cultured goat adopted freeze dried
Adm.	SC
@	1ml Immunity 3 years immunity
Pres.	Freeze dried in ampoules 10 doses

Tissue Culture RP Vaccine	**BVPDIVRI Izat Nagar**
Comp	Living tissue culture of Rinderpest virus
Adm.	SC
@	1 ml annually
Pres.	100 doses

Tissue Culture RP Vaccine	**IAHVB Banalore**
Comp	Living tissue culture of Rinderpest virus
Adm.	SC
@	1ml annually
Pres.	100 doses

Tissue Culture RP Vaccine	**IVPM Ranipet**
Comp	Living tissue culture of Rinderpest virus
Adm.	SC
@	1 ml annually
Pres.	100 doses

Tissue Culture RP Vaccine	**IVBP Pune**
Comp	Living tissue culture of Rinderpest virus
Adm.	SC
@	1 ml annually
Pres.	100 doses

Tissue Culture RP Vaccine	**IAHVBP Mhow**
Comp	Living tissue culture of Rinderpest virus
Adm.	SC
@	1 ml annually
Pres.	100 doses

Tissue Culture RP Vaccine	**APVBRI Hyderabad**
Comp	Living tissue culture of Rinderpest virus
Adm.	SC
@	1 ml annually
Pres.	100 doses

RP Vaccine	Biomed
Comp	Freezed dired tissue cell culture goat adopted tissue live
Adm.	SC
@	2ml repeat annually, dissolve 200ml water in 100 doses
Pres.	100 doses

FD G TV	HVVI Hisar
Comp	Living and freezed dried goat adopted tissue vaccine
Adm.	SC
@	1ml life long immunity. Grind the content of 1 ampoule in sterlised mortar and pestle, dissolve in 100ml normal salina water
Pres.	100 dose ampoule

Anti Rinderpest Serum	IVPM Ranipet
Comp	
Adm.	Details not available
@	
Pres.	

Swine Fever

Swine Fever Vaccine	Intervet
Comp	Contains highly immunogenic attenuated strains of swine fever virus propagated in tissue culture stablised in a freezed dried form
Adm.	IM
@	1 ml Primary at 6 weeks. Revaccination annually
Pres.	5 ml

Swine Fever Vaccine	HVVI Hisar
Comp	It is Lapanised strain of swine fever virus living
Adm.	SC
@	1 ml Immunity for 1 year
Pres.	10 ml

Swine Fever Vaccine	BVDNRI Izat Nagar
Comp	It is Lapanised strain of swine fever virus living
Adm.	SC
@	1 ml Immunity for 1 year
Pres.	10 ml

Swine Fever Vaccine	**PVVI Ludhiana**
Comp	It is Lapanised strain of swine fever virus living
Adm.	SC
@	1 ml Immunity for 1 year
Pres.	10 ml

Swine Fever Vaccine	**IAHBP Mhow**
Comp	It is Lapanised strain of swine fever virus living
Adm.	SC
@	1 ml Immunity for 1 year
Pres.	10 ml

Swine Fever Vaccine	**IBVP Pune**
Comp	It is Lapanised strain of swine fever virus living
Adm.	SC
@	1ml Immunity for 1 year
Pres.	10 ml

Swine Fever Vaccine	**BPI Lucknow**
Comp	It is Lapanised strain of swine fever virus living
Adm.	SC
@	1 ml Immunity for 1 year
Pres.	10 ml

Swine Fever Vaccine	**BPS Calcutta**
Comp	It is Lapanised strain of swine fever virus living
Adm.	SC
@	1ml Immunity for 1 year
Pres.	10 ml

Swine Fever Vaccine	**IVB Guwahati**
Comp	It is Lapanised strain of swine fever virus living
Adm.	SC
@	1 ml Immunity for 1 year
Pres.	10 ml

Swine Fever Vaccine	IVPM Ranipet
Comp	It is Lapanised strain of swine fever virus living
Adm.	SC
@	1ml Immunity for 1 year
Pres.	10 ml

Protozoan Diseases Vaccine

Raksha Vac T	Indian Immunological
Comp	Live schizont grown in lymphoblast cell culture attenuated by prolonged in vitro passage
Adm.	SC
@	3 ml 1st vaccination 2 months and above. Revaccination every 3 years
Pres.	50 doses vial + diluent

Combined vaccine

HS and BQ combined vaccine	Intervet
Comp	Inactivated Pasteurella multocida and Clostridium chauvoei antigens with Aluminium hydroxide gel
Adm.	SC
@	LA 4 ml SA 2 ml. Primary at 6 months age then annually
Pres.	100 ml

HS BQ Vaccine	Biomed
Comp	Inactivated Pasteurella multocida and clostridium Chauvoei antigens with Aluminium hydroxide gel
Adm.	SC
@	LA 4 ml SA 2 ml. Primary at 6 months age then annually
Pres.	25 doses

HS & BQ Vaccine	Brilliant
Comp	Inactivated Pasteurella multocida and clostridium Chauvoei antigens with Aluminium hydroxide gel
Adm.	SC
@	LA 4 ml SA 2 ml. Primary at 6 months age then annually
Pres.	100 ml

Raksha HSBQ Vaccine	Indian Immunological
Comp	Inactivated Pasteurella multocida and clostridium chauvoei antigens with Aluminium hydroxide gel
Adm.	SC
@	LA 4 ml SA 2 ml. Primary at 6 months age then annually
Pres.	30 doses

Raksha Biovac	Indian Immunological
Comp	Combined oil adjuvant vaccine FMD virus antigen OAC & Asia I strain HS component containing formaldehyde inactivated Pasteurella multocida culture
Adm.	IM
@	LA 3ml SA 1ml. Primary at 4 months age Booster 9 month later then annually
Pres.	30 ml

Raksha Triovac	Indian Immunological
Comp	Combined oil adjuvant vaccine FMD virus O A C, Asia I strains as inactivated antigen and component containing formaldehyde inactivated Pasteurella multocida culture and BQ component of formaldehyde inactivated Clostridium chauvei culture
Adm.	IM
@	LA 3ml SA 1ml. Primary at 4 months age Booster 9 month later then annually
Pres.	30 ml, 90 ml

Miscellaneous

Antivenum	Serum Institute India
Comp	Lyophilized antivenum polyvalent serum
Adm.	IM, SC, IV
@	1ml
Pres.	1 dose with 10 ml diluent

□□□

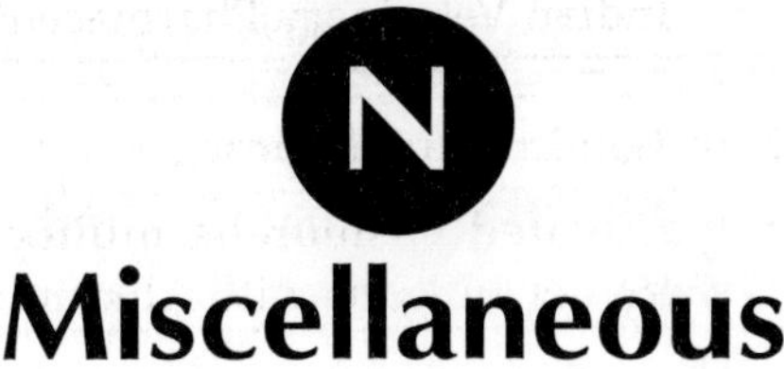

Miscellaneous

Antiseptics - Disinfectants

These are the agents which inhibit or kill microbes on contact. Agents used on living surfaces are called antiseptics while those used for inanimate objects are called disinfectants. There is a considerable overlap and many agents are used in either way. Majority of these have wide spectrum. These are germicidal and kill by oxidation of bacterial protoplasm, denaturation of proteins or detergent like action. There are various groups under this as per their action. Now mostly combinations of various group members are used.

Acids

Some acids are used as bacteriostatic and weak antiseptics.

Boric acid: It is minimally effective but non-irritating so can be used for delicate structures. Used for irrigating eyes, mouth wash, douche etc. By adding glycerine it can be used for stomatitis and glossitis. It is included in prickly heat powder & ear drops. Boro-glycerine is renowned product for human use. Available in pack of 100g, 500g.

Acetic acid: It is a relatively weak antiseptic and bactericidal. It is occasionally used for burn dressing and douche. It is available in 450ml bottles.

Alcohols

Many alcohols are germicidal. Most commonly used as disinfectants and antiseptics. These are lipid solvent and protein denaturants. Thse kill organism by solubilizing the lipid cell membrance. These are most effective when diluted with water. These act rapidly. A cotton swab soaked in 70% of these kills 90% bacteria in 2 minutes. Used before infections and minor cuts. Due to irritation should not be used on mucous membrance or delicate skin like scrotum. It does not kill spores and promotes rusting. It is a poor disinfectant. These are (commonly used are)-

(i) Ethanol (ii) Isopropanol

Aldehydes

These have wide spectrum. Due to irritation their use as antiseptics is restricted. These are

(i) **Formaldehyde:** It is gas and used for fumigation. Its 4% solution called Formaline is used as preservative for tissues. Its action is slow. Those who handle it can develop eczematoid reaction.

(ii) **Glutaraldehyde:** It is less volatile, less pungent, less irritating & better sterilizing agent than formaline. Solutions made have a short life of 2 weeks unless stabilizing agents are added.

Quarternary Ammonium Compound

These are detergents, cidal to bacteria, fungus and virus. Some bacterial spores specially Gram-ve are relatively resistant. These act on cell wall and alter permeability. They spread through oil and grease. They have cleansing and emulgent properties. These are non-irritating and germicidal action is slow. Pus, debris and porous material like cotton polyethylene reduce their activity. These are used as sanitizer and antiseptic.

Benzalkonium chloride: Highly soluble in water used in dilution for douche & irrigation.

Cetrimide: Scapy powder with a faint fishy odour. Good cleansing action, efficiently remove dirt, grease tar and congealed blood from wounds. Alone or in combination it is the most popular hospital antiseptic.

Cetylpyridinium chloride: As cetrimide used as mouth wash and in lozenges.

Dequallrilum chloride: Used as gum paint and in lozenges.

Aldehyde and Quartenary Ammonium Compounds

Aldepol A H	**Wockhardt**
Comp	Each 100 ml contains Benzalkonium chloride 5 ml Gluterldehyde 7.5 ml Formaldehyde 7.5 ml
Adm.	Directly used
@	As per need
Pres.	IL, 5 L

Attak	**Venky's**
Comp	Each 100 ml contains Benzalkonium chloride 5 ml Gluterldehyde 7.5 ml Formaldehyde 7.5 ml
Adm.	Directly used
@	As per need
Pres.	I L, 5 L, 30 L, 35 L

Dis N Det Liq	**Polchem**
Comp	Gluteraldehyole, Benzalkonium chloride, Ionic compound
Adm.	Directly used
@	As per need
Pres.	I L, 5 L, 35 L, 50 L

Diskol Liq	**Polchem**
Comp	Each 100 ml contains Benzalkonium chloride 5 ml Gluterldehyde 7.5 ml Formaldehyde 7.5 ml
Adm.	Directly used
@	As per need
Pres.	IL, 5L

Kohrosln-TH	**Virbac**
Comp	Each 100 ml contains Gluteraldehyde 7 g 1-6 dihydroxy 2-5 diohexane 9.5 g Polymethylurea derivative 16.3 g
Adm.	Direct
@	As per need
Pres.	100 ml, 500 ml, 5 L

Protekt	**Venky**
Comp	Each 100 ml contains Gluteraldehyde sol 7.5 ml Benzalkonium chloride 5 ml Non ionic surfactant 1 g Stabilizer 1 g
Adm.	Direct
@	As per need
Pres.	IL, 5L

Halogens

These have activity against Gram+ve, Gram-ve bacteria, bacterial spores, fungi and most viruses. It exerts these lethal effects by diffusing into the cell and interfering metabolism and disrupting protein and nucleic acid synthesis. These are:

1. **Iodine:** Rapidly acting broad spectrum microbicidal agent. Being used for more than a century acts by Iodinating and oxidizing. Solid Iodine is corrosive and strong solution cause burning and blistering of skin. It is used on cuts and as counter-irritant.
2. **Iodophores:** These are soluble complexes of Iodine which release Iodine slowly. Povidone is the most popular non-irritating, non-toxic, non-staining and exerts prolonged germicidal action. No risk of blistering. It is used in boils, burns, otits externa, ulcers, non-specific vaginitis and for surgical scrubbing.
3. **Chlorine:** Highly reactive element and potent germicide kills most pathogens in 30 seconds. Used to disinfect urban water supply.
4. **Chlorophores:** these are compounds that slowly release hypochlorous acid.
   (a) Chlorinated lime and Bleaching Powder- Obtained by action of chlorine on lime. Used to disinfect water, swimming pools.
   (b) Sodium hypochloride sol- Contains Sod hypochlorite. Powerful disinfectant used in dairies for milk cans and equipments. It is unstable and irritant. It is also used by Dentists for root canal therapy.
   (c) Halozon- Chloramine used as sanitizer.

Halogens and combinations

Polidone Liq or Poliphor Liq	**Polchem**
Comp	Alkylphene polyglycol ether Iodine complex providing 1.6% Iodine
Adm.	Direct
@	As per need
Pres.	IL

Pollunex Sol	**Neospark**	
Comp	Iodophor compound	2%
	Elemental potassium	0.18%
	Caesin protein	1000 ppm
Adm.	Direct	
@	As per need	
Pres.	IL, 5L	

Saofkit Liq	Indian Immunology
Comp	Iodine 0.71%
Adm.	Direct
@	As per need
Pres.	200 ml

Sapegard sol	Venky's
Comp	Iodine 1.6% ptt stabilizer 16%
Adm.	Direct
@	As per need
Pres.	I L, 5 L, 30 L, 35 L

Santiech sol	Cargill (Vetcare)
Comp	Stabilized chlorine dioxide 2%
Adm.	Direct
@	As per need
Pres.	IL, 5L

Wokadine scrubs	Wockhardt
Comp	Povidone Iodine 5%
Adm.	Local
@	As per need
Pres.	500 ml

Oxiding Agents

These liberate oxygen which oxidizes bacterial protoplasm. Solution gets decolourised. Action is slow. If used in higher concentration cause burns & blistering.

1. **Potassium Permaganate:** Used for gargling, douching, irrigating Cavities, Urethra and Wounds. Also used to disinfect water.
2. **Hydrogen Peroxide:** It speeds up decomposition resulting in foaming helps in removing slough, air, wax etc. it loses potency on keeping.
3. **Benzoyl Peroxide:** Gradually liberates oxygen (with the presence of water) used specially for acne. Adverse effects are excessive dryness of skin, marked scaling.

Oxypur P	Generic
Comp	Stabilized Hydrogen peroxide
Adm.	Water purifier
@	As per need
Pres.	500 g, 1 kg, 30 kg

Dyes

Various dyes are also used as disinfectant. Staining is disadvantage with all dyes.

(i) **Gentian violet or Crystal violet:** It is a rosaniline dye active against Gram+ve bacteria & fungi. Not active against Gram-ve or Mycobacteria. Aqueous or alcoholic solution are used in ring worm.

(ii) **Acriflavin & Proflavin:** These are orange yellow acridine dyes active against Gram+ve and Gonococci. Efficacy is not reduced by organic matter. Solution loose efficacy on exposure to light so store in amber bottle. These are non-irritant & suitable for chronic ulcers & wounds. Bandage impregnated with acriflavin Vaseline is used for burn dressing.

Furan Derivatives

Nitrofurans are bactericidal for both Gram+ve & Gram-ve, aerobic and anaerobic bacteria even in high dilution. Activity is reduced in presence of serum. Acts by inhibiting enzyme necessary for carbohydrate metabolism in bacteria. It is highly efficacious in burns & for skin grafting.

Metallic Salts

Some metallic salts and compounds are used as bacteriostatic.

(i) **Mercury Compounds:** These inactivate enzymes but inhibition is often reversible, spores survive even after prolonged action. Poor antiseptic.

(a) Ammoniated Mercury

(b) Phenyl mercuric nitrate

Used for first aid kits for application to skin and eyes.

(ii) **Silver Compounds:** These are astringent and caustic water stored in silver vessels is said to become sterile.

(a) Silver Nitrate: Kills microbes rapidly. Because of slow release action persists. Tissues get stained black.

(b) Silver sulfadiazine: Active against a large number of bacteria & fungi & even those resistant to sulfa drugs. It is slow releasing & most effective drug for prevention of infection in burnt surfaces & chronic ulcers. Itching & burning sensation is there.

(iii) Zinc Salts: These are also astringents and mild antiseptics.

(a) Zinc Sulphate: Highly water soluble. Applied to skin. It decreases perspiration.

(b) Zince Oxide and Calamine: These are insoluble and mild antiseptic. These are popular protective and adsorbants.

Biguanide combination

Chlorhexidine is a biguanide which is powerful non-irritating antiseptic that disrupts bacterial cell membrane. It persists on skin. Used for neonatal bath, mouthwash, obstetrics and general skin antiseptics.

Savlon Sol	**Hind lever**
Comp	Chlorhexidine gluconate 7.5% Cetrimide 15.0%
Adm.	Direct
@	As per need
Pres.	150 ml, I L

Phenol Derivatives

Phenols are the earliest used antiseptics and still the standard for comparing other germicides. These are weak & have poor action on bacterial spores. Higher concentrations can cause skin burns and is a caustic. These are now not used as antiseptics but are used to disinfect Urinals/ Toilets/ Hospitals.

(i) Phenol or Carbolic acid.

(ii) Methyl Phenol or Cresol: Potent less irritating and non-staining. Used in acne ring worm & eczema.

(iii) Hexyl resorcinol: Odourless, non-staining used as mouth wash, lozenges.

(iv) Chloroxylenol: Non-Corrosive, non-irritant to intact skin.

(v) Hexachlorphene: it inhibits enzyones, Odourless, non-irritating and does not stain. It deposits on skin and form a film. It is a good deodrant used in toilet products.

Phenol and other combinations

Disfect S	**Zydus (Pfizer)**
Comp	Polyalkyl monohydric phenol 40% Dodecyl Benzene sulphonic acid 24% Metacresal 5%
Adm.	Direct
@	As per need
Pres.	100 ml, I L, 5 L

Qualitrot sol	**Ranbaxy**
Comp	Orthophenyl phenol 12% Orthobenzyl chlorphenol 10% Paratertiary amyl phenol 4%
Adm.	Direct
@	As per need
Pres.	500 ml, 5 L

Virkon S Pow	**Pfizer**
Comp	Sodium chloride 1.5% containing Potassium monopersulphate and Potassium hydrogen sulphate and Potassium sulphate 49.8%
Adm.	Direct
@	As per need
Pres.	50 g, 500 g

Miscellaneous

Aktichlor T Pow	**Neospark**
Comp	Sodium N chloroparatoluene Sulphonamide/ Chloramine T
Adm.	application
@	As per need
Pres.	50 g, 100 g, 250 g, 500 ,

Bromosept 50	**Zydus**
Comp	Didecyl dimethylammonium bromide 50 g/100ml
Adm.	Applied
@	As per need
Pres.	IL, 5L

Chloramine T Pow	**Polchem**
Comp	Sodium polduene sulfone chloramide cent 20-25%
Adm.	Applied direct
@	As per need
Pres.	90 g, 500 g

Sikrena WS	**Virbac**
Comp	Didecyldimethyl ammonium chloride 7g/100 ml
Adm.	Direct
@	As per need
Pres.	500 ml, 5 L, 100 ml

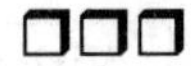

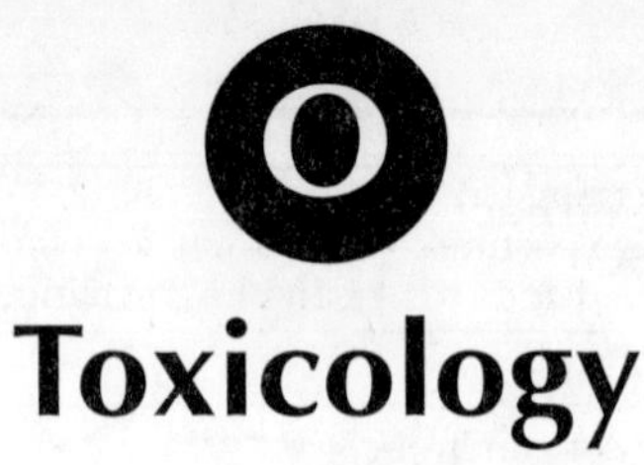

Toxicology

Toxicity of Chemical Origin

Toxic		Source	Manifestations	Treatment
1.	ACIDS	Feed containing acid phosphate	Severe colic, visible damage of oropharyngeal membranes,	2% sodium bicarbonate orally, analgesics sedatives to quieten the animal
2.	ALKALIES	Feed containing excess Calcium hydroxide	Servere colic, damage of oropharrryngeal membranes	5% Acetic acid (Vinegar) orally, analgesics
3.	ARSENIC	Insectcides, herbicides, rodenticides, haemoprotozoan, detergents	Servere colic staggering, collapse, paralysis, fast and weak pulse	B.A.L injection @ 4-5mg/kg I/M, tid for 3 days mineral oils oraly, gastric lavages.
4.	ATROPINE	Atropine containing plants, Datura, Hyoscyamus	Drymouth, thirst, constipation, tachycardia, restlessness, muscle, trembling, respiratory depression	Gastric lavage with Potassium permanganate, Saline purgatives
5.	CADMIUM	Plastics, batteries, rubber tyres, industrial effluents	Acute irriatation, salivation, colic, diarrhea and myalgic pains	Calcium-sodium EDTA
6.	CARBAMATES	Pesticides	Profuse salivation, lacrimaition. Nasal discharge increased respiratory sounds, colic, diarrhea, sweating, vomiting, cough, frequent urination, tremors, twitching, spasm, dyspnea, cyanosis	Atropine 0.2-0.5mg/kg BW Diuretics
7.	CHLORINATED HYDROCARBONS	Insecticides/ pesticides eg. DDT, Aldrin	Abnormal posturing, mania, spasm of cervical, fore quarter and hind quarter muscles, profuse salivation, diarrhea, urination, stiff gait	Saline purgatives, gastric, lavage, Activated charcoal
8.	COAL TAR	Tarred wall/ floors	Anorexia, depression, jaundice, swollen lymph nodes, anaemia	Removal of the cause, gastric lavage

9.	**COPPER**	Contaminated forage/pasture sprayed with Copper, anthelmintics in over dose and footbath	Colic, vomiting, salivation, anorexia, trembling, swaying back, acute dirrhoea	B.A.L injection supportive symptomatic therapy. Ascorbic acid
10.	**CYANIDE**	Cyanide containing fumigants, fertilizers	Excitement, Staggering, Tremors, dyspnoea. Salivation, lacrimation, urination, defecation, severe colic	Inhalation of 5-8 drops of Amyl nitrate. Sodium thiosulphate 600mg/kg. BW as slow IV (20% solution 40-80ml)
11.	**FORMALIN**	Fumigants, disinfectants	**Inhalation** Rhinitis, lacrimation, dyspnea, bronchitis **Ingestion** Severe colic, vomiting, haematuria, anuria	Gastric lavage, Sodium bicarbonate orally
12.	**FLUORIDE**	Rodenticides, insecticides and ectoparasiticides	Excitability, muscle tremor, urination, defecation, severe colic, salivation, sudden collapse	Gastric lavage, fluid therapy with normal saline, Aluminium sulphate @ 30g/day orally
13.	**LEAD**	Lead based paints, building materials, industrial effluents	Hyper excitability, rolling of eyes, pressing of head against wall, sudden jumping in air mania, nervous symptoms like muscle spasms	Ca-Na2EDTA 110 mg/kg/day I/V B.A.L. injection 2-3mg/kg BW IM. Thiamine 2-4 mg/kg/day S/C
14.	**MERCURY**	Industrial effluents	Incordination, salivation, lacrimation, gingivitis with urinary incontinence, haematuria, diarrhea with blood, epistaxis, dyspnoea	Proteins (milk, raw egg), emetics, chloral hydrate, gastric lavage, cathartics
15.	**NITRATES/ NITRITES**	Excessive nitrate containing pasture, feed and water, fertilizer	Rapid respiration, frequent urination, vomiting, diarrhea, colic, dyspnoea, bluish discolouration of mucous membrane	Methylene blue 1% slow IV in isotonic saline (cattle, sheep-10mg/kg BW and other species 5 mg/kg BW)
16.	**ORGANO COMPOUNDS**	Insecticidies/ pesticides	Profuse salivation, lacrimation, nasal dischare, dyspnoea, colic, sweating, constriction of pupil, vomiting, frequent urination, tremors	Atropine sulphate 0.25mg/kg BW (Cattle), supportive therapy like emetics, respiratory stimulants sedatives etc.
17.	**SALT**	Excessively salted feed, salt lick	**Water deprivation syndrome** Salivation, serous nasal discharge, urinary incontinence leading to anuria, colic, emesis, nervous symptoms	Removal of the cause, provide water ad libitum

18.	**SELENIUM**	Insecticides, selenium containing medicaments	**Acute** Lowered head and ears, polyuria, blood tinged froathy nasal discharge, emesis, diarrhea, lethargy, ataxia, paresis, bloat	**Acute** Saline purgatives, oxygen therapy, removal of the cause
19.	**UREA**	Excessively urea treated feed, urea fertilizers	Severe colic, excitement, termors, neuro muscular spasms , ammonical odour from rumen	2% Acetic acid (Vinegar) orally @ 0.5-1 Litre, sedatives/ tranquilzers
20.	**ZINC PHOSPHIDE**	Rodenticides	Lethargy, increased rate and depth of respiration, colic bloat in ruminants	Gastric lavage with 5% soda bicarb Anticonvulsants

Toxicity of Plant Origin

Toxic		Source	Manifestations	Treatment
1.	**BETEL-NUT PALM**	Acrecoline	Colic, diarrhea, restlessness, convulsions	Atropine sulphate 0.044mg/kg BW
13.	**BLACK NIGHTS**	Solanine	Servere colic, salivation, dysponea, trembling, paralysis, diarrhea	Symptomatic treatment, gastric lavage
2.	**BLUE GREEN**	Feed containing excess Calcium hydroxide	Servere colic, damage of oropharrryngeal membranes	5% Acetic acid (Vinegar) orally, analgesics
3.	**CASTOR BEAN**	Ricin	Severe colic, salivation, diarrhea, CNS, depression, colic	Gastric, Lavage, Saline purgatives
4.	**COFFEE WEED**	Saponine	Severe colic, depression, salivation	Symptomatic treatment
5.	**COTTON SEED**	Gossypol	Gastro enteritis, dyspnea	Fluid therapy, vitamin, A supplemention
9.	**DHATURA**	Atropine like alkaloid, Hyoscyamine	Delirium, vocalization	Control convuisions by anaesthesia
6.	**FOX GLOVE**	Digitalis	Loose stool, vomiting, cardiac arrhythmia	Rest, control arrhythmia with anti arrythmics
7.	**HORSE TAIL**	Thiaminase	Excitement, nervous signs, weakness, diarrhea	Thiamine paranterally
8.	**INDIAN TABACCO**	Lobeline	Depression, diarrhea, oral ulcers, hemorrhage, coma	Treat symptomatically
10.	**LOCO WEED**	Locoine	Dyspnoea, excitement, paralysis	Symptomatic treatment only

11.	**LUCENIA**	Mimosine	Loss of hair, reddening, sub cutaneous oedema, necrosis and sloughing of light skinned areas, dark green, dirrhoea, hypothermia	Removal of the cause, keep away from direct sunlight, fluid therapy, antihistamines
12.	**MIMOSA PLANT**	Mimosine	Loss of hair, reddening, sub cutaneous oedema, necrosis and sloughing of light skinned areas, dark green dirrhoea, hypothermia	Removal of the cause, keep away from direct sunlight, fluid therapy, antihistamines
14.	**OAKS & ACORNS**	Tannic acid	Severe colic, diarrhea with blood, depression, ataxia,	Symptomatic treatment only
15.	**OLEANDER**	Nerodorin	Diarrhoea, colic, swealing, cold extremities	Symptomatic treatment only
16.	**ONION**	N-preopyl disulphide	Anaemia	Treat symptomatically
17.	**POPPY PLANT**	Morphine	Seizures, gastro intestinal disturbances	Sedatives
19.	**POTATO**	L-chaloconine, solanidine, solanicin	Severe colic, salivation, paralysis, coma	Gastric lavage, symptomatic treatment
20.	**PRECATORY BEAN**	Abrin	Colic, salivation, depression, diarrhea, tetanic spasm	Symptomatic treatment
18.	**SATYANASHI**	Sanguianarine	Ascites, cardiac, hypertrophy	Diuretics
21.	**SWEET CLOVER**	Dicumarol	Sub-cutaneous haemorrhages	Vitamin K
22.	**SWEET PEA**	Betaine	Leg weakness leading to paralysis	Symptomatic treatment, calcium supplementation
23.	**STRYCHNOS**	Strychnine	Tightened facial muscles, muscular twitch, stiff gait, defecation, seizures, dyspnea, vocalization	Barbiturates IV
24.	**TAPIOCA**	Hydrocyanic acid	Anxiety, salivation, tremors, urination, defection, severe, colic	Inhalation of 5-8 drops of Amyl nitrate, sodium thiosulphate 600 mg/ kg BW as slow IV (20% solution 40-80 ml)
25.	**TABACOO**	Nicotine	Convulsions, depression	Caffeine, oxygen therapy

Toxicity of Mould Origin (Mycotoxin)

Toxic		Source	Manifestations	Treatment
1.	**AFLATOXIN**	Feed	Anorexia, dyspnea, cough, nasal discharge, anaemia, blood in faeces	Remove contaminated feed, low fat diet containing sufficient protein, oxytetracycline 10 mg/kg BW daily as IM for 5 days, supportive multi vitamin and fluid therapy
2.	**ERGOT ALKALOIDS**	Feed contaminated by fungi	Weakness, tremors, hyper excitability, ataxia, posterior paresis	Withheld the contaminated feed, sedatives/ tranquilizers to control nervous signs, Magnesium sulphate orally, antibiotics
3.	**F-TOXIN**	Feed	Vulvo vaginitis, oedematus swelling	Withheld contaminated feed, treat symptomatically
4.	**RUBRATOXIN**	Feed	Anorexia, dehydration, diarrhea	With-held contaminated feed symptomatic treatment

Toxicity of Animal Origin

Toxic		Source	Manifestations	Treatment
1.	**BEE**	Melletin, histamine	Local oedema, irritation, pain	Apply bicarbonate solution locally, antihistamines
2.	**BEETLE**	Canthridine	Blistering, necrosis	Symptomatic treatment
3.	**CENTIPEDE**	Phenols	Inflammation, oedema, spasmogenic effects	Anti histamines, analgesics
4.	**SCORPION**	Neurotoxin	Local inflammation, excitement, shivering, tremors, paralysis	Pressure bandage, anti toxin, symptomatic treatment
5.	**SNAKE**	Neurotoxins	Pain and inflammation at site, excitement followed by depression, paralysis, unconsciousness	Antivenom, anti inflammatory drugs, analgesics, anti tetanus, antibiotics, supportive therapy, fluids and corticosteroids
6.	**SPIDER**	Neurotoxin	Pain, rashes at the site, colic restlessness, crying, ascending paralysis	Anti venom, calcium gluconate slow, IV (10-20ml)
7.	**TICK**	Neurotoxin	Itching, dermatitis, flaccid paralysis, anaemia	Ectoparasiticides, anti histamines, supportive therapy
8.	**TOAD**	Bufotoxin	Cardiac arrhythmia, dyspnea, hypertension	Symptomatic treatment
9.	**WASP**	Histamine	Local pain, swelling at the site	Apply weak acids locally

❑❑❑

CANINE SECTION

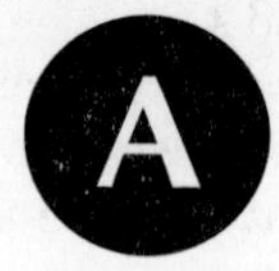

Alimentary System

Terms and Diseases

Amebiasis: Caused by Entamoeba histolytica. It causes inflammation of large intestine which leads to persistent diarrhea. There is weight loss, loss of appetite, straining to defecate and diarrhea.

Anal sac disease: It is caused by clogging or infection of glands called anal sacs located on each side of anus. There is pain, discomfort associated with sitting. Dog may scoot its buttocks on ground lick and bite at anal area and have painful defecation with straining.

Bilous vomiting syndrome: Vomiting in response to bile induced inflammation of stomach. Bile salts interfere with gastric mucosal barrier allowing acid to irritate the stomach lining and cause gastritis.

Bloat: It is caused by twisting of stomach along its axis and the accumulation of gas with or without fluid in stomach. Usually it is caused by eating large meal followed by exercise and repeated attempts of vomiting. Signs include restlessness, discomfort, rapid breathing,abdominal pain and swelling, repeated dry retching and excessive drooling.

Campylobacter Infection: It is a bacterial disease. It is transmitted to human being also by exposure to feces or food of infected dog. Signs include mucus laden, watery or bile streaked diarrhea with fever.

Canine chronic hepatitis: It is longterm inflammation of liver. There is copper accumulation.

Cheek biting: A wound along the side of the cheek caused by self trauma when tissue becomes trapped between teeth during chewing.

Cheilitis: Inflammation of lips. Licking areas of bacterial dermatitis or infected wounds may spread the infection to lips, lipfolds.

Cholocystitis: Inflammation of gall bladder and is usually caused by bacterial infection starting from intestine. There is loss of appetite, abdominal pain, fever, Jaundice and vomiting. Dog may be in state of shock.

Chronic ulcerative stomatitis: Involves inflammation of mucous membrane of the mouth. Signs include severe gum inflammation, receding gums in several sites and large sores on the mouth surface.

Circopharyngeal Achalasia: The circopharyngeal muscle opens and closes to allow food and liquids from mouth into oesophagus. In it achalasia muscle does not adequately relax. This can lead to inability to swallow food or liquid.

Coccidioidomycosis: It is fungal disease of liver caused by the fungus Coccidiodes immitis. Basically it is a respiratory disease with fever and intermittent diarrhea. There can be ascites and enlarged liver.

Coccidiosis: Invasion and destruction of tissue of intestine causing illness. Common signs are diarrhea sometime bloody, weight loss and dehydration.

Colonitis: Swelling of colon. It strains to defecate and may pass mucus laden feces sometimes containing blood.

Copper associated hepatopathy: It is a defect that causes copper accumulation in the liver resulting chronic hepatitis and cirrhosis of liver.

Drool: Saliva or Liquid coming from mouth.

Epulides: Benign oral tumor of dogs most frequently seen at 6 month of age. These are firm masses involving the tissue of the gum.

Exocrine Pancreating Insufficiency: It is a syndrome caused by insufficient production and secretion of digestive enzymes by pancreas. Signs are excessive eating, weight loss and diarrhea. Sometimes vomiting and loss of appetite are seen. Feces are pale, loose and voluminous may be foul smelling.

Fungal stomatitis: It is caused by overgrowth of Candida albicans fungus. Main sign is the appearance of creamy white flat plaques on the tongue or mucous membrane.

Gall stone: Disease is in older dogs especially females. There are stones in the gall bladder. Signs are vomiting, abdominal pain fever and Jaundice.

Gall bladder mucocele: Gall bladder becomes extended with bile and mucous which can lead to blockage of bile out flow from liver.

Gastric dilation volvulus or bloat: Stomach swells with air urinary and reproductive disease.

Gastritis: Swelling of stomach caused by eating something that injures lining of stomach vomiting is usually sign.

Gastrointestinal ulcers: These are caused by drugs, tumors, injections or generalized diseases. These develop by break down of normal stomach lining. There can be vomiting with fresh or digested blood and abdominal discomfort.

Giardiasis: It is longterm protozoal infection caused by Giardia species. They produce cysts that are passed in feces. It causes weight loss and long term diarrhea which can be watery.

Gingival fibroma: A benign growth on the gum that originates near gum line. Growth is insensitive and tough and usually the colour resembles normal colour of gum. It may enlarge and can cover surfaces of several teeth.

Glycogen storage disease: Glycogen is stored sugar. It is caused by deficiency of certain enzymes and result in failure of glycogen not released from cells and its accumulation in liver, outlook of dog is poor.

Haemorrhagic Gastroenteritis: It is characterised by sudden onset of bloody diarrhea in healthy dog. Cause is not known.

Helicobacter infection: It is caused Helicobacter pylori bacteria. There is mild inflammation of stomach with ulcers.

Hepatic amyloidosis: Amyloid is a protein. In this it is misfolded and causes damage to liver cells. Signs include loss of appetite, excessive thirst and urination, vomiting, Jaundice and enlarged liver. Affected animals have pale mucous membrane and may collapse.

Hepatic cyst: It is liver developmental anomaly which generally cause no signs of illness. Hepatic cysts mostly occur with Polycystic kidney diseases.

Hepatic encephalopathy: A syndrome of neurologic problems caused by poor liver function. Signs include circling, head pressigns, aimless wandering, weakness and poor coordination, blindness, excessive drooling, aggression, dementia, seizures and coma.

Hernia: It is protrusion of a portion of an organ or tissue through an abnormal opening.

Hiatal hernia: It involves extension of part of the stomach through the diaphragm with sign of loss of appetite or drooling or vomiting.

Histoplasmosis: It is a fungal disease caused by fungus Histoplasma. Symptoms are similar to other fungal infections.

Idiopathic liver fibrosis: Fibrosis is accumulation of tough scar tissue that replace normal liver tissue. Signs are fluid accumulation in abdomen/ weight loss, vomiting and diarrhea.

Infections canine hepatitis: It is longterm inflammation and scarring of liver along with death of liver tissue.

Inflammatory Bowel Disease: It is a group of digestive system problems Signs are inflammation without a cause. There can be diarrhea.

Intestinal incarceration: Digested food is trapped in intestine. It has abdominal pain that rapidly progresses to shock.

Intussusception: It is problem of intestine which may cause vomiting abdominal pain and scant bloody diarrhea.

Leptospirosis: It is bacterial infection of Leptospira interrogans that cause liver disease.

Lip fold dermatitis: Chronic skin inflammation in breeds of dog with drooping upper lips and lower lips folds. These lips accumulate moisture causing inflammation to develop.

Malabsorption: It occurs when nutrients are not properly absorbed into the blood stream.

Maldigestion: A condition in which certain foods are not digested.

Malocculusion: It is dental problem when the bite is uneven.

Megaesophagus: abnormal dilation or stretching of oesophagus.

Mouth burns: Thermal, chemical or electrical burns involving the mouth. It is minor injury usually but discomfort. It may lead to loss of tissue scar formation or even tissue loss.

Nodular hyperplasia: It is nonspreading age related condition in dogs. It is form of cancer.

Pancreatic adenoma: It is an abcess in which there is collection of pus. Signs may include vomiting, abdominal pain, depression, fever, loss of appetite, diarrhea and dehydration. A mass in abdomen can be felt.

Pancreatic pseudocast: Collection of sterile pancreatic fluid enclosed by a wall of tissue. Signs are similar to pancreatitis but vomiting is the most consistent sign. Cysts can be seen by ultrasound usage.

Pancreatits: Swelling of pancreatic tissue. It can be short term or longterm. Both form are severe. In the beginning pancreatic juices decrease, loss of appetite, vomiting, weakness, abdominal pain and dehydration are common signs.

Papilloma: These are like viral warts but they tend to grow more slowly and are mostly found in groups.

Periodontitis: There is severe tissue damage including gums, ligament and bone. It is seen after long year of development of plaque, tartar and gingivitis. It results permanent loss of tooth.

Ptyalism or Sialosis: Excessive salivation caused either by excessive production or the dog can not swallow effectively the produced saliva Animal drools. Mostly it happens in rabies.

Pyloric stenosis: It results from muscular thickening of pyloric sphincter (the exit of stomach). This thickening blocks the flow of digested food from stomach to intestine

Recta tear: A tear in the rectum or anus can be caused by a dog swallowing a sharp object. Signs include constipation, rectal bleeding and reluctance to defecate.

Rectal and Anorectal Stricture: These are narrowing caused by scar tissue. Scarring may be the result of injury from foreign object or a bite, wounds or accident.

Rectal Polyps: Growth called rectal polyps are benign. Signs include straining to defecate, blood in feces and diarrhea.

Rectal Prolapse: Protrusion of layers of rectum involving one or more layers. It may be incomplete protrusion or complete protrusion. Signs are severe diarrhea and strain to defecate.

Regurgitation: Coming back of swallowed food from alimentary canal into mouth.

Salivary fistula: Fistulas are abnormal paths or opening between 2 organs in the body. Cause may be injury to salivary gland in lower jaw cheeks or pace or under the tongue.

Salmonellosis: It is gastro intestinal illness caused by Salmonella. It can cause severe septicemia and inflammation of intestine.

Tartar: Technically it is calculus on or inside the teeth by continuous accumulation of minerals or food particles due to unhygienic conditions of mouth.

Tooth decay: Pits on the bite surfaces or on the sides of molar teeth near gum line.

Toxoplasmosis: It is a parasitic disease that can kill liver cell and cause sudden liver failure, Jaundice, fever, lethargy, vomiting and diarrhea. Nervous system and eye can also be involved. It is caused by protozoa Toxoplasmagondii.

Trench mouth: It is severe inflammation of gums, ulceration and death of tissue lining the mouth. There is reddening and swelling of gum edges which are painful and bleed easily.

Tyzzer's disease: Infection caused by Clostridium piliforme. Signsinclude decreased activity, loss of appetite, fever, Janudice and diarrhea.

Umblical hernia: It involves abdominal wall and depending upon location near umblical area.

Viral warts: These are non cancerous growths caused by virus. The mouth lining and corners of the lips are affected. Back and roof of mouth can also be involved.

Xerostomia: It is decreased secretion of saliva which causes a dry mouth. It causes significant discomfort and difficulty with eating.

Antiemetic

Anicalm inj/Tab	**Generic**
Comp	20mg of Triflupromazine per ml Tablet of 5mg or 10mg
Adm.	Inj IM, IV Tablet oral
@	Inj 2-4mg/ kg B.wt IM 1-2 mg/kg B.wt IV Tablet 2-4mg/ kg B.wt oral
Pres.	5ml vial

Cimetidine CHC Tab	**Cadila Health care**
Comp	Cimetidine 200mg Tablet
Adm.	Oral
@	5-10mg/ kg B.wt 2-4 times daily
Pres.	10's

Avomine Tab	**Rhone Poulenc**
Comp	Promethazine 25mg Tab
Adm.	Oral
@	1.5-2.5mg/ kg B.wt oral
Pres.	10's

Phenergan Inj	Primavet care
Comp	Promethazine 25mg/ml
Adm.	IM/ IV
@	1.5mg-2mg/ kg B.wt
Pres.	2ml ampoule

Siquil Inj/ Tab	Sarabhai Zydus
Comp	Triflupromazine Inj 20mg/ml 10mg Tablet
Adm.	IM/ IV Tab oral
@	Inj 2-4mg/kg B.wt IM 1-2mg/kg B.wt IV Tablet 2-4mg/kg B.wt
Pres.	5ml inj, 10's Tablet

Anti-diarrhoel

Antrima Tab	Rhone Poulenc
Comp	Sulphadiazine 1g Trimethoprim 0.2g – 1.2g Tab
Adm.	Oral
@	30mg/ kg B.wt od
Pres.	4's strip

3 Care Bolus	Cargill (Vetcare)
Comp	Halquinol 1.5g
Adm.	Oral
@	1/4-1/2 Bol bid for 4-5 days
Pres.	30's bottle

Dependal M Susp	Glaxo	
Comp	Each 5ml contains Furazole 25mg	Metronidazole 75mg
	Pectin 50mg	Kaolin 1g
Adm.	Oral	
@	5ml bid for 5-7 days	
Pres.	60ml	

Diamukt Syp Dry	Ayurvet
Comp	Ayurvedic formulation
Adm.	Oral

@	5ml upto 10kg B.wt 10ml above 10kg B.wt tid for 2-3 days by adding water upto mark
Pres.	15g

Diardon Pow	**Vets Farma**
Comp	Ayurvedic formulation
Adm.	Oral
@	15-20g bid for 3 days
Pres.	150g

Duaprim Bol/Pow	**Brihans**
Comp	Bolus Trimethoprim 400mg Sulpha methoxazole 2g Pow 5g contains as in 1 Bolus
Adm.	Oral
@	30mg/kg B.wt od for 5 days
Pres.	2.4 g bolus, 15g

Duocidal Bol	**KAPL**
Comp	Bolus Trimethoprim 400mg Sulpha methoxazole 2g-Pow 5g contains as in 1 Bolus
Adm.	Oral
@	30mg/kg B.wt od for 5 days
Pres.	2.4 g Bol, 150 g

Flagyl Tab/ Susp	**Rhone Poulenc**
Comp	Tab 200mg of Metronidazole Susp 200mg in 5 ml
Adm.	Oral
@	20mg/kg B.wt for 5-7 days od
Pres.	Tab 10's, Susp 30ml

Gramogyl Pow	**Ranbaxy**
Comp	Each ml contain Nalidixic acid 300mg Metronidazole 200mg
Adm.	Oral
@	2.5ml qid for 5 days
Pres.	150g

Megadox Sol/Pow	**Neospark**
Comp	Doxycycline 2.5% per g.
Adm.	Oral
@	1-2g per 25kg B.wt bid
Pres.	50g

Megadox N Sol. Powd	**Neospark**
Comp	Each gm contain Doxycycline 100mg Neomycine sulphate 100mg
Adm.	Oral
@	10-20mg/kg B.wt bid for 3-4 days
Pres.	50g

Neblon Pow	**Natural Remedies**
Comp	Ayurvedic ingredients
Adm.	Oral
@	2-3g bid with rice or curd for 2-3 days
Pres.	100g

Pesulin Liq	**Sarabhai Zydus**
Comp	15 ml contains Kaolin 3g Pectin 150g Phthalysulpha thiazole 1g
Adm.	Oral
@	15ml bid
Pres.	100ml

Unimezole Susp/ Tab	**(Unichem) Cargill**
Comp	Tab Metronidazole 200mg Susp 200mg Metronidazole per 2ml
Adm.	Oral
@	20mg/kg B.wt bid for 5 days for both
Pres.	Tab 10's Susp 60ml

Antispasmodic

Atropine Sulphate inj	**Generic**
Comp	Atropine sulphate 1mg per ml
Adm.	IM/ IV
@	1mg/kg B.wt
Pres.	10ml

Spasmovet inj	**Wockhardt**
Comp	Dicyclomin hydrochloride 10mg/ml
Adm.	IM
@	0.5-2ml
Pres.	30ml

Ridalpin inj	**KAPL**	
Comp	Analgin	500mg
	Pitofenon hydrochloride	2mg
	Fenpeverinium bromide	0.01mg/ml
Adm.	IM	
@	1-2ml	
Pres.	10ml	

Valginate	**TTk**
Comp	Each ml contains Valethamale 2 mg gamide Analgin 500 mg Chlorontol 0.4%
Adm.	IM
@	3-5 ml
Pres.	10 ml

Baralgan	**Novartis**
Comp	Each ml contains Analgin 500 mg Pitofenon hydrochloride 0.05 mg
Adm.	
@	IM or IV
Pres.	3-5 ml

Antacids – ulcerhealing

Acicloc Tab/ inj	**Cadila Pharma**
Comp	Ranitidine hydrochloride 150mg, 300mg
	50mg/ml in inj
Adm.	Oral, IM
@	2mg/kg B.wt oral and injection bid
Pres.	Tab 10's 2ml inj

Histac Tab/inj	**Ranbaxy**
Comp	Ranitidine hydrochloride 150mg, 300mg Tab 50mg/ml in inj
Adm.	Oral IM
@	2mg/kg B.wt oral and injection bid
Pres.	Tab 10's 2ml inj

R-Loc Tab/inj	**Cadila Healthcare**
Comp	Ranitidine hydrochloride 150mg, 300mg Tab 50mg/ml in inj
Adm.	Oral IM
@	2mg/kg B.wt oral and injection bid
Pres.	Tab 10's 2ml inj

Zintec Tab	**Glaxo**
Comp	Ranitidine hydrochloride 150mg, 300mg Tab
Adm.	Oral
@	2mg/kg B.wt oral bid
Pres.	Tab 10's

Ultact Tab	**Cipla**
Comp	Ranitidine hydrochloride 150mg, 300mg Tab
Adm.	Oral
@	2mg/kg B.wt oral bid
Pres.	Tab 10's

Tagamed Tab/ inj	**Glaxo**
Comp	Cimetidine Tab 200mg, 400mg, 800mg
Adm.	Oral
@	5-10mg/kg B.wt bid or qid. Inject 5-10mg/kg B.wt bid
Pres.	Tab 10 inj – 2ml amp

Appetie Stimulant

Unienzyme Syrup	**Unichem**
Comp	5ml contains Fungal diastase 50mg Papain 60mg
Adm.	Oral
@	5-10ml bid
Pres.	200ml

Festal Tab	**Hoechst**
Comp	Pancreatin 192mg Bile constituent 25mg Hemicellulase 50mg
Adm.	Oral
@	1-2 Tab tid
Pres.	10's

Brotone liq	**Glaxo**
Comp	10 ml contains Yeast extract 400mg Thiamine 2.5g Nicotinic acid 24mg Liver fraction 1.25g (with B_{12} activity 7.5mcg of cyanocobalamin)
Adm.	Oral
@	5-10ml bid
Pres.	120ml

Digyton Drops	**Himalya**
Comp	Herbal formulation
Adm.	Oral
@	Dogs S.breed 1-2ml bid, L breeds 10-15mg bid
Pres.	100 ml

Laxative

Agarol	Generic	
Comp	Liq. Paraffin 9.5ml	Phenolphthalein 400mg
	Agar 60mg/ 30ml	
Adm.	Oral	
@	5-10ml od	
Pres.	120ml	

Pursennid-in Tab	Novartis
Comp	Sennaglycosides 18mg dioctyl sodium sulfosuccinate 50mg/ tab
Adm.	Oral
@	1-2 Tab od
Pres.	10's

Senade Tab	Cipla
Comp	Standardized senna extract (Sennosides A & B as calcium salts) 13.5mg/ Tablet
Adm.	Oral
@	1 Tab od
Pres.	10's

Mag hydroxide or Milk of magnesia liq	Generic
Comp	Magnesium hydroxide
Adm.	Oral
@	15-20ml/kg B.wt
Pres.	100ml

Magnesium citrate Sol	Generic
Comp	Magnesium citrate
Adm.	Oral
@	2-4ml/kg B.wt
Pres.	20ml

Digestive Enzymes

Digeplex Drops Liq	Rallis	
Comp	Each ml contains	
	Diastase 31.25mg	Pepsin 10mg

	Cardamum 0.4mg Cinnamon oil 0.4mg
Adm.	Oral
@	10 drops- 5ml bid
Pres.	15ml

Provisacc Pow	**Venky Petcare**
Comp	Culture of Sacchromyces cervisae strain 5x10 billion live cells/g
Adm.	Oral
@	S. breeds 2.5g od L. breed 5g od
Pres.	200g

Hepato protective

Beekom L inj	**Wockhardt**
Comp	
Adm.	Refer Livestock section
@	
Pres.	10ml

Belamyl inj	**Zydus**
Comp	
Adm.	Refer Livestock section
@	
Pres.	10ml

Detox FS Powder	**Neospark**
Comp	Herbal formulation
Adm.	Oral
@	3-5g od
Pres.	50g

Liv 52 Drops/ Tab	**Himalya**
Comp	Herbal formulation
Adm.	Oral
@	Drops S.breeds 5-8 drops bid L.breeds 10-15 drops bid Tabets S.breeds 1-2 tab bid L.breeds 2-3 tab bid
Press	30 ml Tabs 10

Livjivan drops/Tab	Ayurvet
Comp	Herbal formulation
Adm.	Oral
@	Dogs upto 10kg 0.5ml tid 1 tab od. Dogs above 10kg 1ml tid 2 tab od
Pres.	Drops 20 ml tab 10

Livogen inj	Glaxo
Comp	
Adm.	Refer livestock section
@	
Pres.	

Livol Pow	Natural Remedies
Comp	Herbal formulation
Adm.	Oral
@	3-5g bid
Pres.	100g

Livron Pow	Vets Farma
Comp	Herbal formulation
Adm.	Oral
@	5-10g od
Pres.	100g

Zigup Sys	Natural Remedies
Comp	Herbal formulation
Adm.	Oral
@	Pups 2.5mg od Adult 1-2 teaspoon full
Pres.	60 ml

Pepsin inj	Concept
Comp	
Adm.	Refer Livestock section
@	
Pres.	10ml

Pinkojet	**Brihans**
Comp	
Adm.	Refer Livestock section
@	
Pres.	10ml

Hepaplex inj	**Unichem**
Comp	
Adm.	Refer Livestock section
@	
Pres.	10ml

Ripason inj	**TTK**
Comp	Antigen free water soluble anticirrhotic extract of liver 0.026 derived from 15.4g fresh liver per ml
Adm.	IM
@	2-3ml od
Pres.	10ml

Teffroli Syp/ granules	**TTK**
Comp	Herbal formulation
Adm.	Oral
@	Syp. 5-10ml od granule 1-3g od
Pres.	Syp 120ml granule 100g

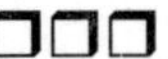

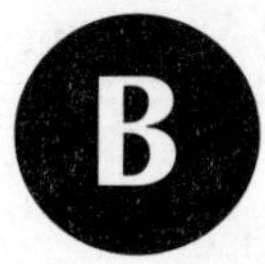

Cardiovascular System

Cardiovascular and Circulatory Diseases

(Special canine terms- not included in Livestock)

ACE inhibitors: These are drugs used in heart failures.

Alloimmune hemolysis: Production of antibodies that are directed against RBC of another individual of same species.

Aneurysm: enlargement of a blood vessel caused by weakening of middle layer of blood vessel.

Aortic stenosis: Obstruction of blood from the left ventricle. If it is within valve leading out of left ventricle it is valvular stenosis.

Aplastic anemia: Anemia in which the ability of bone marrow to generative blood cells cause reduction in number of all types of blood cells. Red, white and platelets.

Arrhythmia: Abnormality of rate, regularity or site of heart beat formation.

Bacteremia: Denotes the presence of bacteria in blood (emia is suffix for denoting the presence of a substance in blood)

Cardiac catheterization: It involves the placement of specialized catheter into, heart, aorta or pulmonary artery to identify abnormalities.

Cardiac tamponade: When increased pressure compresses the heart interfering with its ability to pump blood.

Congestive heart failure: It is the result of any severe, overwhelming heart disease that most commonly results in pulmonary edema (fluid in lungs), pleural effusion (fluid around lungs) ascites (fluid in abdomen). It can be due to any heart defect, pulmonary hypertension, or heart worm. Signs depend on which side of heart is affected. Left side heart failure results in rapid or difficult breathing and sometimes coughing. Right side heart failure results in large liver congestion and buildup of fluid in abdomen and around lungs.

Cortriatriatrum: It is characterised by fibrous division of right artrium into two chambers usually with a hole in between them. It results in right heart failure (ascites).

Cyclic hematopoiesis: Characterised by 12 day cycles during which all types of blood cells including platelets decrease.

Degenerative mitrial valve disease: A heart disease which may cause heart failure. The leaflets of valves become thickened and nodular leading to mitrial valve regurgitation and volume overload of left side of heart.

Digitalis glycosides: These are drugs used to increase the force of heart muscle contraction. Digoxin is also of the same group.

Dilated Cardiomyopathy (DCM): Disease of heart muscle resulting in decreased myocardial contractility. The left ventricle compensates for the disease by growing larger. The left atrial is also dilated when disease is severe.

Dysfibrinogenemia: Abnormally functioning fibrinogen with mild bleeding problems.

Echocardiograph: It is a type of ultrasonography used to evaluate the heart, aorta, pulmonary artery to identify abnormalities.

Electrocardiography: Recording of hearts activity form the body surface with the use of electrodes. It is used to identify heart arrhythma.

Embolus: Part of a clot in the vessel which lodges at a point to narrow the path.

Extra nodal lymphoma: Lymphomas are in extra nodal sites. Symptoms include difficult breathing, kidney failure, blindness and seizures.

Failing heart: Due to insufficient blood flow to supply the organs with oxygenated blood for proper function.

Heart failure: Due to insufficient blood flow to supply the organs with oxygenated blood for proper function.

Hemolysis: Destruction of red blood cells (lysis is suffix for destruction for cells)

Hemolytic anemia: Signs are destruction of RBC due to exposure to toxins such as lead or infections. There can be pica. The dog eats concrete dust, sand tile grout.

Hemophilia: Prolonged bleeding in females mostly from the umblical cord after birth in puppies. Gums may bleed. Lameness due to bleeding into a joint.

Hemostasis: Stablise the blood (stasis is suffix for stop or stable).

Hypofibrinogenemia: Abnormal shortage of fibrinogen in blood accompanied severe bleeding.

Immune mediated hemolytic anemia: It occurs on its own as a result of tumor, infections, drugs, or vaccinations. There is jaundice and fever with enlarged spleen.

Leucocytosis: Increase in WBC.

Lymphocytosis: Abnormal increase in blood level of lymphocytes (osis is suffix for increase in blood level).

Mediastinal lymphoma: When thymus, lymph nodes are enlarged, fluid builds up in chest and there is trouble in breathing.

Microangiopathic hemolysis: When RBC's are damaged due to turbulent flow through abnormal blood vessels usually after strong heart worm infection or tumors of blood vessels.

Multicentric lymphoma: Rapid nonpainful enlargement of lymph nodes. When large there is weakness, lack of energy, loss of appetite and depression.

Myelofibrosis: A progressive disease leading to anemia and enlargement of spleen and liver. It leads to failure of bone marrow.

Myelodysplasia: When the growth and maturation of blood forming cells in bone marrow is defective and leads to non regenerative anemia.

Neutropenia: Decrease in blood level of neutrophils (penia is suffix for decrease in blood level)

Neutrophilia: Increase in blood cell Neutorphils (philia suffix for increase in blood level)

Non regenerative anemia: When bone marrow responds inadequately to the increased need for red blood cells.

Pericardial effusion: It is a collection of fluid in pericardium. It is usually serosanguinous (bloody fluid) caused by cancer. In rare cases it include trauma, clotting disorders and left atrial rupture. It can be caused by infection and congist of pus.

Primary leukemia: A cancer type in which abnormal blood cells replace normal blood cells. This leads to anemia and lack of WBC and platelets.

Pulmonary hypertension: it is high pressure in pulmonary artery. Caused by heart worm, pulmonary thromboembolism or chronic hypoxemia (low oxygen). It can result in right sided heart disease. Signs include difficult breathing, cyanosis and exercise intolerance.

Pulmonary stenosis: Obstruction to the blood flow from right ventricle.

Red cell aplasia: In it only RBC or the elements that produce RBC are affected and characterised by non regenerative anemia.

Regenerative anemia: When bone marrow responds appropriately to the decreased number of RBC by increasing their production.

Rocky Mountain spotted fever: It is caused by Rickettsia transmitted through ticks. These kill blood cells and there is blood vessel swelling. They may bleed through nose, urine, bowel etc.

Sick sinus syndrome: It is characterised by sinoatrial node dysfunction and may include atrioventricular node disease and bundle branch block.

Thrombecytosis: A condition characterised by excess of platelets. Mostly it is caused by exercise or reactive (secondary to cancer, blood loss or some drugs). Platelets may not function and blood may not clot congestive heart failure. It is the result of any severe, overwhelming heart disease that most commonly results in pulmonary edema (fluid in lungs), pleural effusion (fluid around lungs) ascites (fluid in abdomen). It can be due to any heart defect, pulmonary hypertension or heart worm. Signs depend on which sides of heart is affected. Left sides heart failure results or difficult breathing sometimes coughing. Right side heart failure results in a large liver congestion and build up of fluid in abdomen and around lungs.

Thrombocytopenia: Lack of platelets caused by Ehrilichia organism or dysfunctioning of immune system, vaccination or drugs.

Thrombus: A blood clot that may form when the blood flow of an artery or vein is restricted. It caused obstruction of blood vessel.

Trapped Neutrophil Syndrome: It is autosomal recessive disease which results in mature neutrophils being unable to migrate from bone marrow, into blood. These have chronic infection and fail to thrive. Other symptoms are stunted growth and a ferret like facial appearance.

Haematinics

Iron Tablet/ Ferrous sulphate tab	**Generic**
Comp	Ferrous sulphate
Adm.	Oral
@	1 tab od for 20-30 days
Pres.	50's, 100's

Ferrous sulphate Pow	**Generic**
Comp	Ferrous sulphate IP
Adm.	Oral
@	0.5-2g od for 2 weeks or more
Pres.	50g, 100g, 450g

Imferon inj	**Rallis (Intas)**
Comp	Iron dextran (Elemental iron) 50mg/ml
Adm.	IM
@	1ml-2ml depending upon weight
Pres.	2ml, 10ml

Macferon	Macwell
Comp	Iron dextran (Elemental iron) 50mg/ml
Adm.	IM
@	1ml-2ml depending upon weight
Pres.	2ml, 10ml

Haemup Syp	Cadila Pharma
Comp	15ml contains Glycinated haemoglobin 1g Ferric ammonium citrate 100mg Copper sulphate 30mcg Zinc sulphate 30mcg Alcohol 0.87ml
Adm.	Oral
@	5-10ml per dog od
Pres.	200ml

Anti-arrhythmics

These are used in Bradycardia, cardiac arrhythemia and AV block etc.

Atropine sulphate	Generic
Comp	0.6mg/ml of atropine sulphate
Adm.	IM/ IV/ SC
@	0.04mg/kg B.wt tid
Pres.	1ml

Dicard Tab.	Intas
Comp	Diltiazem 30mg, 60mg
Adm.	Oral
@	0.1-1.5mg/kg B.wt tid
Pres.	10's

Diltime Tab	**Cadila Healthcare**
Comp	Diltiazem 30mg, 60mg
Adm.	Oral
@	0.1-1.5mg/kg B.wt tid
Pres.	10's

Lignocaine inj	**Sarabhai**
Comp	Lignocaine hydrochloride 2%
Adm.	IV
@	1-2mg/kg body weight
Pres.	10ml, 30ml

Xylocaine	**Novartis**
Comp	Lignocaine hydrochloride 2%
Adm.	IV
@	1-2mg/kg body weight
Pres.	10ml, 30ml

Lopresor Tab	**Novartis**
Comp	Metoprolol 50mg, 100mg
Adm.	Oral
@	0.5-1mg/kg B.wt
Pres.	10's

Espolin inj	**Cadila Healthcare**
Comp	Phenytoin 50mg/ml
Adm.	IV
@	2mg/kg B.wt
Pres.	2ml

Ciplar Tab	**Cipla**
Comp	Propranolol hydrochloride 10mg, 40mg, 80mg
Adm.	Oral
@	100mcg/kg B.wt tid
Pres.	10's

Haemostatics

Adrenalin inj	**Generic**
Comp	Epinephrin hydrochloride or Adrenalin 1mg/ml
Adm.	IV or Intracardiac
@	0.1-0.3mg/kg B.wt
Pres.	1ml, 2ml, 5ml

Adchrome	**G.Loucatos**
Comp	Adrenochrome monosemi carbazone
Adm.	IM/ IV
@	5-10mg
Pres.	10ml

Haemocoagulase inj	**Generic**
Comp	Haemocoagulase 1unit
Adm.	IM
@	0.5-1ml total
Pres.	1ml

Maclote inj	**Macnor**
Comp	
Adm.	Refer Livestock section
@	
Pres.	

Styplon Tab	**Himalya**
Comp	
Adm.	Refer Livestock section
@	
Pres.	

Cardiac Stimulant

Digox Tab	**Zydus**
Comp	Digoxin 0.25mg
Adm.	Oral
@	10mcg/kg B.wt bid
Pres.	10's

Digoxin Paed Elixir	**Glaxo**
Comp	Digoxin 0.05mg/ml
Adm.	Oral
@	10mcg/kg B.wt bid (Maximum 750mcg/day)
Pres.	30ml

Lanoxin Tab	**Glaxo**
Comp	Digoxin 0.25mg
Adm.	Oral
@	10mcg/kg B.wt bid
Pres.	10's

Lanoxin inj	**Glaxo**
Comp	Digoxin 0.5mg per 2ml
Adm.	IM
@	10mcg/kg B.wt bid (Maximum 750mcg/day)
Pres.	2ml

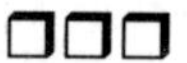

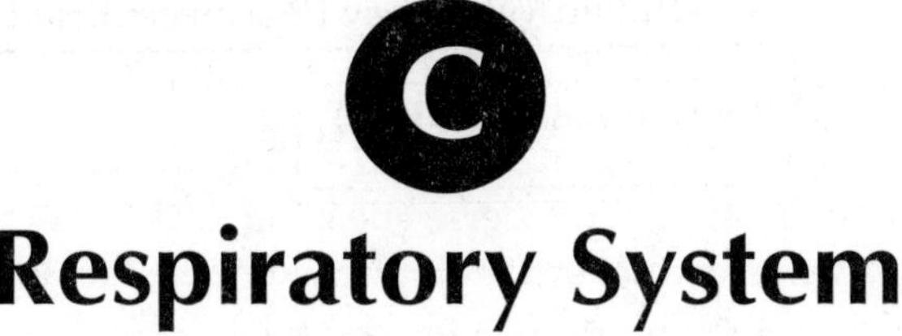

Respiratory System

Terms Related to Respiratory System
(Other than included in live Stock section)

Allergic pneumonitis: Acute or chronic allergic reaction of lungs and small air ways. Lungs over-react and then are inflammed

Alveolar emphysema: There is abnormal permanent enlargement of alveoli

Aspiration pneumonia: A lung infection caused by inhalation of foreign material. Severity depends upon material inhaled. Signs are lethargy, loss of appetite, deep cough, rapid breathing, blowing of lips and bluish mucous membrane and fever.

Bronchoscopy: Examination of airways with an endoscope.

Chronic obstructive Pulmonary Disease (COPD): There is enlargement and destruction of air spaces.

Chylothorax: Accumulation of high triglyceride lymphatic fluid in pleural cavity

Congenital lobar emphysema: It occurs because of incomplete development of bronchial cartilage.

Fungal Pneumonia: It is also called Mycotic pneumonia caused by fungi of various type or inhalation of spores. There is thick discharge of mucous from nose may be seen.Later on there is general weakness, weight loss, labored breathing with short moist cough.

Grunting: Noise associated with breathing

Hemothorax: Accumulation of blood in the pleural (chest) cavity

Hydrothorax: Accumulation of clear fluid in the pleural (chest) cavity

Interstitial emphysema: There is presence of air within the supporting connective tissue of the lungs.

Kennel Cough: It is also known as Infectious tracheobronchitis. It is the result of inflammation of upper airways. It spreads quickly and caused by viral and bacterial organisms. There is spasm of harsh dry coughing followed by retching and gagging.

Labored breathing: Shortness of breath

Metastatic Lung tumors: It is tumor that originates in another part of the body and spreads to lungs through blood or lymph system.

Nasal mite: Mite Pneumonyssoides caninum is mite live in nasal passage and sinuses. All breed, age and sex of dogs can suffer but usually in old age dogs. Bleeding from the nose, sneezing, reverse sneezing, facial itching, nasal discharge, labored breathing, headshaking and high pitched noisy breathing are symptoms

Oropharynx: The middle part of the pharynx and far back of the mouth.

PIE Syndrome: Pulmonary infiltration with Eosinophilia. It is infiltration of lungs with thick fluid and WBC. It is caused by allergens, parasites and viral. There is difficult in breathing and lethargicity

Pneumothorax: Accumulation of air in plural cavity

Pulmonary nodular eosinophilic granulomatous syndrome: It is severe allergy reaction and mostly associated with heart worms, chronic cough is main symptom.

Reverse sneeze: It is aspiration reflex which is a short rapid inhalation in an attempt to clear the nose.

Rhino: Pertaining to nose

Sneezing: Attempt to clear the upper airways of discharge.

Tonsillitis: Inflammation of tonsils, usually caused by bacterial infection. There is localized swelling or abcess. Poor appetite, listlessness, salivation and difficulty in swallowing and high pitched noisy breathing

Tracheal collapse: Dogs have dry, honking, chronic cough and labored breathing.

Expectorants

Piriton Expectorant	**Glaxo**	
Comp	Chlorpheniramine maleate	2.5mg
	Ammonium chloride	125mg
	Sodium citrate	55mg in 5ml
Adm.	Oral	
@	½ + tsp tid	
Pres.	115ml	

Koflix Electuary	**Charak**
Comp	Herbal formulation
Adm.	Oral
@	4g bid
Pres.	90g

Avil Expectorant	Hoechst	
Comp	5ml contains	
	Pheniramine maleate 15mg	
	Ammonium chloride125mg	Menthol 1.14mg
Adm.	Oral	
@	5ml tid	
Pres.	100ml	

Respiratory Stimulant Bronchodilators

Adrenalin inj	Generic
Comp	1ml contains Adrenalin acid tartrate 1800mcg
Adm.	IV/ IM
@	0.2-0.3ml
Pres.	10ml

Brincanyl Tab	Brihans
Comp	Terbutaline sulphate 2.5mg, 5mg
Adm.	Oral
@	1.25-5mg tid
Pres.	10's

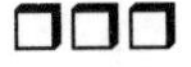

Central Nervous System

Terms related to Nervous System

Acquired laryngeal paralysis: Signs include voice change, noisy breathing and dry cough. Tongue and gums may turn bluish later.

Acquired myasthenia gravis: It is a disease of connections between nerve and muscles. Signs are stiffness, tremors and weakness that improve with rest.

Acute Idiopathic polyradiculoneuritis: Inflammation of peripheral nerves signs develop 7-14 days after a raccoon bite or scratch.

Auto immune disorders: when problems are caused by the body's own overactive immune system.

BAER: Brainstem Auditory evoked response: It records the electrical activity in the pathway from sound receptors in ear to brain stem and cerebrum.

Canine cognitive dysfunction: It is a progressive disease in older dogs which is similar to dementia in human.

Canine distemper encephalomyelitis: It is a viral disease. There is swelling of brain and spinal cord. Signs are fever, pain and loss of motor control or develop paralysis.

Canine dysautonomia: It is disorder of autonomic nervous system which controls many reflexes and neurologic functions. Signs are pupillary light reflex loss, eyelids may drop or protrude abnormal and position of eyeball is normal. Painful and difficult urination and lose anal sphincter.

Cauda equine syndrome: Also known as degenerative lumbosacral stenosis. It is a compression of cauda equine by narrowing of the lumbosacral vertebral canal. Signs include pain, weakness and rear limb muscle atrophy.

Cerebellar hypoplasia: Incomplete development of cerebellum. Cause is an in utero infection with canine herpesvirus.

Coenurosis: Also called gid, sturdy or stagger. It is caused by Taenia multiceps an intestinal tape worm. There is loss of muscle control, blindness, head tilting, stumbling and paralysis.

Coonhound paralysis: It is a type of poly radiculoneurtis seen in coonhounds cause is related to raccoon bite. Signs include rear leg weakness progressing rapidly to paralysis and decreased reflexes.

Dancing Doberman disease: It is a type of myopathy that primarily affects the gastrocnemius muscle in Dobermans. One rear leg will flex while standing. In next few months it affects other rear leg.

Delayed organophosphate intoxication: After ingestion or skin contact with insecticide or pesticide that contains organophosphate develops. Partial paralysis of hind leg progresses to 4 legs later.

Diskospondylitis: Inflammation of disk between two vertebrates by bacterial infection. There is spinal pain, fever, depression and weight loss. Blood and urine test confirms infections.

Electroencephalogram: It records electrical activity in the brain

Electromyogram: It records the electrical activity in muscles and nerves

Epilepsy: It can be primary, idiopathic disorder secondary to previous head trauma or CNS infections. The most common signs are recurring general seizures.

Facial nerve paralysis: It is mainly caused by trauma otitis media or as an idiopathic conditions. Signs include an inability to blink, dropping of ear and drooping of lips on affected side. In chronic conditions flbrosis occurs and the ear and lips may appear to be in abnormal position.

Granulomatous meningoencephelitis GME: It is an inflammatory disease of central nervous system. Disease is more in female.

Hepatic encephalopathy: Abnormality of blood vessels within the liver. It results from enzyme deficiency in liver. Signs are staring into space, improper barking and aggression then depression, blindness, seizure and coma.

Hydrocephalus: Excess of fluid that puts pressure on the brain and may damage cerebrum. Signs are blindness or impaired vision.

Hypothyroid neuropathy: It is a thyroid condition. Signs vary including partial paralysis, weakend reflexes, loss of paw position sense in 4 legs, loss of balance, inability to swallow and vomiting.

Idiopathic epilepsy: Refers to epileptic seizures of unknown cause

Intervertebral disk disease: A degenerative disease of spinal column that results in compression of spinal cord and spinal nerves.

Laryngeal paralysis: It is unilateral or bilateral paralysis of larynx. It can be congenital or acquired, idiopathic disease. Signs include change in voice and difficult breathing.

Motion sickness: Seen during travel by land, sea or air. Signs are nausea, excessive drooling, vomiting and sometimes poor appetite for several hours. Animal may whine, shows uneasiness or has diarrhea disease.

Motor neurons: These carry responses to sensory information from spinal cord and brain to the rest of the body.

Myelography: A special dye that is visible on x-rays is injected into the cerebrospinal cord to find out spinal problem like slipped disk or tumors

Myiasis: Development of larval dipteran flies (bot and warbles) within tissue or organs.

Neosporosis: It is a protozoan disease caused by Neospora caninum. There is inflammation of brain and spinal cord in young puppies. There is paralysis with muscle rigidity is one or both hind legs.

Nephroblastoma: Tumor found in the middle or lower back causing partial paralysis in hind legs.

Neurotransmitters: it is chemical released by axon of neurons. These pass signals to the dendrites of other neurons to muscles or glands.

Polyneuropathy: Is a collection of peripheral nerve disorders. It indicates that multiple nerves are involved.

Puppy hypoglycemia: Low blood sugar in small toy breeds in first 6 months of age.

Rabies: It is caused by viral infection spreads to CNS from peripheral nervous system. Signs slowly lead to loss of motor control and progressive paralysis. Dogs die within 2-7 days of signs.

Rocky Mountain spotted fever: There is swelling in spinal cord due to Rickettsial infection.

Scotty cramp: It causes spasms and hyerflexion and hyperextension of legs. It is caused by disorder in serotonin metabolism that causes a deficiency of available serotonin.

Sensory neurons: These nerve cells carry information on from body to the spinal cord and then on to cerebellum and cerebrum for interpretation.

Slipped disk: It causes several signs. There is degeneration of disk. Most common is in the neck leads to neck pain, stiffness and muscle spasm. If it is in the middle of back then back pain and dog is reluctant to move. There may be paresis and incontinence.

Syringomyelia: It is a condition where a fluid sac develops in spinal cord. It can be due to under developed occipital bone which interferes with spinal fluid circulation and results in fluid accumulation in cervical spinal cord.

Tick paralysis: It is caused by neurotoxin found in salvia of female ticks. There is gradual onset of signs which include incoordination progressing to paralysis and decreased reflexes.

Toxoplasmosis: It is caused by protozoa Toxoplasma gondii. It can cause inflammation of brain and spinal cord. It can lead to canine distemper.

Trigeminal neuritis: Inflammation and damage of Trigeminal nerve causing sudden onset of Jaw paralysis. Animal is unable to close mouth and has difficulty in eating and drinking.

Verminons myelitis: Inflammation of spinal cord caused by parasite round worm Ascaris. Signs of spinal cord inflammation is there.

White dog shaker syndrome: It causes full body tremors in small white dog breeds.

Wobbler disease: It is cervical instability. It is a condition of cervical vertebrae that causes unsteady gait and weakness in dogs.

Analgesics – Antipyretics

Analgin inj	**KAPL/ TTK**
Comp	Analgin 500mg/ml
Adm.	IM/ IV
@	1-5ml
Pres.	30ml

Banpin inj	**Brihans**
Comp	Analgin 500mg/ml
Adm.	IM/ IV
@	1-5ml
Pres.	30ml

Novalgin inj	**Hoechst**
Comp	Analgin 500mg/ml
Adm.	IM/ IV
@	1-5ml
Pres.	30ml

Ronalgin inj	**Ranbaxy**
Comp	Analgin 500mg/ml
Adm.	IM/ IV
@	1-5ml
Pres.	30ml

Bolin inj	**Wockhardt**
Comp	Each ml contain Paracetamol 150mg Analgin 150mg
Adm.	IM/ IV
@	2-5ml
Pres.	10ml

Valginate inj	**TTK**
Comp	Each ml contains Analgin 500mg Valethamate bromide 2mg
Adm.	IM
@	5-10ml
Pres.	30ml

Polygesic inj	Unichem
Comp	Each ml contains
	Analgin 500mg Pitofenone hydrochloride 2mg Fenpiverinium bromide 0.02mg
Adm.	IV/ IM
@	2ml
Pres.	10ml

Paracetol inj	Zydus
Comp	Paracentamol 150mg/ ml
Adm.	IM
@	10-20mg/kg B.wt
Pres.	30ml

Herbina Cap	Natural Remedies
Comp	Herbal formulation
Adm.	Oral
@	1 cap bid
Pres.	12 cap

Forturin inj	Ranbaxy
Comp	Pentazocine lactate 30mg/ml
Adm.	IM
@	2mg/kg B.wt
Pres.	1ml ampule

Inflagin inj	Neospark
Comp	Analgin 500mg/ml
Adm.	IM/ IV
@	1-5ml
Pres.	30ml

Petofen inj	Marc
Comp	Each ml contains Analgin 500mg Pitofenone hydrochloride 2mg Fenpiverinium bromide 0.02mg

Adm.	IV/ IM
@	2ml
Pres.	10ml

Ridalpin inj	**KAPL**	
Comp	Each ml contains	
	Analgin	500mg
	Pitofenone hydrochloride	2mg
	Fenpiverinium bromide	0.02mg
Adm.	IV/ IM	
@	2ml	
Pres.	10ml	

Norswel Tab	**Cadila Healthcare**
Comp	Ibuprofen Tab 400mg
Adm.	Oral
@	10mg/kg B.wt od
Pres.	10

Tabalon Tab	**Hoechst**
Comp	Ibuprofen Tab 400mg
Adm.	Oral
@	10mg/kg B.wt od
Pres.	10

Melonex Inj	**Intas**
Comp	Meloxicam 5mg/ml
Adm.	IM/ IV/ SC
@	0.5mg/kg B.wt
Pres.	15ml

Artagen Tab	**Ranbaxy**
Comp	Naproxen 250mg
Adm.	Oral
@	5mg/kg B.wt Primary dose 2mg/kg B.wt maintenance
Pres.	250mg 10's

Algesin inj	**Alembic**
Comp	Phenyl butazone 200mg/ml
Adm.	IV
@	22mg/kg B.wt
Pres.	3ml

Ibugin Tab	**Glaxo**
Comp	Ibuprofen Tab 400mg
Adm.	Oral
@	10mg/kg B.wt od
Pres.	10

Steroidal Anti Inflammatory Drugs

Betnesol	**Glaxo**
Comp	Betnesol 4mg/ml
Adm.	IM/ IV
@	0.5-2mg
Pres.	1ml

Muscle Relaxant

Scoline inj	**Glaxo**
Comp	Each ml contains 50mg/ml of succinylcholine
Adm.	IV
@	0.3mg/kg B.wt
Pres.	2ml vial

Sedatives – Tranquilizers

Largactil inj/Tab	**Rone Poulenc**
Comp	Chlorpromazine hydrochloride 2.5% inj, 25mg, 50mg, 100mg Tab
Adm.	Inj IM/ IV Tablet oral
@	Oral 5mg/kg B.wt od, Inj 1-2mg/kg B.wt
Pres.	1ml, 2ml, Tab 10's

Promethazine hydrochloride inj	**Primavet**
Comp	5% Promethazone hydrochloride
Adm.	IM
@	1.5-2mg/kg B.wt
Pres.	10ml

Siquil inj/ Tab	**Sarabhai**
Comp	Triflupromazine Tab 10mg inj 20mg/ml
Adm.	Tab oral inj IM/ IV
@	Oral 2-4mg/kg B.wt inj 1-2mg/kg B.wt IV, 2-4mg/kg B.wt IM
Pres.	5ml, 10 Tab

Anicalm inj	**Intas**
Comp	Triflupromazine Tab 10mg inj 20mg/ml
Adm.	Tab oral inj IM/ IV
@	Oral 2-4mg/kg B.wt inj 1-2mg/kg B.wt IV, 2-4mg/kg B.wt IM
Pres.	5ml, 10

Bomazine	**Sarabhai**
Comp	Xylazine hydrochloride 20mg/ml
Adm.	IV
@	0.25-0.5ml/5kg B.wt
Pres.	10ml

Izine	**Intas**
Comp	Xylazine hydrochloride 20mg/ml
Adm.	IV
@	0.25-0.5ml/5kg B.wt
Pres.	10ml

Anoxocare Tab	**Himalya**
Comp	Herbal formulation
Adm.	Oral
@	S.breed 1-2 tab bid L.breed 2-3 tab
Pres.	60

Phenergan inj	**Rhone Poulenc**
Comp	5% Promethazone hydrochloride
Adm.	IM
@	1.5-2mg/kg B.wt
Pres.	5ml

Xylaxin	**Indian Immunology**
Comp	Xylazine hydrochloride 20mg/ml
Adm.	IV
@	0.25-0.5ml/5kg B.wt
Pres.	2ml, 10ml

Xylocad inj	**CadilaPharma**
Comp	Xylazine hydrochloride 20mg/ml
Adm.	IV
@	0.25-0.5ml/5kg B.wt
Pres.	5ml

Megatil Tab/ inj	**Intas**
Comp	Chlorpromazine hydrochloride 2.5% inj, 25mg, 50mg, 100mg Tab
Adm.	Inj IM/ IV Tablet oral
@	Oral 5mg/kg B.wt od Inj 1-2mg/kg B.wt
Pres.	1ml, 2ml, Tab 10's

Rompun inj	**Bayer**
Comp	Xylazine hydrochloride 20mg/ml
Adm.	IV
@	0.25-0.5ml/5kg B.wt
Pres.	15ml

Anti-convulsant

Calmpose Tab	**Ranbaxy**
Comp	Diazepam 2mg, 5mg, 10mg
Adm.	Oral
@	5-10mg
Pres.	10's

Calmpose Susp	**Ranbaxy**
Comp	Diazepam 2mg/5ml
Adm.	IV
@	5-50mg. Slow infusion in Dextrose
Pres.	60ml

Calmpose inj	Ranbaxy
Comp	Diazepam 5mg/ml
Adm.	IV
@	5-50mg
Pres.	2ml

Gardenal Tab	Rhone Poulenc
Comp	Phenobarbitone 30mg, 60mg
Adm.	Oral
@	1.5mg-5mg bid
Pres.	10

Luminal	Bayer
Comp	Phenobarbitone 30mg, 60mg
Adm.	Oral
@	1.5mg-5mg bid
Pres.	30ml

Epsolin Tab/inj	Cadila Healthcare
Comp	Phenytoin 100mg Tab 50mg/ml inj
Adm.	Inj IM tab oral
@	15mg/kg B.wt oral 8mg/kg B.wt inj
Pres.	Tab 100, inj 2ml

Valtril Tab	Wockhardt
Comp	Sodium valproate 200mg, 500mg
Adm.	Oral
@	60mg/kg B.wt tid
Pres.	10

Anaesthetics

Local

Lidocaine (Lignocain)

Novocaine Hoechst

Refer Livestock Section

Bupivacaine

Refer Livestock Section

General

Refer Livestock Section

Antidepressant Euthanasia

❑❑❑

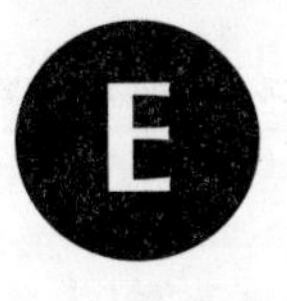

Dermatology

Terms Related to Skin Disorders

Acquired aurotrichia: The hair along the middle of the back above associated with thinning of hair coat.

Albinism: It is a skin colour abnormality with pink or pale irises and visual defects.

Amputation neuromas: These develop as growth form after amputation or traumatic injury (e.g docking of tail) Neurofibromas grow in connective tissue around a nerve. These appear as white firm lumps. These can be benign or malignant.

Aplasia cutis: Missing or absent skin.

Appocrine gland cysts: These are found in middle aged dogs and occur either in or outside of hair follicles. These appear mostly on head and neck One or more cysts appear in middle to upper layer of skin with a loose association of hair follicles.

Apocrine gland tumor: These appear in deep firm masses near anal sac. These compress rectum and cause constipation. These can spread to lymph nodes and other organs.

Atopy: Airborne allergies. Allergy due to material in the air.

Basal cell Tumors: these are benign cancer tumor lie at the base of top layer of skin (epidermis). These appear as firm, solitary, dome shaped elevated masses mostly hairless or ulcerated.

Black hair follicle dysplasia: It develops earlier with more complete hair loss in black coloured areas.

Canine Demdicosis: It is caused by mites live in hair follicles and sebaceous glands cause is Demodox canis. There is inflammation and hair loss. It can be localized and generalized. Affected areas are hairless red or densely pigmented raised lumps look like acne. There may or not itching. In generalized there are inflamed foot pads, enlarged lymph nodes, lethargy, fever and pus filled inflammation of deeper layer of skin.

Canine extramedullary plasmacytomas: Skin tumors frequently on ears lips mouth and legs of mature to aged dogs. Tumors are generally small and narrow.

Canine ichthyosiform dermatoses: Body is covered with large scales that may flake off in large sheets. Due to discomfort there is swelling or thickening of nose and paws.

Canine Scabies or Scarcoptic mange: It is caused by sarcoptes scabiescanis mite. They have intense itching suddenly caused by sensitivity to mites droppings. Skin erupt with small bumps. When dog scratches or bites the skin around bump is damaged causing thick crusted sores. Secondary yeast infection develop in damaged skin. Usually sores appear on abdomen chest, ears, elbows and legs.

Canine warty dyskeratomas: These grow near hair follicles or sweat glands. These are bumps with a dark dot in centre.

Cheyletiellosis: It is known as walking dandruff and caused by Cheyletiella yasguri mites. It is very contagious. Scaling of skin along the back, intense itching frequently.

Collagenous nevi: These are benign fibrous protein on the legs, head, neck and areas prone to trauma. These are flat to raised lumps develop in the skin or fat beneath the skin.

Collie nose: Nasal solar dermatitis.

Colour dilution alopecia: In this the colour of hair changes from black to blue, beige or fawn.

Contagious Ecthyma: Infectious skin disease caused by parapox virus. It occurs by contact with symptoms Sore develop on skin of lips and inside the mouth. They can be found on feet Scales drop off within 4 weeks and tissues heal without scarring.

Contagious Pustulardermatitis: Contagious Ecthyma

Cornifying epitheliomas: It is benign tumor. These are growths, tough layered lumps stick up from skin surface. These look like a horn or cornified cysts. These mostly arise from a hair follicle.

Cutaneous angiosarcomas: these develop on the underside of trunk, hip, thigh, and lower legs. First these are benign but later on become malignant. These spread to lungs and liver.

Cutaneous asthenia: Condition in which skin does not produce enough collagen. This causes loose stretchy Fragile skin. Skin hangs from body cysts and bruising may develop. This becomes fatal.

Cutaneous lymphosarcoma: A type of skin cancer and primary lumphoid tumor involvement. It can be epitheliotropic and Nonepitheliptropic. In first type of lymphosarcoma tumor or tumor like growth appears on lips, eyelids or foot pads and in the beginning confused with allergies. Nonepitheliotropic are multiple tumors. These spread to other organs.

Cutaneous mucinosis: A condition in which mucus is so excessive that skin exhibits pronounced folding and blisters.

Cuterbriasis: Infestation of parasite cuterbra as known as Rabbit bot flies. There are boils around head neck or trunk. Hair is often matted and skin is swollen.

Dermatomyositis: Inflammatory disease of skin and muscles of young dogs. There can be ulcers, crusting and hair loss on the face, eartips, tailtips and legs. Heat, sun exposure and wounds worsen the condition.

Dermatophytosis: It is ringworm infection of skin, hair or claws caused by fungus Microsporum canis, M.gyseum and Trichophyton mentagrophytes. It is spread by contact. There are bald scaly patches with broken hairs in rings like whirls. Mostly it affects face, eartips, tail and feet.

Dermatosparaxia: cutaneous asthenia

Dermoid cysts: These are skin pockets in which dander, hair, oil and other debris accumulate. They are found on skin above the backbone.

Diffuse lipomas: In this type of lipoma entire skin is affected resulting in prominent folds in skin and neck and trunk.

Ectoparasitis: Mosquitoes, some flies, stable flies and Tsetse flies are other external parasites. Female mosquitoes feed on blood They annoy animal. They spread heart worms. Sandflies female have piercing mouthparts and feed on the blood. These are active during nights. These are intermediate flies and intermediate host of Trypanosoma causing a fatal disease. Dogs show nervous system signs, blindness and die.

Eosinophilic granuloma complex: It is disorder associated with unusual reactions to insect bite or hypersensitive reaction. There are bumps or nodules anywhere on the body which can be ulcerated or crusted.

Epidermal hamartomas: these are dark pointy bumps on the skin usually arranged in a line. Some form pimples, dark, thick skin folds and are benign.

Epidermolysis bullosa syndrome: There is problem between outer and inner layer of the skin resulting blistering of skin. It is in many forms Blister may rupture leaving glistening flat ulcersEpitheliogenesis imperfecta: Missing or absent skin part of layers or all of layers of skin.

Ethlers Danlos syndrome: Cutaneous asthenia.

Eye gnats: These are eyeflies. These congregate around eyes. Some species are attracted to genitalia.

Familial footpad hyper keratosis: A syndrome in which there is increased thickening of hard layer of skin. All footpads are involved. In severe cases horns, cracks and secondary infection cause pain and lameness.

Fibromas: These resemble Collagenious nevi or skin tags. These are tumors appear as isolated generally raised hairless lumps originating under skin surfaces. It can be fibroma durum if firm and rubbery and can be fibroma molle if soft and mushy.

Fibromatosis: It is thickening and invasive growth in tendon sheath seen on heads of dogs. These are also called lumpy fasciitis. These are small lymphoid lumps scattered throughout tissue. These can spread through blood stream to distant organs.

Fibrosarcoma: These are fast growing malignant tumors located in trunk and legs. These vary in size and appearance. These are firm and fleshy appear deep in skin and fat underneath or soft tissue and look like lump. They spread only within same area.

Firbrous histiocytomas: These are inflammatory reactions like tumor Some of these can be malignant form. These are firm, lumpy to diffuse swelling that may bleed.

Flea Allergy dermatitis: Fleas inject their saliva on which they are living Dogs itch intensely in some or all area of body. They are restless and incomfortable scratch, lick, rub, chew and even nibble their skin. This may lead to hair loss, scabbing and even anemia.

Fly strike: Maggot infestation or Myiasis is caused by house flies, blow flies, bottle flies and flesh flies. These lay egg in the skin wounds. These produce maggots that move rapidly invade surrounding tissue.

Granulomatous sebaceous adenitis: There is destruction of oil glands with severe oil discharge and hair loss.

Hair coat: Outer covering of hair is known as hair coat. This protects its skin from physical and ultraviolet damage and helps regulate body temperature. It helps to cool the skin.

Hair follicles: These are compound in dogs. These have a central hair surrounded by 3-15 smaller hairs all exiting from one pore. Dogs are born with simple hair follicle that develop into compound hair follicles.

Hemangiomas: These are benign tumors common on head, legs and abdomen. These can be single or multiple, compressible red to black lumps look like blood blister.

Hemangiopericytomas: These develop mostly on lower legs and chest of older dogs more often in females. These sarcomas are firm, solitary with irregular looping borders occurs in fat under the skin.

Hepatoid gland tumor: It is also tumor found near the anus in dogs. These may occur along the abdomen from anus to base of skull and tail. It occurs mostly in male dogs in ageds. These commonly form, ulcers and bleed, cause difficult defecation.

Histiocytoma: It is skin tumor usually in younger age of dogs and involve head, ear and limbs. These are solitary, raised, ulcerated lumps that are freely movable.

Hygroma: It is a fluid filled sac that develops over bony prominences and pressure point. Repeated trauma and lying on hard surface leads to inflammation. This leads to soft, flexible fluid filled painless swellings especially in leg joints.

Hyperpigmentation: It is darkening and thickening of skin of dog. It is due to a reaction of dog's body to certain condition. There is appearance of light brown to black, velvety rough areas of thickened hairless skin in legs and groin areas.

Hypopituitarism: It is a disease characterised by short stature and hairloss, seborrhea and calcium deposits in skin. Scratching is very common.

Infiltrative lipoma: It affects chest and legs. These are soft and lumpy swelling in the fat layer under the skin. It spreads to underlying tissue

Infundibular Kerato canthoma: Cornifying epithelioma or Influndibuler Keratinizing acanthoma.

Interdigital furunculosis: Abcess or localized infection of the skin between the toes.

Invasive lipomas: These are partially malignant sarcoma

Itching: It is known as pruritis. It is an unpleasant sensation within skin that provokes the desire to scratch. Itching is a sign usually seen in parasite infestation, infections and allergies. Dogs scratch, bite or lick skin.

Keratinization: In this process new skin cells are created near the base of epidermis and migrate upward. This produces a complex layer of dead cells on the skin surface. Later on top layer is shed and replaced by cells from lower layers.

Keratinized Skin cysts: these are cysts filled with Keratin. They are hard or solid core. These can be isthmuscatagen cysts, matrix cysts, hybrid cysts or panfollinlar cysts and demoid cysts. These are benign single or multiple.

Keritinocytes: Cells found in epidermis which provide a protective layer and is constantly renewed by a process called Keratinization.

Langerhans cells: These are part of immune system and are in epidermis. These cells are damaged when exposed to excessive ultra violet rays and anti-inflammatory drugs. These help skin to development of rashes when animal is exposed to any irritant material.

Lipoma: Benign tumor of adipose tissue or fat generally occur in old dogs on trunk and near the top of legs. These are soft, thin and discreet lumpy masses move freely.

Liposacromas: It occurs in older male dogs on chest and legs. These are lumpy and can be soft or firm.

Lumpy skin syndrome: It is associated with kidney cysts. There is testicular tumor, widespread hairloss and occasional itching with skin rash.

Lupoiddermatosis: It is condition shown by scaling and rusting on the head and upper parts of body and legs. This leads to generalized scaling of skin accompanied by redness and it becomes painful or itchy. There may be fever and enlarged lymph nodes.

Malignant histocytosis: This is histoycytosis, appears in internal organs and lungs causing illness, pain and death.

Mange: It is caused by mites and is highly contagious. It is of many types.

Merkel cells: These are specialized cells in epidermis and associated with senory organs in the skin. These help animals with sensory information from whiskers and deep skin are called tylotrich pads.

Melanocytes: These are cells located at the base of epidermis the outer root sheath of hairs and ducts of glands. These produce colouring pigments called melanin. Melanin helps protect the cells from damaging rays of the sun.

Melanomas: these are dark pigmented skin tumors benign or malignant. These develop on head, and forelimbs in middle aged dogs. These can appear spots or patches or raised or flat masses. Mostly they have dark surface. Malignant melanomas develop in old age. Nailbeds lips and mouth are common sites. These are not on haired skin and found in lower abdomen and scrotum. These appear as ulcerated lump and variably darkened. When appear on lips or in the mouth tumor appears as dark to light gray or pink raised lump.

Mite infestation: Mange is caused by microscopic mites that invade skin and cause irritation of skin, itching, hair loss and inflammation.

Nasal solar dermatitis: It is caused by many diseases. These may affect the bridge of nose or nose. Sometimes muzzle is crusted. Nasal dermatitis is caused by solar radiation. There is inflammation and become ulcerated. There is redness and sometimes fluid discharge.

Nevus: Area where skin is malformed including pigmented spots.

Oily glands or Sebacious glands: These are present in large numbers near the paws, back of the neck, rump, chin and tail area. These secrete an oily substance called sebum into hair follicle and on to the skin.

Otodectic mange: This is caused by Otodectes cynotis mites. These mostly infest external ear causing inflammation of ear canal (otitis) Dog shake its head and scratch its ears.

Papillomas: These are also known as warts. These are caused by papilloma virus by contact. Multiple warts of skin or mucous membranes are generally seen in younger dogs. In older dogs these are single warts mostly. These are 3 kinds of warts Mucous membrane appillomatosis, skin warts and skin inverted papilloma. First type affects mouth from lips to oesophagus skin warts are around mucous membrane and solitary found on skin. Skin inverted papillomas warts develop on lower abdomen. They can go themselves.

Pelodera dermatitis: It is a skin worm infestation of Pelodera strongyloides. They are infested by contact. There are sores on parts of body such as legs, groin, abdomen and chest. Skin becomes red, and partially hairless. There may be lumps in the skin, lumps filled with crust or ulcers. There is even itching and animal scratch, bite or rub the affects area.

Perianal gland adenocarcinoma: these are found in male dogs mostly. These spread to draining lymph nodes located along the lower back.

Photosensitization: It is a clinical condition in which skin is over sensitive to sunlight. (Not sun burn). It can be Photosensitization type. I and II chemical in plants, fungi, bacteria may act as photosensitization agents. They feel discomfort in sunlight. There can be changes in skin. Redness and swelling develop. If exposure is prolonged fluid discharge, scab formation and skin death is there.

Pseudomyiasis: When fly maggots have been consumed and are found in digestive tract. These pass through feces undigested.

Pyoderma: It means pus in skin caused by inflammation, infection and cancer. Mostly it is superficial. There is excessive scaling. Scales are often pierced by hairs. Itching is variable. It occurs as bold patches, welts around hairs and scabbing.

Screw worms: Filth breeding flies are named screw worms as their shape resemble a wood screw.

Sebaceous gland adenocarcinoma: These are malignant form of tumor occur in middle aged dog. These spread within skin.

Sebaceous gland adenoma: These overgrowths tend to be larger and are in multiple and may occur anywhere on the body. These are covered with a crust and filled with pus.

Sebaceous gland haematomas: These are solitary tumor elongated and circular usually appear after birth. Simple lumps can be sebaceous gland overgrowth also.

Sebum: Secretion of oil gland is sebum. It keeps skin soft, moist and pliable. Sebum gives hair coat sheen and has antibiotic properties.

Seborrhoea: It is characterised by a defect in Keratinization or cornification of outer layer of skin, hair follicles and claws. It results in increased scale formation, greasiness of skin and hair coat. Often secondary infection and inflammation is there. Mostly caused by hormonal disorders and allergies Keratinization abnormalities cause is also there.

Skin tags: These are distinctive benign skin lumps on older dogs. These can be single or multiple. These look like stalk like growth covered by a wart like surface.

Solar keratosis: It is thickened discolouration of skin.

Sore month: contagious ecthyma.

Subcutis: It is inner most layer of skin subcutis means beneath the skin.

Subungual Squamous cell carcinoma: These are tumors that originate under a nail (clow). These arise on multiple toes and solitary also. These appear as raised, irregular on toes with ulcers or pimples. Dogs show lameness.

Sweat glands: These produce sweat. In dogs these are found on the feet and have a minor role in cooling the body.

Systemic histocytosis: It is an aggressive skin disease that causes multiple skin lesions that wax and wane.

Tick Paralysis: It is progressive motor paralysis caused by salivary toxin released by ticks. Otobius megnini is the tick species causing it.

Tricholemmomas: Hair follicle tumor found on head. These appear as oval masses and gradually grow. When funnel shaped called trichofolliculomas and when multiple small lumps called Trichoepitheliom. In later form hair follicle is filled with condensed, yellow, granular cheesy material. When it becomes malignant and spread to skin surface known as malignant trichoepithelioma.

Trombiculosis: It is a type of mange caused by parasitic larval stage of mites of family Trombiculidae. Larvae attach to the host feed for a few days and leave when enlarged. These look like tiny orange red oval dots that do not move. Signs include redness, bumps, hair loss and crusts. Intense itching even when they leave the dog. These are found in clusters on the head, ears, feet or belly.

Twitch muscle: It is major muscle immediately beneath the skin.

Urticaria: there are hives of skin rashes, localized patches of red usually itch skin. They develop and disappear suddenly. These are caused by insect bites or stings, shampoos and medication. These can be due to contact with toxic plant or chemical. Sunlight, heat, exercise, stress may intensify condition.

Vasculopathy: It is a problem and sets in first vaccination in puppies. Signs are footpad swelling and loss of colour and ulcers. Crusting and ulcers on ear and tail tips and loss of colour on the bridge of muzzle.

Vitiligo: There is bleached splotches of skin that also affect the hair coat and claws. Most of them are on face especially on the bridge of muzzle around the eyes.

Weather coat: This is also hair coat but with shorter, thicker hairs and fewer secondary hairs. These are warm weather coats.

Zinc Deficiency syndrome: Lethal acrodermatitis. There are signs of retarted growth, thickened skin on legs and pustules around mucous membrane. Later on there can be diarrhea, pneumonia and death.

Anti-infective Topical

Antifungal

Canesten Sol/ cream	**Bayer**
Comp	Clotrimazole 1% Sol 10mg/g cream
Adm.	Local application
@	As per need
Pres.	Sol – 15ml cream 15g

Imidil Pow/ cream/ Sol	**Lyka**
Comp	Clotrimazole 1% in all
Adm.	Local
@	As per need
Pres.	Sol 15ml cream 15g Pow 30g

Myconil Pow	**Ranbaxy**
Comp	Clotrimazole 1% in all
Adm.	Local
@	As per need
Pres.	100g

Micogel Cream	Cipla
Comp	Miconazole nitrate 2%
Adm.	Local application
@	As per need
Pres.	Sol – 15ml cream 15g

Canesten S. Cream	Bayer
Comp	Clotrimazole 10mg and Beclomethazone dipropionate 0.25mg/10g
Adm.	Local
@	As per need
Pres.	10g

Betnovate GM cream	Glaxo
Comp	Miconazole nitrate 2% Betamethasone 0.12% Gentamicine sulphate 0.1%
Adm.	Local
@	As per need
Pres.	20g

Betnovate M. Cream	Glaxo
Comp	Miconazole nitrate 2% Betamethasone valerate 0.12%
Adm.	Local
@	As per need
Pres.	20g

Spectrazole Cream	Ranbaxy
Comp	Miconazole 2% Gentamicine 0.1% clobetasol 0.1%
Adm.	Local
@	As per need
Pres.	20g

Kenacomb oint	Sarabhai
Comp	Nystatin 100000 unit Triamcinolone aetate 0.1% Neomycin 2.5mg Gramicidin 0.25mg
Adm.	Local
@	As per need
Pres.	10g

Canisep Cream	**Himalya**
Comp	Herbal
Adm.	Local
@	As per need
Pres.	30g

Dermocept Cream	**Concept**
Comp	Herbal
Adm.	Local
@	As per need
Pres.	25g

Himax Lotion	**Natural Remedies**
Comp	Herbal
Adm.	Local
@	As per need
Pres.	100ml

Melicon v oint	**Zydus**
Comp	Melia azadirachta 10% combined extract of Lawsonia inermis and Swertia chirata 15% Cedraus deodara 3% Gardenia gummifera 2%
Adm.	Local
@	As per need
Pres.	15g

Mycostatin oint	**Zydus**
Comp	Nystatin 100000 IU per g
Adm.	Local
@	As per need
Pres.	10g

Newcharm gel	**Ayurvet**
Comp	Herbal
Adm.	Local
@	As per need
Pres.	25g

Kiskin Lotion	Intas
Comp	Miconazole nitrate 2% clobetasol propionate 0.025% Gentamicin 0.1%
Adm.	Local
@	As per need
Pres.	30ml, 100ml

Antimicrobial Topical

Gentim Spray	Wockhardt
Comp	Gentamicin sulphate 5%
Adm.	Local
@	As per need
Pres.	100g

Gentamicine Sulphate Pow	Lyka
Comp	Gentamicin sulphate 0.1%
Adm.	Local
@	As per need
Pres.	100gsa

Vetbacin oint	Glaxo
Comp	Each gm contains Neomycin Sulphate 5mg Zinc bacitracin 500 IU
Adm.	Local
@	As per need
Pres.	20g

Cambison oint	Hoechst
Comp	Each g contains Neomycin hydrochloride 1.6mg Prednisolone 5mg Surfen 3mg
Adm.	Local
@	As per need
Pres.	5g

Bactoban Cream	**Glaxo**
Comp	2% Mupirocin
Adm.	Local
@	As per need
Pres.	5g

Dermocure oint	**Pranav**	
Comp	Gamma benzene hexachloride	0.1%
	Cetrimide	0.45%
	Proflavin hemisulphate	0.1%
Adm.	Local	
@	As per need	
Pres.	100g	

Flurry Liquid	**Sarabhai**
Comp	Ayurvedic Herbal
Adm.	Local
@	As per need
Pres.	120g

Furacin cream/ oint/ Pow	**Pfizer**
Comp	Nitrofurazone 0.2%
Adm.	Local
@	As per need
Pres.	20g, 25g oint, 10g Pow

Lorexane cream	**Virbac**
Comp	Gamma benzene hexachloride 0.1% Cetrimide 0.45% Proflavin hemisulphate 0.1%
Adm.	Local
@	As per need
Pres.	100g

Terramycin oint/ Liq	**Pfizer**
Comp	Oxytetracycline hydrochloride 50mg/ml or/g
Adm.	Local
@	As per need
Pres.	60ml, 15g

Utrox Top Liq	Neospark
Comp	Oxytetracycline hydrochloride 50mg/ml or/g
Adm.	Local
@	As per need
Pres.	60ml, 100ml

OTC Dusting Pow	Cipla
Comp	20mg/g of oxytetracyclin Hydrochloride
Adm.	Local
@	As per need
Pres.	100g

M. Lorex oint	Marc
Comp	Gamma benzene hexachloride 0.1% Cetrimide 0.45% hemisulphate 0.1%
Adm.	Local
@	As per need
Pres.	25g, 100g

Antiscabies

Benzene Hexachloride	Generic
Comp	1% Gamma Benzene hexachloride
Adm.	Local
@	As per need
Pres.	100ml, 450ml

Scabicip Lotion	Cipla
Comp	Gamma Benzene hexachloride 20%
Adm.	Local
@	As per need
Pres.	100ml

Doline Sol	Ranbaxy
Comp	0.1% Gamma Benzene hexachloride 0.1% Proflavin hemisulphate 0.45% cetrimide
Adm.	Local
@	As per need
Pres.	100ml

Coolmac Spray	**Macnor**
Comp	0.1% Gamma Benzene hexachloride 0.1% Proflavin hemisulphate 0.45% cetrimide
Adm.	Local
@	As per need
Pres.	100ml

M. Lorex oint	**Marc**
Comp	0.1% Gamma Benzene hexachloride 0.1% Proflavin hemisulphate 0.45% cetrimide
Adm.	Local
@	As per need
Pres.	100ml

Eumosone G cream	**Glaxo**
Comp	Gentamicine sulphate 0.1% clobetasone 0.05%
Adm.	Local
@	As per need
Pres.	10g

Nebasulf Powder/ oint	**Pfizer**
Comp	Each g contains Neomycin sulphate 5mg Bacitracin 250 units Sulphacetamide 60mg
Adm.	Local
@	As per need
Pres.	Pow 10g, Oint 15g

Megasunt dusting Powder	**Bayer**
Comp	Each g contains Coumaphos 30mg Propoxur 20mg Sulphanilamide 50mg
Adm.	Local
@	As per need
Pres.	40g

Petbacin oint	Glaxo
Comp	Each g contains Polymixin B sulphate 5000 IU Zinc bacitracin 400 IU Neomycin sulphate 3400 IU
Adm.	Local
@	As per need
Pres.	20g

OTC Spray	Cipla
Comp	Oxytetracycline hydrochloride 5g + Gentian violet 0.7g
Adm.	Local
@	As per need
Pres.	5.7g

Healup Spray	Century
Comp	Ayurvedic Herbal
Adm.	Local
@	As per need
Pres.	250ml

Dermanol Cream	Venky
Comp	Herbal
Adm.	Local
@	As per need
Pres.	25g

Antiseptics

Sterdin oint/ sol	Sterling Lab
Comp	Povidone Iodine 5% in both
Adm.	Local
@	As per need
Pres.	Oint 15g, 100g, 250g Sol 100ml, 500ml

Cipladine sol/ oint	**Cipla**
Comp	Povidone Iodine 5% in both
Adm.	Local
@	As per need
Pres.	100ml, 100g

Wokadin oint/Sol/ Pow/cream/spray	
Comp	Povidone Iodine 5% in all
Adm.	Local
@	As per need
Pres.	Oint 15g, 125g, sol 100ml Pow 10g, cream 15g spray 50ml

Sulphoben Sol	**Ranbaxy**
Comp	Sulphur 2% Benzyl Peroxide 2.5% Zincoxide 0.25%
Adm.	Local
@	On all over body 2-3 times per week
Pres.	100ml, 185ml

Charmil	**Ayurvet**
Comp	Herbal
Adm.	Local
@	As per need
Pres.	25g, 50g, 1kg

Iopaint Sol/Oint/	**Venky**
Comp	Povidone Iodine 5% in both
Adm.	Local
@	As per need
Pres.	100ml, 100g

Dermanol	**Indian Herbs**
Comp	Herbal
Adm.	Local
@	As per need
Pres.	25g

Dressol oint/Lotion	Cattle Remedies
Comp	Herbal
Adm.	Local
@	As per need
Pres.	Oint 50g Lotion 100ml, 450ml

Melcon V oint	Cadila Pharma
Comp	Herbal
Adm.	Local
@	As per need
Pres.	50g

Scavon Cream	Himalya
Comp	Herbal
Adm.	Local
@	As per need
Pres.	50g

Veto Max oint	Rakesh
Comp	Herbal
Adm.	Local
@	As per need
Pres.	50g, 1kg

Wisprec Pow	Natural Remedies
Comp	Herbal
Adm.	Local
@	As per need
Pres.	25g

Topicure Liq	Natural Remedies
Comp	Herbal
Adm.	Local
@	As per need
Pres.	250ml

Samodin spray	Wockhardt
Comp	5.5% Povidone Iodine
Adm.	Local
@	As per need
Pres.	80ml

Coat Conditioners & Cleaners

Various preprations are used for cleaning, grooming and conditioning the hair coat and skin hygiene of pets. There are nutritional coat and skin conditioner which help to correct all type of skin and coat conditions like dull coat, flaky skin, excess shedding and scratching caused by deficient diet. These are also used as supportive treatment in various skin diseases. Apart from hair coat conditioning and skin, these also prevent dandruff, ectoparasitic infections, insect repellant, insect growth inhibitor and deodorizer. Some are medicated with antiscptic properties and control bacterial contamination. Some relieve itching and soothes sensitive skin. Some are used topically and some are taken orally. Regular use of such coat conditioners prevent hair loss and promotes the growth of hair. It also helps to keep the coat healthy and shining. It makes the pet odour free. Topical application conditioners are applied against the lay of the hair and make sure that the entire coat of the animal is wetted. Ruffle the coat specially with long hair of animals so that the product penetrates down to the skin allow to dry naturally. After a few minutes comb. Some can be rinsed with water. With some products one has to work up a rich lather and massage thoroughly. Later on drying with towel, brush and comb the hair thoroughly. Take care to avoid eyes, ears and mouth. Repeat the treatment at 4-5 days interval or as directed by veterinarian or manufacturer.

Coat conditioners

Conifer Liq	**Sarabhai**
Comp	Herbal
Adm.	Bath to ensure wetting Rub
@	10-20g
Pres.	120g

Canifur AZ	**Zydus**
Comp	Herbal
Adm.	Bath to ensure wetting Rub
@	10-20g
Pres.	120g

Erina Coat cleanser	**Himalya**
Comp	Herbal
Adm.	Bath
@	As per need
Pres.	120g

Loamglo	**Ayruvet**
Comp	Herbal
Adm.	Bath
@	As per need
Pres.	100ml

Nutri Coat oral Liq	**Petcare**
Comp	Linolinic acid 3000mg, Lecithin 50mg, Vt B_6 400mcg Zinc 4.5mg A 1000 IU, E 10IU, D3 100 IU selenium 2mcg
Adm.	Oral
@	2.5-5g od
Pres.	100ml

Samfur F.S	**Wockhardt**		
Comp	10g contain		
	Protein 15%	Fat 6%	Fibre 0.9%
	Calcium 48mg	Phosphorous 25mg	
	Iron 20mg	Vit D_3 33.33mcg	
	Biotin 0.3mg + 24 essential amino acid		
Adm.	Oral		
@	10g od		
Pres.	100g		

Samglow PV coat conditioner	**Wockhardt**
Comp	Not given
Adm.	Local
@	As per need
Pres.	12ml sache, 185ml

Vitacharm Liq	**Ayurvet**
Comp	Herbal with evening primrose and Vit A D E
Adm.	Local
@	As per need
Pres.	100ml

Laurell	**Natural Remedies**
Comp	Herbal
Adm.	Bath
@	As per need
Pres.	125g

Splenderm	**Indian Herbs**
Comp	Herbal
Adm.	Bath
@	As per need
Pres.	100g

Shampoos / Soaps

Various preprations are used as shampoos which clean and condition the hair coat and skin. Skin is the most challenged organ in animal body which is exposed to extremes of environment changes, parasites, virus,bacteria, etc. Whereas hair or hair coat provides some protection to the skin but still continuous care of skin is must otherwise it leads to various skin disorders. Hair coat also provides a good look & help in overall outlook of the animal. Different shampoos are used for different objectives in mind. Some are antidandruff, some make coat shining silky and glossy, some protect skin from various microorganisms and a few skin diseases, scales and crusts on the skin are controlled. These relieve itching, inflammation of skin & coat and keep skin smooth, shiny, some also provide fragrance to the coat and soothen skin.

These are applied by wetting the hair coat thoroughly with warm or cold water depending upon climate. Shampoos are applied and worked into the skin of entire body. More water is added to get good lather and left for a few minutes. Body is rinsed and dried.

Shampoos

Arnibax Shampoo	**Ranbaxy**
Comp	Herbal
Adm.	Shampoo coat, rinse with water and dry
@	As per need
Pres.	250ml

Clinal Pet	**Glaxo**
Comp	Cypermethrin 1% with glycerine
Adm.	Local
@	As per need
Pres.	100ml

Dermeez Shampoo	**Ranbaxy**
Comp	Bronopol 0.2% dichlorobenzyl alcohol 0.5%
Adm.	Local
@	As per need
Pres.	100ml

Seledruff Shampoo	Petcare
Comp	Selenium sulphide 2.5%
Adm.	Local
@	As per need
Pres.	12ml, 150ml

Ichgon	Glaxo
Comp	Bronopol 0.2% dichlorobenzyl alcohol 0.5%
Adm.	Local
@	As per need
Pres.	100ml

Tetmosol Soap/ sol/ cake	(ICI) Glaxo
Comp	Tetra ethyl thiuram monosulphide 5%
Adm.	Local
@	As per need
Pres.	50ml sol, 75g cake

Blaze	Indian Herbs
Comp	Cypermethrin 1% with glycerine
Adm.	Local
@	As per need
Pres.	100ml

Pedigri Soap	Glaxo
Comp	Tetra ethyl thiuram monosulphide 5%
Adm.	Local
@	As per need
Pres.	50ml sol, 75g cake

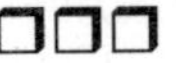

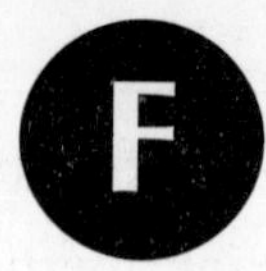

Infection and Infestation

Bacterial Diseases

Borreliosis (Lyme disease): Cause is Borrelia burgodorferi, a spirochaete transmitted through ticks. Symptoms are unspecific. These include fever, fatigue and loss of appetite. There are painful inflamed joints. Dog is lime or exhausted.

Brucellosis: It is sexually transmitted that cause uveitis, abortion and orchitis.

Clostridiasis: It is caused by Clostridia perfringens and C difficle symptoms are diarrhea.

Colibacillosis: Cause is Escherichia coli or enterococci. Bacteria enter through contaminated water or licking of anus. It can lead to serious intestinal or urinary tract infection. Painful urinary tract infection diarrhea and vomiting. Puppies are particularly at risk. In rare cases in puppies it can lead to meningitis.

Ehrlichiosis: It is caused by Ehrlichia canis and spread by brown dog tick. Signs include fever, vasculitis and low blood counts.

Kennel cough or canine tracheobronchitis: Cause can be viruses or Bordtella bronchiseptica a bacteria. It occurs in dogs in confinement of Kennels. It is mainly transmitted from dog to dog. Major signs are protracted harsh cough which sounds as though the dog has a bone stuck in its throat. It remains cheerful and continue eating. In puppies it is complicated by secondary infection and pneumonia causing death.

Leptospirosis (Spicrochaete): It is also known as Stuttgart Dog disease or Lamppost disease. It is caused by Leptospira canicola from contaminated plants or ponds or through urine of wild animals or rodents. It is highly contagious. Symptoms can be different. Some do not show any external signs. Mostly fatigue, appetite, vomiting also occur. If untreated it can cause irrepairable liver and kidney damage which can be fatal, specially in puppies.

Salmonellosis: It is caused by Salmonella pathogen. Signs range from mild diarrhea to severe vomiting and diarrhea with blood, fever and formation of abceses on internal organs. These can lead to jaundice, lung or joint inflammation and nervous system disorder.

Staphylocci: This infection affects, skin causing bacterial dermatitis Usually visible signs are on stomach. Symptoms include itching, red skin hairloss, ulcers and boils. Inflammation can spread to heart, bones and joints.

Viral Infections

Canine Coronovirus: It is called Feline infectious peritionitis or pleuritis caused by corona virus. Transmission is through ingestion of virus and close contact with infected cat or excreta and saliva. Primary infection is asymptomatic then conjunctivitis, upper respiratory sign and diarrhea may occur. There is weight loss and major organ failure.

Canine distemper: It is caused by myxovirus with 7-21 days incubation period. There is fever accompanied by loss of appetite. It can be (a) cutaneous form and (b) oculo nasal form in which there is discharge from eyes and nose (c) Pulmonary form with coughing laboured breathing (d) Gastro enteric- constipation followed by diarrhea and vomiting (e) nervous form with ecliptic fits, blindness and paralysis of hind legs with twitching of jaws and limbs. It is accompanied by thickening of pads and nose.

Canine herpesvirus: It causes fatal haemorrhage diseae in newborn pups. It affects 7-12 days old puppies. Generalised necrotizing vasculitis is accompanied by perivascular haemorrhage and mild rhinitis. It is a fatal disease and puppy dies within 24 hours. Transmission is through contact, oral, nasal and vaginal secretion.

Canine minute virus: It is also known as minute virus of canine MVC It causes inapparent to severe illness in neonatal pups. They have bronchitis and pneumonia with various degree of lymphoadenitis. There is lethargy, loss of weight, abdominal pain, dehydration, fever and death.

Canine Parvovirus: Incubation period is 7 days. It is transmitted from dog to dog via virus excreted in feces human footwear. 2 forms (i) Canine parvovirus myocarditis in which heart muscles become weak and destroyed. Puppies suddenly collapse at 4-10 week of age. They die after play or feeding (ii) Canine parvovirus intestinal form. It affects 4 weeks of age to old dog. It is fatal. Signs are vomiting, depression diarrhea with blood. Puppy may be bald.

Infectious Canine hepatitis: Also known as canine viral hepatitis. It is caused by canine adenovirus. Incubation period is 8 days. Early signs are illness lack of appetite with pale conjunctiva and gums, high temperature, vomiting, diarrhea abdominal pain. There can be Jaundice. Recovering animal show blue clouding over cornea. Dogs of all ages suffer.

Parainfluenza: It is caused by RNA virus. It is usually associated with mild to subclinical infection. Clinical signs include pyrexia, cough, serous nasal and lachrymal discharge, increased respiratory rate and breath sounds. Severity of signs worsen with onset of bacteria pneumonia.

Pseudo rabies or Aujeszky's disease: It is caused by herpes virus Infection, is usually fatal. Signs are coughing, sneezing, fever, depression, seizure circling and excess salivation. There is itching and pregnant can abort or reabsorb their foetus.

Rabies: It is a fatal disease transmitted through saliva of many animals. Incubation period is very long 2-3 weeks. It is of 2 form Dull or furious rabies. Ferocious animals becomes affectionate and seek human company and quiet animals become furious and can make unpredictable attacks on human and animals. Facial expression changes. Eyes become staring, jaws fixed and paralised with drooling copious saliva. Dogs tend to hide away from light and are very dangerous to approach. There is coma and death but it may take 15 days. Affected dogs may develop difficulty in swallowing and do not go into spasms at the sign of water.

Canine Fungal Infection

Aspergillosis: Caused by Aspergillus fumigatus- infections is in nasal cavity. Signs are sneezing, nasal discharge, bleeding from nose and its ulceration, decreased appetite.

Blastomycosis: Caused by Blastomyces dermatitidis. It affects eyes, brain, lungs, skin or bones. Signs are coughing, weight loss and lameness. It may result in pneumonia.

Caccidioidomycosis: Caused by cocciodioides immitis or C posadasi. It can cause cough, fever weight loss, anorexia and lethargy. It can cause lameness, seizers and localized swellings.

Cryptococcosis: Caused by Cryptococcus neoformans. It affects lungs and skin but more commonly eyes and central nervous system. Signs include coughing, imbalance gait, circling, seizures, inflammation of eyes, blindness and swollen lymph nodes.

Histoplasmosis: Caused by Histoplasma capsulatum. It affects lungs and small intestine.

Mycomycosis: It is collection of fungal and mould disease. It affects gastro intestinal tract and skin.

Pythosis: Caused by water mould of Pythium insdiosum. It affects gastro intestinal system, lymph nodes and rarely skin.

Ringworm: Cause is Microsporum canis or Microsporum gypseum and Trichophyton mentagrophytes. There is hair loss and scaly skin in form of rings.

Sporotrichosis: Cause Sporothrix schenckii. There are nodular skin lesions of head and trunk.

Protozoan Diseases

Amebiasis: It is caused by Entamoeba histolytica. It causes inflammation of large intestine which leads to persistent diarrhea. Diarrhea becomes severe and leads to weight loss. Loss of appetite, straining to defecate.

Babesiosis: It is spread by hard ticks. Babesia canis and Babesia gibsoni. These cause hemolytic anemia. Dogs have fever anorexia and depression.

Coccidiosis: Caused by variety of coccidion protozoa commonly Isospora. There are usually no symptoms but diarrhea and weightloss may occur. There can be dehydration.

Giardiasis: Caused by Giardia lambia symptoms are diarrhea, sometimes there are no signs. It causes weight loss and longterm diarrhea which can be continual or intermitted. Faces are soft, poorly formed pale and foul smelling. It is neither watery nor bloody.

Hepatozoon infection: It is caused by ingestion of ticks Hepatozoon canis. Symptoms are lethargy, myalgia, muscle wasting. It also infects skeletal and cardiac muscles.

Leishmaniasis: It is spread by sandfly. It is cutaneous and asymptomatic or can develop severe chronic disease involving muscle wasting ocular signs, renal disease, alopecia and other skin lesions.

Neosporosis: Caused by Neospora caninum. Dogs usually do not show and symptoms and signs can be seen in some puppies and adult dogs. Typically animal develops partial paralysis of legs particularly hind legs. This can lead to rigid contracture of muscles. There can be skin inflammation with sores.

Protothecosis: It is caused by green algae. Symptoms include weight loss, uveitis, retinal detatchment and anal seepage, diarrhea, ataxia and seizures. Treatment is difficult. Algae enters the body through mouth or nose.

Trypanosomiasis: It is caused by Trypansoma cruzi transmitted from kissing bugs. Symptoms are generalized lymphoadenopathy, lethargy, enlarged liver and spleen and myocarditis.

Antibacterial

Aerosporin inj	**Glaxo**
Comp	Polymyxin B sulpha 500000 IU
Adm.	IM
@	15000-25000 IU/kg bwt
Pres.	500000 IU vial

AC Vet inj	**Intas**
Comp	Ampicillin Sodium
Adm.	IM IV
@	6-10mg/kg B.wt
Pres.	1g, 2g, vial

Alcephin Susp	**Alembic**
Comp	Cephalexin 125mg/5ml
Adm.	Oral
@	10-15mg/kg B.wt bid
Pres.	40ml

Alcyclin O inj	**Alembic**
Comp	Oxytetracyclin 50mg/ml
Adm.	IM, IV, SC
@	1ml/10kg B.wt
Pres.	30ml

Althrocin liq	**Alembic**
Comp	Erythromycin 125mg/5ml
Adm.	Oral
@	10mg/kg B.wt od
Pres.	60ml

Aminocin inj	**Neospark**
Comp	Gentamycin sulphate 40mg/ml
Adm.	IM, SC
@	1-2mg/kg B.wt tid
Pres.	30ml

Ampisyn liq	**Cipla**
Comp	Ampicillin 125mg/5ml
Adm.	Oral
@	4-20mg/kg B.wt
Pres.	40ml

Ampi Vet	**Lyka**
Comp	Ampicillin Sod
Adm.	IM IV
@	6-10mg/kg B.wt
Pres.	2g

Ampoxin inj	**Unichem**
Comp	Ampicillin 125mg cloxacillin 125mg
Adm.	IM IV
@	6-10mg/kg B.wt od
Pres.	250mg vial, 500mg

Bacipen drops/syp	Alembic
Comp	Ampicillin trihydrate drop 100mg/ml, Syp 25mg/ml
Adm.	Oral
@	4-20mg/kg B.wt tid
Pres.	Drop 10ml, Syrp 40ml

Baxin Dry Syp/Pow	Lyka
Comp	Syp. Ampicillin trihydrate 62.5mg cloxacillin 62.5mg/5ml Pow Ampicillin trihydrate 125mg cloxacillin 125mg
Adm.	Oral
@	Syp 1-2 tsp tid. Pow 4-11mg/kg B.wt
Pres.	Syp 24g, Pow 24g

Benzapen inj	KAPL
Comp	Benzathine Pencillin 24 Lakhs IU
Adm.	IM
@	3-6 L IU/kg B.wt in 6 days
Pres.	24L vial

Bridox / Pow	Wockhardt
Comp	Neomycin sulphate 100mg Doxycyclin 100mg/g
Adm.	Oral
@	10-15g od
Pres.	50g

Bepen 20 inj	KAPL
Comp	Benzyl Penicillin 20L IU
Adm.	IM
@	2-4 Lakhs Units/kg B.wt
Pres.	20L Vial

Betalactin inj	Unichem
Comp	Ampicillin 250mg Cloxacillin 250mg
Adm.	IM, IV
@	5mg/kg B.wt od
Pres.	500mg vial

Biodox Sol granules	**Wockhardt**
Comp	Doxy cyclin hydrochloride 100mg/g
Adm.	Oral
@	1-2mg/kg B.wt bid
Pres.	10g, 50g

Brioxy inj	**Brihans**
Comp	Oxytetracyclin 50mg/ml
Adm.	IM, IV, SC
@	1ml/10kg B.wt
Pres.	10ml

Campicillin Drop/syp	**Cadila**
Comp	Ampicillin Sod 100mg/ml in drops 125mg/5ml in Syp
Adm.	Oral
@	4-20mg/kg B.wt tid
Pres.	10ml, 60ml Syp.

Campicillin inj	**Sarabhai**
Comp	Ampicillin Sodium
Adm.	IM IV
@	6-10mg/kg B.wt
Pres.	500mg, 1g vial

Chloramphenicol inj	**Lyka**
Comp	Chloramphenicol Sod. Succinate
Adm.	IM IV
@	25mg/kg B.wt bid
Pres.	1g, 2g

Chlortec inj	**Neospark**
Comp	Chloramphenicol 100mg/ml
Adm.	IM IV
@	25mg/kg B.wt bid
Pres.	30ml

Cloxacillin inj	KAPL
Comp	Cloxacillin
Adm.	IM
@	10mg/kg B.wt
Pres.	1g

Comoxyl in	Concept
Comp	Amoxicillin
Adm.	IM
@	4-7mg/kg B.wt
Pres.	2g

Conampi inj	Concept
Comp	Ampicillin Sodium
Adm.	IM IV
@	6-10mg/kg B.wt
Pres.	1g

Crys 4 inj	Sarabhai
Comp	Procaine Penicillin 15L IU Penicillin G Sodium 5L IU
Adm.	IM
@	2-4L IU od
Pres.	1 vial

Chlorovet inj	G.Loucatos
Comp	Chloramphenicol 100mg/ml
Adm.	IM IV
@	25mg/kg B.wt bid
Pres.	30ml

Dynacil inj	HAL
Comp	Ampicillin Sodium
Adm.	IM IV
@	6-10mg/kg B.wt
Pres.	1g

Gentabiotic inj	**KAPL**
Comp	Gentamycin sulphate 40mg/ml
Adm.	IM, SC
@	1-2mg/kg B.wt tid
Pres.	10ml

Gentamicin inj	**Wockhardt**
Comp	Gentamycin sulphate 40mg/ml
Adm.	IM, SC
@	1-2mg/kg B.wt tid
Pres.	10ml

Kampibiotic inj	**KAPL**
Comp	Ampicillin Sodium
Adm.	IM IV
@	6-10mg/kg B.wt
Pres.	1g

Keflong inj	**Glaxo**
Comp	Cephaloridine
Adm.	IM IV SC
@	11mg/kg B.wt od
Pres.	0.5g, 1g vial

Klox Dry Syp	**Lyka**
Comp	Cloxacillin 125mg/3g
Adm.	Oral
@	5-10g tsp tid
Pres.	24g

Kloxamp inj	**KAPL**
Comp	Ampicillin 125mg Cloxacillin 125mg
Adm.	IM IV
@	6-10mg/kg B.wt od
Pres.	500mg, 1g

Longacillin inj	**HAL**
Comp	Benzathine Pencillin 24 Lakhs IU
Adm.	IM
@	3-6 L IU/kg B.wt in 6 days
Pres.	6L, 12L

Lykacetin inj	Lyka
Comp	Chloramphenicol Sod. Succinate
Adm.	IM IV
@	25mg/kg B.wt bid
Pres.	1g

Megadox N Sol/Pow	Neospark
Comp	Doxycycline hydrochloride 100mg Neomycin sulphate 100mcg/g
Adm.	Oral
@	10-20mg/kg B.wt od
Pres.	50g

Nepocil Pow	TTK
Comp	Ampicillin 50mg/g
Adm.	Oral
@	4-12mg/kg B.wt bid
Pres.	30g

Novamox Dry Syp	Cipla
Comp	Amoxicillin 125mg/5ml
Adm.	Oral
@	10mg/kg B.wt
Pres.	30ml

Phexin DS syp	Glaxo
Comp	Cephalexin 250mg/5ml
Adm.	Oral
@	10-15mg/kg B.wt bid
Pres.	30ml

Roscillin Drop/Syp	Ranbaxy
Comp	Ampicillin Sod 100mg/ml in drops 125mg/5ml in Syp
Adm.	Oral
@	4-20mg/kg B.wt tid
Pres.	Drops 10ml Syp 40ml

Roscillin Pow	**Ranbaxy**	
Comp	Ampicillin 3g in 30g	
Adm.	Oral	
@	40-120mg/kg B.wt bid	
Pres.	30g	

Rosclox inj	**Ranbaxy**	
Comp	Ampicillin 250mg	Cloxacillin 250mg
Adm.	IM, IV	
@	5mg/kg B.wt od	
Pres.	250mg, 500mg	

Solampi	**Brihans**
Comp	Ampicillin Sodium
Adm.	IM IV
@	6-10mg/kg B.wt
Pres.	500mg, 1g

Stanicllin inj	**Zydus**
Comp	Ampicillin Sodium
Adm.	IM IV
@	6-10mg/kg B.wt
Pres.	250mg

Unimycin inj	**Unichem**
Comp	Neomycin sulphate 140mg/ml
Adm.	IM
@	11mg/kg B.wt
Pres.	10ml

Vetopen inj	**HAL**
Comp	Streptomycin 1g, Procaine Benzyl Penicillin 3L IU, Benzyl Penicillin Sod 1Lac IU
Adm.	IM
@	30-200mg/kg B.wt
Pres.	1 vial 1.0g

Biotrim inj IM	Ranbaxy
Comp	Sulphadiaziine 400mg Trimethoprim 80mg per ml
Adm.	IM
@	1ml/10kg B.wt od
Pres.	10ml

Biotrim inj IV	Ranbaxy
Comp	Sulphadiazine 200mg Trimethoprim 40mg per ml
Adm.	IV
@	1ml/8kg B.wt
Pres.	30ml

Oriprim susp	Cadila
Comp	Sulphamethoxazole 200mg Trimethoprim 40mg/5ml
Adm.	Oral
@	5ml/8kg B.wt
Pres.	50ml

Oriprim inj IM/IV	Cadila
Comp	IM inj Sulphamethoxazole 800mg Trimethoprim 160mg IV inj Sulphamethoxazole 400mg Trimethoprim 80mg
Adm.	IM + IV as vial
@	IM 1ml/20kg B.wt IV 2-5ml od
Pres.	IM 5ml ampoule IV 30ml vial

Anarobin inj	Unichem
Comp	Metronidazole 5mg/ml
Adm.	IM/IV
@	20mg/kg B.wt
Pres.	50ml

Baytril inj	Bayer
Comp	Enrofloxacin 25mg/ml
Adm.	IM
@	5mg/kg B.wt
Pres.	50ml

Cifran inj	**Ranbaxy**
Comp	Ciprofloxacin 2mg/ml
Adm.	IV
@	5-8mg/kg B.wt bid
Pres.	50ml

Ciplox IV inj	**Cipla**
Comp	Ciprofloxacin 200mg/ml
Adm.	IV
@	5-8mg/kg B.wt bid
Pres.	100ml

Conflox inj	**Concept**
Comp	Enrofloxacin 50mg/ml
Adm.	1ml/20kg B.wt od
@	IM
Pres.	30ml

Enrocin inj	**Ranbaxy**
Comp	Enrofloxacin 100mg/ml
Adm.	IM
@	1ml/20kg B.wt od
Pres.	15ml

Quintas inj	**Intas**
Comp	Enrofloxacin 100mg/ml
Adm.	IM
@	1ml/20kg B.wt od
Pres.	30ml

Enrogil inj	**G.Loucatos**
Comp	Enrofloxacin 100mg/ml
Adm.	IM
@	1ml/20kg B.wt od
Pres.	15ml

Enrox inj	**Alembic**
Comp	Enrofloxacin 100mg/ml
Adm.	IM
@	1ml/20kg B.wt od
Pres.	15ml

Flagyl Syp	**Rhone Poulenc**
Comp	Metronidazole 200mg/5ml
Adm.	Oral
@	20mg/kg B.wt
Pres.	30ml

Tinidazole Tab	**Cadila**
Comp	Tinidazole 300mg, 500mg
Adm.	Oral
@	30-50mg/kg B.wt
Pres.	10

Norbid Tab	**Alembic**
Comp	Norfloxacin Tab 100mg/200mg
Adm.	Oral
@	10mg/kg B.wt
Pres.	10

Britax inj	**Brihans**
Comp	Cefotoxamine
Adm.	IM IV
@	25-50mg/kg B.wt
Pres.	250mg, 500mg, 1g

Haltax inj	**HAL**
Comp	Cefotoxamine
Adm.	IM IV
@	25-50mg/kg B.wt
Pres.	250mg, 500mg, 1g

Temobax Sus	**Ranbaxy**
Comp	Amoxyyclin 200mg and clavulanic acid 28.5mg
Adm.	Oral
@	12.5-25mg/kg B.wt
Pres.	30ml

Cefstan inj	**Ranbaxy**
Comp	Ceftriaxone
Adm.	IM
@	20mg/kg B.wt od
Pres.	500mg with 5ml Distt water

Augmentin inj.	**Glaxo**
Comp	Amoxyyclin 200mg and clavulanic acid 28.5mg
Adm.	Oral
@	12.5-25mg/kg B.wt
Pres.	30ml

Ceporan inj	**Glaxo**
Comp	Cephaloridine
Adm.	IM IV
@	15-30mg/kg B.wt
Pres.	500mg, 1g

Antifungal

Fungizone IV	**Sarabhai**
Indi	Histoplasmosis, candidiasis
Comp	Amphotericin B
Adm.	IV in 5% Dextrose
@	0.25-0.5mg/kg B.wt (every 48 hrs)
Pres.	50mg vial

Grisovin Tab	**Glaxo**
Indi	Ringworm, Microsperum
Comp	Griseofulvin
Adm.	Oral
@	20mg/kg B.wt od for 30 days
Pres.	250mg, 500 Tab, 10

Charmaid cap	Ayurvet
Comp	Herbal
Adm.	Oral
@	1 cap od for large dogs 2 cap od
Pres.	30 cap

Teeburb cap	Natural Remedies
Comp	Herbal
Adm.	Oral
@	1 cap bid
Pres.	24

Antiprotozoan

Pronil H	Wockhardt
Indi	Trypanosomiasis
Comp	Diminazone aceturate 0.44g/g
Adm.	IM
@	0.2-0.4g per dog
Pres.	4.8g

Lithiomony inj	Indian Immunology
Comp	Lithium Antimonythiomalate 6%} Indication- Haemoparasite Leishmania
Adm.	IM
@	2-3ml thrice in a week
Pres.	50ml

Antricide Prosalt	Glaxo
Indi	Surra or Trypanosomiasis
Comp	Quinapyramine sulphate, quinapyramine chloride 1g
Adm.	IM
@	Add 15mg water 1-2ml
Pres.	2.5g

Corridan	**HAL**
Indi	Surra or Trypanosomiasis
Comp	Quinapyramine sulphate, quinapyramine chloride 1g
Adm.	IM
@	Add 15mg water 1-2ml
Pres.	2.5g

Tevansi	**Ranbaxy**
Indi	Surra or Trypanosomiasis
Comp	Quinapyramine sulphate, quinapyramine chloride 1g
Adm.	IM
@	Add 15mg water 1-2ml
Pres.	2.5g

Triquin	**Wockhardt**
Indi	Surra or Trypanosomiasis
Comp	Quinapyramine sulphate, quinapyramine chloride 1g
Adm.	IM
@	Add 15mg water 1-2ml
Pres.	2.5g

Gilpol	**G.Loucatos**
Indi	Surra or Trypanosomiasis
Comp	Suramin
Adm.	IV
@	30-50mg/kg B.wt
Pres.	1g vial

Naganol	**Bayer**
Indi	Surra or Trypanosomiasis
Comp	Suramin
Adm.	IV
@	30-50mg/kg B.wt
Pres.	1g vial

Anthiomoline	**Novartis**
Indi	Surra or Trypanosomiasis
Comp	Lithium Antimonythiomalate 6%} Indication- Haemoparasite Leishmania
Adm.	IM
@	2-3ml thrice in a week
Pres.	50ml

Berenil	Intervet
Indi	Trypanosomiasis
Comp	4, 4 diamidino diazomino benzene diceturate
Adm.	IM
@	0.2-0.4g/25kg B.wt
Pres.	22.5g

Parasiticides

Parasites – Endoparasites

Trichinosis: Trichinella spirals heavy infestation may show serious illness and death.

Echinococcosis: Cause infectious disease Echinococcus granulosis. In dogs it is asymptomatic.

Heart worm: Dirofilaria immitis through mosquito. Live in pulmonary artery or right ventricle of heart. Signs are cough, tachycardia and tachypnea.

Intestinal Parasites:

Hook worm- Ancyclostoma caninum cause diarrhea vomiting and weight loss.

Tapeworm- Diphylidium caninum spread by lice and fleas. Signs are irritability, variable appetite, shaggy coat, colic and mild diarrhea.

Round worm or Toxicara- Toxocara canis or Toxascaris leonine. Signs are diarrhea, pot bellied appearance, poor growth and vomiting.

Whipworm- Live in cecum and large intestine. Trichuris vulpis. These can cause diarrhea and weight loss.

Intestinal flukes- These do not cause illness till their number is very high.

Liver fluke- Is found in bile ducts and gall bladder. It causes mild to severe liver disease fibrosis. Dogs develop weakness ending in complete exhaustion and sometimes death.

Strongyloides stercoralis- Symptoms are bloody diarrhea, dehydration and sometimes death

Internal Parasites

Combantrin Tab/Susp	Pfizer
Indi	Nematodes
Comp	Pyrantel pamoate 200mg tab, 25mg/ml susp
Adm.	Oral
@	5mg/kg B.wt
Pres.	2 Tab, 8ml

Curaminth Tab	**Sarabhari**
Indi	Anthelmintic
Comp	Fenbendazole 150mg
Adm.	Oral
@	5mg/kg B.wt or 1 Tab for 30kg B.wt
Pres.	10 tab

Droncit Tab	**Bayer**
Indi	Mature and immature stages of tapeworms
Comp	Praziquantel 50mg
Adm.	Oral
@	5mg/kg B.wt or 1 Tab for 10kg, 11-20kg 2 tab Repeat after 2 week
Pres.	1 Tab

Albenz Tab	**Sterling**
Comp	Albendazole 150mg
Adm.	Oral
@	25mg/kg B.wt od for 5 days
Pres.	150mgX10

Albomar cap	**Glaxo**
Comp	Albendazole 150mg
Adm.	Oral
@	25mg/kg B.wt od for 5 days
Pres.	10

Albomar sus	**Glaxo**
Comp	2.5% Albendazole
Adm.	Oral
@	3-5ml bid for 3 days
Pres.	30ml

Alzonex Tab	**Neospark**
Comp	Albendazole 150mg
Adm.	Oral
@	25mg/kg B.wt od for 5 days
Pres.	10

Analgon sus	Wockhardt
Comp	2.5% Albendazole
Adm.	Oral
@	3-5ml bid for 3 days
Pres.	60ml

Analgon Tab	Wockhardt
Comp	Albendazole 150mg
Adm.	Oral
@	25mg/kg B.wt od for 5 days
Pres.	3x4 strip

Banocide Tab/Syp	Glaxo
Indi	Heartworm
Comp	Diethylcarbamazine citrate 50mg, 100mg Syp 120mg/5ml
Adm.	100mg/10kg B.wt od
Pres.	10 Tab Syp, 15ml

Drontal Plus Tab	Bayer
Indi	Tapeworm
Comp	Praziquantel 50mg, Pyrantel embonate 144mg, febental 150mg
Adm.	Oral
@	1 Tab/10kg B.wt
Pres	20 Tab

Fenomar Tab/Sus	Glaxo
Comp	Fenbendazole 150mg, Suspension 2.5%
Adm.	Oral
@	1 Tab bid x3 days Suspension 3-5ml bid for 5 days
Pres.	10

Fentas Pow/Tab	Intas
Comp	250mg Fenbendazole
Adm.	Oral
@	1g/25kg B.wt for 3 days, 1 Tab bidx3
Pres.	6g pouch

Fenzole 150mg Bol	**KAPL**
Comp	Fenbendazole 150mg
Adm.	Oral
@	75mg/15kg B.wt
Pres.	3x4 strip

Paratak	**Sarabhai**
Indi	Mature and immature stages of tapeworms
Comp	Praziquantel 50mg
Adm.	Oral
@	5mg/kg B.wt or 1 Tab for 10kg, 11-20kg 2 tab Repeat after 2 week
Pres.	1 Tab

Prazipet	**Petcare**
Indi	Mature and immature stages of tapeworms
Comp	Praziquantel 50mg
Adm.	Oral
@	5mg/kg B.wt or 1 Tab for 10kg, 11-20kg 2 tab Repeat after 2 week
Pres.	1 Tab

Interceptor oral	**Novartis**
Indi	Heartworm
Comp	Milbemycin oxine Tab 2.3mg, 5.75mg, 11.5mg, 23mg
Adm.	Oral
@	0.5mg/kg B.wt
Pres.	2.3mg Tab, 5-7mg Tab, 11.5mg Tab 23mg tab x10

Prazi Plus Tab	**Petcare**
Comp	Albendazole 300mg and Praziquintal 25mg
Adm.	Oral
@	1 Tab/10kg B.wt
Pres.	4

Worcid Tab	**Vets Farma**
Indi	Anticestodal (Ascaria – Filaria)
Comp	Dichlorphen 400mg
Adm.	Oral
@	300mg/kg B.wt
Pres.	10 Tab

Fentas Plus	Intas
Comp	Praziquintal 50mg Fenbendazole 50mg in 1 Tab
Adm.	Oral
@	1 Tab/10kg B.wt
Pres.	10

Plozin Tab	Ranbaxy
Indi	Tapeworm
Comp	Praziquantel 50mg, Pyrantel embonate 144mg, febental 150mg
Adm.	Oral
@	1 Tab/10kg B.wt
Pres	10

Prazital Plus	Indian Immunology
Indi	Tapeworm
Comp	Praziquantel 50mg, Pyrantel embonate 144mg, febental 150mg
Adm.	Oral
@	1 Tab/10kg B.wt
Pres	10

Prazifen	KAPL
Indi	Tapeworm
Comp	Praziquintal 50mg Fenbendazole 50mg in 1 Tab
Adm.	Oral
@	1 Tab/10kg B.wt
Pres.	10

Gutomil Bol/ granules	Worckhardt
Indi	Stomach and Intestinal worms
Comp	Levamesol 150mg Bol, 300mg/g granule
Adm.	Oral
@	5mg/kg B.wt
Pres.	10, 10g granule

Gutomil inj	Wockhardt
Indi	Stomuch and Intestinal worms
Comp	Levamisole 150mg/ml
Adm.	SC/ IM
@	5mg/kg B.wt
Pres.	10ml

Helmigard Bol/Granule	**Unichem**
Indi	Stomach and Intestinal worms
Comp	Bol 1.2g, 5% granule Albendazole
Adm.	Oral
@	25mg/kg B.wt
Pres.	1.2g Bol, 30g sachet granule

Kalmisole Tab	**KAPL**
Indi	Stomach and Intestinal worms
Comp	Levamisole 150mg
Adm.	SC/ IM
@	5mg/kg B.wt
Pres.	4

Lemasole Pow	**Ranbaxy**
Indi	Stomach and Intestinal worms
Comp	Levamisole 10%
Adm.	Oral
@	5mg/kg B.wt
Pres.	20g

Lemex Plus Pow	**Novartis**
Indi	Stomach and Intestinal worms
Comp	Levamisole 10%
Adm.	Oral
@	5mg/kg B.wt
Pres.	100g

Mebex Tab/Sus/granule	**Cipla**
Indi	Stomach and Intestinal worms
Comp	Mebendazole Tab 100mg, Sus 100mg/5ml, 200mg/5g granules
Adm.	Oral
@	50mg upto 2 kg B.wt, 100mg above 2kg B.wt bid for 5 days
Pres.	Tab 6, 30ml Susp, 5g granules

Minthal Bol/Susp/Pow	**Alembic**
Indi	Stomach and Intestinal worms
Comp	Albendazole 200mg Bol, Sus 2.5%, 5% Powder
Adm.	Oral
@	25mg/kg B.wt od for 5 days
Pres.	Tab 10, Sus 30ml Pow 10g

Nematex L Pow	Neospark
Indi	Stomach and Intestinal worms
Comp	Levamisole 10%
Adm.	Oral
@	5mg/kg B.wt
Pres.	100g

Nilverm Pow	Glaxo
Indi	Stomach and Intestinal worms
Comp	Tetramesole hydrochloride 30%
Adm.	Oral
@	15mg/kg B.wt of Tetramesole
Pres.	10g

Nilverm Forte pow	Glaxo
Indi	Stomach and Intestinal worms
Comp	Levamisole 10%
Adm.	Oral
@	5mg/kg B.wt
Pres.	10g

Panacur Tab/ Susp/Pow 25%	Intervet
Indi	Stomach and Intestinal worms
Comp	Fenbendazole 150mg, Suspension 2.5%
Adm.	Oral
@	1 Tab bid x3 days Suspension 3-5ml bid for 5 days
Pres.	10

Panfugal Pow	Wockhardt
Indi	Stomach and Intestinal worms
Comp	25% Fenbendazole
Adm.	Oral
@	20mg/kg B.wt od for 5 days
Pres.	6g

Piperazine Adipate Pow	KAPL
Indi	Roundworms
Comp	Piperazine activity 37%
Adm.	Oral
@	1g pow/10kg B.wt
Pres.	5g

Piperazine Hexahydrate Sol	**Wockhardt**
Indi	Roundworms
Comp	Piperazine hexahydrate 40.6g equivalent to 18g Piperazine 100ml
Adm.	Oral
@	2.5ml/10kg B.wt
Pres.	10ml

Piperazine Hexahydrate liq 45%	**TTK/Sterling/Glaxo/KAPL**
Indi	Roundworms
Comp	45% Piperazine hexahydrate
Adm.	Oral
@	5ml
Pres.	30ml

Piperazine hydrate 61%	**Neospark, sarabhai**
Indi	Roundworms
Comp	61% Piperazine hydrate
Adm.	Oral
@	5ml
Pres.	30ml

Piperol Syp	**Indian Immunology**
Indi	Roundworms
Comp	Piperazine hexahydrate 45%
Adm.	Oral
@	5ml every month
Pres.	500ml

Praziplus Tab	**Petcare**
Indi	Stomach and Intestinal worms
Comp	Praziquintal 50mg Fenbendazole 50mg in 1 Tab
Adm.	Oral
@	1 Tab/10kg B.wt
Pres.	10

Prazital Tab	**Indian Immunology**
Indi	Stomach and Intestinal worms
Comp	Each tab contains Praziquintal 50mg Pyrantel pamoate 144mg Fenbendazole 500mg
Adm.	Oral

@	1 tab/10kg B.wt. I dose 2 week Pup, II 1 month then every month upto 9 month
Pres.	

Suprazole Sus	**Ranbaxy**
Indi	Stomach and Intestinal worms
Comp	2.5% Albendazole
Adm.	Oral
@	3-5ml bid for 3 days
Pres.	30ml

Valbazen Tab	**Pfizer**
Indi	Stomach and Intestinal worms
Comp	Albendazole 150mg
Adm.	Oral
@	25mg/kg B.wt od for 5 days
Pres.	150mgX10

Valbazen Susp	**Pfizer**
Indi	Stomach and Intestinal worms
Comp	2.5% Albendazole
Adm.	Oral
@	3-5ml bid for 3 days
Pres.	60ml

Vetalben Susp/ Pow	**Indian Immunology**
Indi	Stomach and Intestinal worms
Comp	Susp 2.5%, Pow 5% Albendazole
Adm.	Oral
@	25mg/kg B.wt bid x5 days
Pres.	100ml susp, 50g Pow

Vibex Susp	**Wockhardt**
Indi	Stomach and Intestinal worms
Comp	2.5% Albendazole
Adm.	Oral
@	3-5ml bid for 3 days
Pres.	30ml

Wormin Tab/Susp/Pow	**Zydus**
Indi	Stomach and Intestinal worms
Comp	Mebendazole Tab 100mg, Sus 100mg/5ml, 200mg/5g granules

Adm.	Oral
@	50mg upto 2 kg B.wt, 100mg above 2kg B.wt bid for 5 days
Pres.	100mg Tabx6, Syp 30ml, Pow 50g

Zomar Susp	**Cadila**
Indi	Stomach and Intestinal worms
Comp	2.5% Albendazole
Adm.	Oral
@	3-5ml bid for 3 days
Pres.	60ml

External Parasites

Fleas: Cause itching and hair loss. Mostly cat flea, dog flea.

Ticks: External parasite spread Lyme disease, Rocky mountain spotted fever, babesiosis, and ehrlichiosis, tick paralysis.

Mosquitoes: Spread heart worm. Which can cause cough, difficult breathing and death.

Mites:-

Earmite- Otodectes cynotis mite.It causes itching, inflammation and black debris in ear.

Cheyletellosis- Mild pruritic skin disease caused by Cheyletiella yasguri

Chiggers- Harvest mite causes itching, redness and crusting of skins.

Demodicosis- Demodectic mange caused by Demodex canis causes inflammation and hair loss, secondary infection with fever, mange, lethargy and enlarged lymph nodes.

Sarcoptic mange- Sarcoptes scabie canis. Signs are itching and scaling.

Lices: Three types of lices are found on dogs. Sucking lices, biting lices and biting louse that feeds on blood.

Neocidol Liq	**Novartis**
Comp	Dizinon 20%
Adm.	Spray/ wash
@	2-3ml in 1L
Pres.	30ml, 100ml

Asuntol Pow	Bayer
Comp	50% coumafos
Adm.	Spray by adding
@	2-3g/ litre
Pres.	15g

Arunima Pow	Ayurvet
Comp	Herbal
Adm.	Dust on entire coat
@	As per need for 30 minutes
Pres.	120g

Asuntol Medicated soap	Bayer
Comp	Coumaphas 10mg/g
Adm.	Wash
@	As per need
Pres.	75g cake

Balfo spray	Bayer
Comp	Propoxur 1%
Adm.	Spray
@	As per need
Pres.	250ml

Butox Liq.	Intervet
Comp	Deltamethrin 12.5%
Adm.	Spray
@	2ml/Litre of water
Pres.	15ml

Canifer Liq	Sarabhai
Comp	Herbal
Adm.	Rub
@	10-20g
Pres.	120g

Cisaflux Liq	**Ranbaxy**
Comp	Cypermethrin 1%
Adm.	Wet the coat
@	As per need
Pres.	100ml

Cyperin 100 EC liq	**Wockhardt**
Comp	Cypermethrin 100g/Litre
Adm.	Wet the coat
@	As per need 20ml/Litre
Pres.	15ml

Flematic Skin oil	**TTK**
Comp	Herbal
Adm.	Bath after application
@	As per need
Pres.	100ml

Keetout Liq.	**Ayurvet**
Comp	Herbal
Adm.	Drops on coat
@	As per need
Pres.	10ml

Killtix collar	**Bayer**
Comp	Propoxur 10% flumethrin 2.25%
Adm.	Band on neck for 24 hrs
@	1 collar for 6-7 month
Pres.	1 collar

Negasunt dusting Pow	**Bayer**
Comp	Coumaphos 30mg Propoxur 20mg Sulpanilamide 50mg/g
Adm.	Dusting on coat
@	As per need
Pres.	40g

Notix Scrub Liq Talc Pow	Petcare
Comp	Liq carbaryl 10% Pow 5%
Adm.	Local dusting or wetting
@	As per need
Pres.	30g, 150g liquid and 150g Pow

Notix CP liq	Petcare
Comp	Cypermethrin 100mg/ml
Adm.	Wetting/ spray
@	As per need
Pres.	15ml

Pectocide Liq.	Sarabhai
Comp	Cypermethrin 100mg/ml
Adm.	Wetting/ spray
@	As per need
Pres.	15ml

Pestoban Liq.	Natural Remedies
Comp	Herbal
Adm.	Wetting
@	As per need
Pres.	100ml

Petmosol Soap	Glaxo
Comp	Monosulfiram 5%
Adm.	Application
@	As per need
Pres.	75g cake

Preventic Antitick collar	Ranbaxy / Virbac
Comp	Amitraz 9%
Adm.	Apply on neck
@	For 2 months
Pres.	Collar

Program Tab	**Novartis**
Comp	300mg/g Lufenuron
Adm.	Oral
@	1 Tab monthly
Pres.	Strip of 6

RIDD Sol	**Petcare**
Comp	Amitraz 12.5%
Adm.	Application
@	2ml/Litre of water
Pres.	6ml

RIDD Tick and Flea collar	**Petcare**
Comp	Amitraz 9%
Adm.	Apply on neck
@	For 2 months
Pres.	Collar

Tactic Sol	**Intervet**
Comp	Amitraz 5%
Adm.	Wetting
@	6ml/Litre
Pres.	25ml

Ticomax Sol.	**Ranbaxy**
Comp	Fenvalerate 20%
Adm.	Wetting
@	2ml/Litre
Pres.	15ml

Tikkil Pow	**Indian Immunology**
Comp	Cypermethrin 100mg/ml
Adm.	Wetting/ spray
@	As per need
Pres.	5g pouch

Zero keet liq	**Ayurvet**
Comp	Herbal
Adm.	Local application

@	1:4 dilution or 1:2 dilution
Pres.	100ml

Ectozee spray	**Indian Herbs**
Comp	Herbal
Adm.	Local
@	As per need daily
Pres.	200ml

Ectosep oint	**Zydus**
Comp	Herbal
Adm.	Local
@	As per need
Pres.	50g

HSD oint	**Alembic**
Comp	Herbal
Adm.	Local
@	As per need daily
Pres.	200ml

Maggacide Lotion	**Cattle Remedies**
Comp	Herbal
Adm.	Local
@	As per need daily
Pres.	50ml, 100ml, 450ml

Ostaderm oint	**Vets Farma**
Comp	Herbal
Adm.	Local
@	As per need
Pres.	50, 500g

Magout Lotion	**zydus**
Comp	Herbal
Adm.	Local
@	As per need
Pres.	40ml, 100ml

Defendog spray	**Ranbaxy**
Comp	Permethrin 2%
Adm.	Local
@	As per need
Pres.	100ml

Notix Green Pet Soap	**Petcare**
Comp	Neem oil 10% coconut oil
Adm.	Local for washing
@	As per need
Pres.	70g soap cake

Canifur AZ Liquid	**Cadila Pharma**
Comp	Herbal
Adm.	Local
@	As per need
Pres.	120g

Endectocide

Endact inj	**Wockhardt**
Indi	External and internal parasites
Comp	Ivermectin 10mg/ml
Adm.	IM/ SC
@	0.5-1ml
Pres.	1ml vial

Exinot Sol	**Cadila Pharma**
Comp	Closantel 15%
Adm.	Oral
@	0.5-0.7ml/ 10kg B.wt
Pres.	30ml

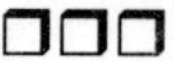

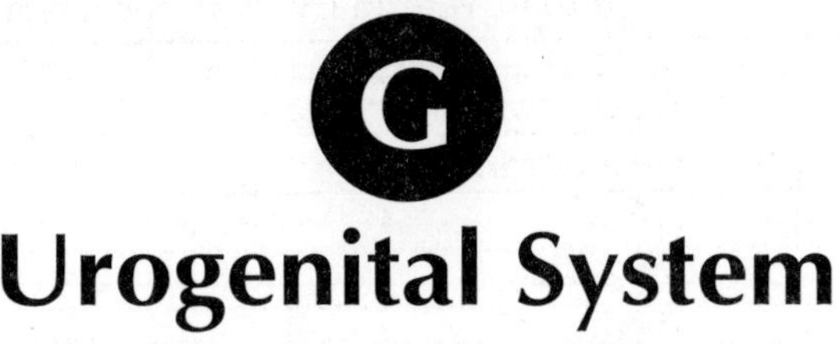

Urogenital System

Urinary and Reproductive Disease

Cryptorchidism: When one testicle is retained in abdomen or inguinal canal.

Glomerulonephritis: Leakage of protein in urine. It can be caused by cancer, heartworm, pyometra, rickettsial infections. It can result chronic kidney failure, hypoalbuminemia causigns ascites and peripheral edema.

Inguinal hernia: It is protrusion of abdominal contents through the inguinal canal.

Prostatitis: Inflammation of prostate due to infection, cysts, cancer and abcesses.

Pseudocyesis: It is false pregnancy. Signs include swelling of mammary glands, lactation, not eating and mothering small objects.

Umbical hernia: Failure of umblical ring of abdominal wall to close.

Urine incontinence: Leakage of urea due to incontinence of urethral sphincter and ectopic ureter.

Uroliths: These are common in dogs (stones in bladder)

Urinary System

Diuretics

Lasix Tab/ inj	**Hoechst**
Ind.	Decrease oedema and urinary flow
Comp	Frusemide 40mg tab, 10mg/ml inj
Adm.	Oral inj IM or IV
@	5mg/kg B.wt for both
Pres.	Tab 10, Inj 10ml

Ridema inj	**wockhardt**
Comp	Frusemide 50mg/ml
Adm.	IM IV
@	0.25-0.5ml/5kg B.wt
Pres.	10ml

Nephtone Cap	**Indian Herbs**
Comp	Herbal
Adm.	Oral
@	2 cap
Pres.	40

Esidrax Tab	**Novartis**
Comp	Hydrochlorthiazide 50mg
Adm.	Oral
@	1-2mg/kg B.wt
Pres.	10

Urolithiasis

Mandalamine Tab	**Generic**
Indi	urinary antiseptic
Comp	Methenamine mandelate
Adm.	Oral
@	1g Tab od
Pres.	1g Tab x20

Oricitral liq	**TTK**
Comp	Disodium hydrogen citrate
Adm.	Oral
@	1 Tab bid
Pres.	100

Bangshil Tab	**Alarsin**
Comp	Herbal
Adm.	1 Tab oral
@	1-3 tab od
Pres.	100

Genital System

Drugs acting on uterus

Picorex inj	**Pranav**
Indi	Antispasmic for uterus and urinary tract
Comp	Dicyclomine hydrochloride 10mg/ml

Adm.	IM
@	1ml
Pres.	10ml

Spas	**G Loucatos**
Indi	Antispasmic for uterus and urinary tract
Comp	Dicyclomine hydrochloride 10mg/ml
Adm.	IM
@	1ml
Pres.	10ml

Spasmovet	**Wockhardt**
Indi	Antispasmic for uterus and urinary tract
Comp	Dicyclomine hydrochloride 10mg/ml
Adm.	IM
@	1ml
Pres.	10ml

Jospas inj	**Animax Heathcare**
Indi	Antispasmic for uterus and urinary tract
Comp	Dicyclomine hydrochloride 10mg/ml
Adm.	IM
@	1ml
Pres.	10ml

Chorulon inj	**Intervet**
Comp	Chorionic gondao trophin (Leutinising hormone) 1500 IU per vial
Adm.	IM
@	100-500 units single dose
Pres.	1500 IU vial

Epidosin inj	**TTK**
Indi	Expulsion of foetus in dystocia
Comp	Valethamate bromide 10mg/ml
Adm.	IM
@	2.5-5ml
Pres.	5ml

Drugs acting on Ovary and Uterus

Fertomid Tab	**Cipla**
Indi	Induce ovulation
Comp	Clomiphene citrate 25mg and 50mg
Adm.	Oral
@	25mg Tab od x5 days
Pres.	10, 5

Folligon inj	**Intervet**
Indi	Induce oestrus
Comp	Serum Gonadotripin 1000 IU
Adm.	IM
@	400-1000 IU repeated twice weekly
Pres.	1000 IU vial

Myron Tab	**Alarsan**
Comp	Herbal
Adm.	Oral
@	2-3 Tab bid for 2-3 weeks
Pres.	100

Tropnovet inj	**Indian Immunology**
Indi	Induce oestrus
Comp	Pregnant mare serum gonadotropin (MSG) 1000 IU
Adm.	IM IV
@	400-700 IU
Pres.	1000 IU vial with 5ml diluent

Utertone liq	**Cattle Remedies**
Comp	Herbal
Adm.	Oral
@	10-25ml od x5 days
Pres.	225ml

Heat up cap	**Century**
Comp	Herbal
Adm.	Oral
@	2 cap od x3 days
Pres.	6

Sajani	**Sarabhai**
Comp	Herbal
Adm.	Oral
@	2 cap od x2 days
Pres.	6

Miscellaneous

Fortege	**Alarsin**
India	Male infertility
Adm.	Oral
@	2 tab bid
Pres.	100

Drugs acting on Uterus and Vagina

Terramycin liq	**Zydus**
Comp	Oxytetracyclin hydrochloride 50mg/ml
Adm.	IU
@	5ml x3 days
Pres.	60ml

Ultrox IU Insert	**Neospark**
Comp	Oxytetracyclnie hydrochloride 500mg
Adm.	IU
@	½ - 1 tab od x3
Pres.	4's

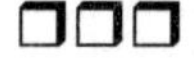

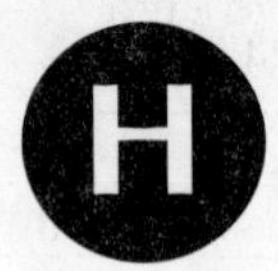

Musculo Skeletal System

Skeletal and Muscular Disorders

Back pain: Usually caused by in vertebral disk disease. It is caused by degeneration and protrusion of disk and compression of spinal cord. It usually occurs in cervical and thoracolumbar regions. Signs are back pain, hindlimb weakness and paralysis.

Hypertopic osteopathy: Bone disease secondary to disease in lungs. Signs are new bone formation on the outside of long bones.

Hypertropic osteodystrpy: It is a bone disease. Signs include swelling of metaphysis (part of bone adjacent to joint) pain, depression, loss of appetite and fever. Usually it is bilateral in limb bone.

Leg calve Perthes syndrome or Perthes disease: It is avascular necrosis of femoral head and characterised by deforming of head of femur and hip pain.

Masticatory muscle myositis: MMM is an inflammatory disease affecting the jaw muscles. Signs are swelling of jaw muscles and pain on opening the mouth. In chronic MMM there is atrophy of jaw muscles and scarring of masticatory muscles due to fibrosis and may result in inability to open the mouth.

Osteoarthritis: Known as degenerative arthiritis. It is characterised by progressive deterioration of articular cartilage in joints of limbs. There is pain and lameness.

Osteochondritis dissecans: Separation of immature articular cartilage from underlying bone. It is caused by osteochondrosis. Mostly seen in stifle, elbow, shoulder and hock.

Panosteitis: A disease of unknown cause that causes pain and a shifting leg lameness. It affect long bones of hind and forelimbs.

Spondylosis or Spondylosis deformans: It is growth of osteophytes on the ventral and lateral surfaces of vertebral bodies.

Steroidal Anti-inflammatory Drugs (SAID)

Betacortril Tab/inj	**Pfizer**
Comp	Betamethasone 0.5mg tab, 4mg/ml inj
Adm.	IM/IV inj Tab oral
@	Tab 25mcg/kg B.wt 40-80mcg/kg B.wt inj
Pres.	Tab 10 inj 2ml

Betnesol Tab/inj	**Glaxo**
Comp	Betamethasone 0.5mg tab, 4mg/ml inj
Adm.	IM/IV inj Tab oral
@	Tab 25mcg/kg B.wt 40-80mcg/kg B.wt inj
Pres.	Tab 10 inj 2ml

Betnesol oral drop	**Glaxo**
Comp	Betamethasone phosphate 0.5mg/ml
Adm.	Oral
@	25mcg/kg B.wt
Pres.	15ml

Brisone inj	**Brihans**
Comp	Dexamethasone sodium phosphate 4mg/ml
Adm.	IM, IV
@	0.5-2mg od
Pres.	2ml

Curadex inj	**Concept**
Comp	Dexamethasone sodium phosphate 4mg/ml
Adm.	IM, IV
@	0.5-2mg od
Pres.	2ml

Dexavet inj	**Wockhardt**
Comp	Dexamethasone sodium phosphate 4mg/ml
Adm.	IM, IV
@	0.5-2mg od
Pres.	2ml

Dexona inj	**Sarabhari**
Comp	Dexamethasone sodium phosphate 4mg/ml
Adm.	IM, IV
@	0.5-2mg od
Pres.	2ml

Rancortin inj	**Ranbaxy**
Comp	Dexamethasone sodium phosphate 4mg/ml
Adm.	IM, IV
@	0.5-2mg od
Pres.	2ml

Vector inj	Alembic
Comp	Dexamethasone sodium phosphate 4mg/ml
Adm.	IM, IV
@	0.5-2mg od
Pres.	2ml

Ketocart inj	Intas
Comp	Dexamethasone sodium phosphate 4mg/ml
Adm.	IM, IV
@	0.5-2mg od
Pres.	2ml

Dexona Tab/ oral Drop	Cadila Heathcare
Comp	Dexamethasone 0.5mg tab, 0.5mg/ml drop
Adm.	Oral
@	0.25-0.5mg od
Pres.	Tab 10 drops 10ml

Deltacortril Tab	Pfizer
Comp	Prednisolons 5mg, 10mg
Adm.	Oral
@	0.5-2.5mg od
Pres.	10's

Prednisolone inj	Intervet / Wockhardt
Comp	Prednisolone 10mg/ml
Adm.	IM
@	1-3ml od
Pres.	10ml

Vetalog inj	Sarabhai
Comp	Triamcinolone 10mg/ml
Adm.	IM
@	6-8mg od
Pres.	6mg/ml- 5ml vial, 10mg/ml-1ml vial

B V Log Inj	Venky
Comp	Triamcinolone 10mg/ml
Adm.	IM
@	6-8mg od
Pres.	5ml

Hostacartin H Inj.	Hoechst
Comp	Prednisolone 10mg/ml
Adm.	IM
@	1-3ml od
Pres.	10ml

B.V.cort	Venky
Comp	Prednisolone 10mg/ml
Adm.	IM
@	1-3ml od
Pres.	10ml

Non Steroidal Anti-inflammation Drugs (NSAID)

Novalgin inj	Novartis
Comp	0.5g/ml Analgin
Adm.	IM/ IV
@	1-3ml
Pres.	30ml

Vetalgin inj	Intervet
Comp	0.5g/ml Analgin
Adm.	IM/ IV
@	1-3ml
Pres.	30ml

Inflagin inj	Neospark
Comp	0.5g/ml Analgin
Adm.	IM/ IV
@	1-3ml
Pres.	30ml

Banpin inj	Barihans
Comp	0.5g/ml Analgin
Adm.	IM/ IV
@	1-3ml
Pres.	30ml

Algesin inj	**Alembic**
Comp	Phenylbutazine Sodium 250mg/ml
Adm.	IV
@	2-20mg/kg B.wt Max 800mg
Pres.	3ml

Paracetol inj	**Cadila Heathcare**
Comp	Paracetamol 150mg/ml
Adm.	IM
@	20mg/kg B.wt
Pres.	10ml

Melonex inj	**Intas**
Comp	Meloxicam 5mg/ml
Adm.	IM
@	0.3mg/kg B.wt
Pres.	15ml

A3 Vet inj	**Brihans**
Comp	Meloxicam 5mg/ml
Adm.	IM
@	0.3mg/kg B.wt
Pres.	30ml

Melaxone inj	**Venky**
Comp	Meloxicam 5mg/ml
Adm.	IM
@	0.3mg/kg B.wt
Pres.	30ml

Painkind inj	**Vetkind**
Comp	Meloxicam 5mg/ml
Adm.	IM
@	0.3mg/kg B.wt
Pres.	30ml

Diclovet inj	**Alembic**
Comp	Meloxicam 5mg/ml
Adm.	IM
@	0.3mg/kg B.wt
Pres.	30ml

A3 Vet Plus inj	**Brihans**
Comp	Each ml contains Meloxicam 5mg, Paracetamol 150mg Lignocain1%
Adm.	IM
@	2-3ml od
Pres.	30ml

Melonex Plus inj	**Intas**
Comp	Meloxicam 5mg/ml + Paracetamol 150mg.
Adm.	IM
@	0.3mg/kg B.wt
Pres.	30ml

Pyrecalm inj	**Carevet Pharma**
Comp	Piroxicam 20mg/ml
Adm.	IM
@	1mg/kg B.wt or 1ml
Pres.	30ml

ROC Plus inj	**Macwell**
Comp	Piroxicam 20mg, Paracetamol 75mg
Adm.	IM
@	1ml
Pres.	30ml

Nimpyrin inj	**Carevet Pharma**
Comp	Nimuslide 200mg/ml
Adm.	IM
@	1ml
Pres.	15ml

ROC-NP Plus inj	**Macwell**
Comp	Each ml contains Nimuslide 100mg Paracetamol 150mg
Adm.	IM
@	1ml
Pres.	20ml

Portrio inj	**Wellcon**	
Comp	Each ml contains	
	Nimuslide 100mg	Paracetamol 150mg
Adm.	IM	
@	1ml	
Pres.	10ml	

Rest inj	**Pail**	
Comp	Each ml contains	
	Nimuslide 100mg	Paracetamol 150mg
Adm.	IM	
@	1ml	
Pres.	10ml	

Anip C inj	**Animax Healthcare**	
Comp	Each ml contains	
	Nimuslide 100mg	Paracetamol 150mg
Adm.	IM	
@	1ml	
Pres.	10ml	

Ketop inj	**Alembic**
Comp	Ketoprofen 100mg/ml
Adm.	IM/ IV
@	2-4mg/kg B.wt
Pres.	15ml

Vetoprofen	**Merial**
Comp	Ketoprofen 100mg/ml
Adm.	IM/ IV
@	2-4mg/kg B.wt
Pres.	15ml

Topically used Products

Arjet spray	**Cadila**	
Comp	50ml contains	
	Methyl salicylate	875mg
	Menthol	1600mg

	Camphor	1500mg
	Benzyl nicotinate	20mg
	Squalane	250mg
	Glycol salicylate	875mg
Adm.	Spray on affected area	
@	As per need	
Pres.	50ml	

Iodex oint	**SKF**
Comp	Iodine 4% Methyl Salicylate 5%
Adm.	Local
@	As per need
Pres.	25g

Pirox Gel	**Cipla**
Comp	Piroxicam 0.5%
Adm.	Local
@	As per need
Pres.	30g

Rumalya Vet	**Himalya**
Comp	Herbal
Adm.	Local
@	As per need
Pres.	50g

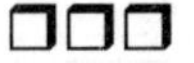

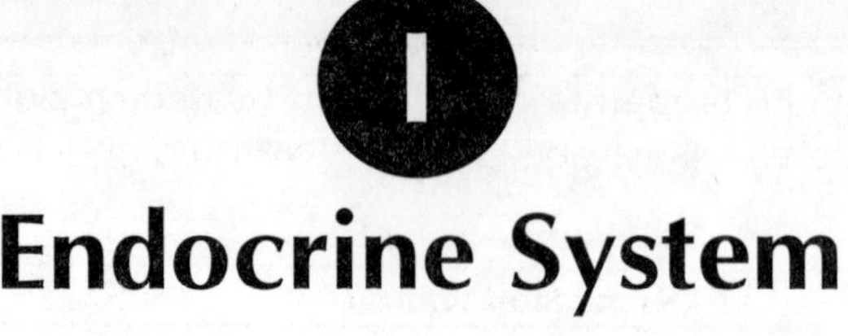

Endocrine System

Disease related to Endocrine System

Acromegaly: Hormonal condition resulting from over secretion growth hormone somatotropin from pituitary gland. Symptoms include overgrowth or enlargement of gums with wide spaces between teeth, increased drinking, urination, thickening of skin and skin fold, enlargement of tongue and excessive panting.

Addison's disease or Hypoadrenocorticism: Reduction on the production of glucocorticoids and mineral corticoids by adrenal glands. Signs include increased drinking and urination, vomiting, diarrhea, Collapse, shivering and weight loss.

Cushing syndrome: Or Hyperadrenocorticism is characterised by increase in glucocorticids secreted by adrenal glands. Signs include increased appetite, increased drinking and urination, pot bellied appearance, muscle weakness and lethargy. It is caused by overuse of steroid.

Diabetes insipidus: It is caused by lack of antidiuretic hormones. Signs are inability to concentrate urine, increased drinking and urinating

Diabetes mellitus: Also known as Type 1 or insulin dependent diabetes. There is lack of insulin production due to destruction of pancreatic beta cells.

Hypothyroidism: Reduced thyroid or atrophy of thyroid gland. Signs include decreased appetite, weight gain, hair loss dry skin or coat, skin cold to touch, recurring skin infections and lethargy.

Antidiabetic

Chlorpropamide

It is sulphonlurea acting primarily by stimulating the release of insulin and inhibit the release of glucose by liver and increase sensitivity of peripheral tissue. It is indicated in the treatment of insulin. It can cause GI upset, rashes, skin eruptions and anemia.

Copamide Sol.	**Dey's**
Comp	Chlorpropamide 250mg
Adm.	Oral
@	5-10mg per day
Pres.	10

Glibenclamide

It provokes a brisk release of insulin from pancreas. It acts on Beta cell membrane leading to enhanced calcium flux across it, hence degranulation. Then improvement in glucose intolerance is maintained. It is indicated in noninsulin dependent Diabetes dogs. Side effects can be nausea, vomiting, anorexia, urticaria pruritis and leucopenia.

Euglucon Tab	**Nicholas Piramal**
Comp	Glibenclamide 5mg
Adm.	Oral
@	0.5mg od
Pres.	5mg tab x10

Betanase Tab	**Cadila Healthcare**
Comp	Glibenclamide 5mg
Adm.	Oral
@	0.5mg od
Pres.	5mg tab x10

Glinil Tab	**Cipla**
Comp	Glibenclamide 5mg
Adm.	Oral
@	0.5mg od
Pres.	5mg tab x10

Glipizide

It is one of the second generation Sulfonylurea having similar pharmacological profile as that of Glibenclamide

Glipy 5 Tab	**Alembic**
Comp	Glipizide 5mg
Adm.	Oral
@	0.5mg od
Pres.	5mg tab x10

Glucolip Tab	**Wallace**
Comp	Glipizide 5mg
Adm.	Oral
@	0.5mg od
Pres.	5mg tab x10

Glynase Tab	USV
Comp	Glipizide 5mg
Adm.	Oral
@	0.5mg od
Pres.	5mg tab x10

Insulin

Secretion of Insulin from B cells of pancreas which has an overall effects to favour storage of fuel. Insulin also facilitates glucose transport across cell membrane and glycogen synthesis from glucose in liver, muscle and fat by stimulating the enzyme glycogen synthetase. It inhibits glyconeogenesis in liver and lipolysis in adipose tissue and favours triglyceride synthesis.

Insulatard Inj.	Abbot
Comp	Isophane insulin (NPA) procine 40 IU/ml
Adm.	IV
@	50mg
Pres.	10ml vial

Lentisulin HPI Inj	Cadila
Comp	Isophane insulin (NPA) proine 40 IU/ml
Adm.	IV
@	50mg
Pres.	10ml vial

Mixtard Inj	Abbot
Comp	Biphasic insulin porcrine containing a mixture of 30%
	Nordisulin 70% Insulatard 40 IU/ml
Adm.	IV
@	50mg
Pres.	10ml vial

Rapisulin Inj	Cipla
Comp	Biphasic insulin porcrine containing a mixture of 30%
	Nordisulin 70% Insulatard 40 IU/ml
Adm.	IV
@	50mg
Pres.	10ml vial

Antithyroid

Carbimazole

It acts in 3 steps in the synthesis of thyroid hormone inhibits oxidation of iodide, iodination of thyrosin residues coupling of iodotyrosine residue to form T3 and T4. It does not interfere with trapping iodide and do not modify the action of T3 and T4. TSH release are consequence of reduction in feed back inhibition. Side effects can be bone marrow depression, mouth ulcers, rashes, nausea, loss of hair and fever.

Neomercazole Tab	**Cipla**
Comp	Carbimaxole Tab 5mg, 10, 20mg
Adm.	Oral
@	5mg od
Pres.	100

Thyrozole Tab	**Cadila**
Comp	Carbimazole tab 5mg
Adm.	Oral
@	5mg od
Pres.	100

Methimazole

It is anththyroid drug which inhibits the enzyme thyroperoxidase, a necessary step in synthesis of triiodothyronine T3 and thyroxine T4. It is indicated in hyperthyroidism or toxic goiter. Stomach upset, nausea, vomiting, rashes can be side effects.

Methimazole Tab	**Sun Pharma**
Comp	Methinmazole 5mg, 10mg
Adm.	Oral
@	5-8mg and daily
Pres.	5mg 10, 10mg 10

Growth Hormone Elevator

Clonidine

It acts on the pituitary to stimulate growth hormone production. It may be used to assess the ability of pituitary to produce growth hormone. It is also used to treat high blood pressure. Side effects are dry mouth, nausea, fatigue and constipation.

Catapres Tab	German Remedies
Comp	Clonidine hydrochloride
Adm.	Oral
@	0.05mg tds
Pres.	150mcg tab x10

Xylazine

Though it is a potent sedative but it also stimulates growth hormone production and used to assess growth deficiency.

Xylazine inj	Indian Immunology
Comp	Xylazine hydrochloride 20mg/ml
Adm.	IM
@	1-3mg/kg B.wt
Pres.	2ml, 10ml

Bomazine Inj	Sarabhai
Comp	Xylazine hydrochloride 20mg/ml
Adm.	IM
@	1-3mg/kg B.wt
Pres.	10ml

Hypothalamic/ Pituitary

Buserlin

It is a synthetic releasing hormone analogue for lutenising hormone and follicle stimulating hormone. It is indicated in ovulation failure or induce lactation in post partum. In males it may stimulate the secretion of testosterone to reduce libido.

Receptal	Intervet
Comp	Buserelin acetate .0042mg/ml
Adm.	IM
@	4µg repeat after 24hrs, 48hrs
Pres.	10ml vial

Desmopressin

It is analogue of vasopressin an antidiuretic hormone. It is used to treat hyperactive excitable young dogs.

D Void	Sun
Comp	Desmopressin 0.1mg/ml
Adm.	Intra nasal
@	20mcg
Pres.	5ml

Oxytocin

It is a synthetic oxytocin. It stimulates smooth muscle contraction in uterus and is used to induce parturition when uterine inertia is there. It is used to evacuate uterine contents following parturition.

Oxytocin inj	Generic
Comp	Oxytocin 10 IU/ml
Adm.	IM/ Sc
@	5-20 IU
Pres.	1ml, 10ml

Syntocinon Inj	Novartis
Comp	Oxytocin 5 IU/ml
Adm.	IM
@	5-25 IU
Pres.	1ml

PMSG

It is derived from serum of pregnant mares. Its action is similar to follicle stimulating hormone (FSH). It is indicated for the indication of oestrus and to increase spermatogenesis.

Folligon Inj	Intervet
Comp	1000 IU of PMSG/ml
Adm.	IM/ SC
@	50-200 IU
Pres.	1000 IU vial with solvent

Trophovet Inj	Indian Imunology
Comp	1000 IU of PMSG/ml
Adm.	IM/ SC
@	50-200 IU
Pres.	1000 IU vial with solvent

Sex Hormones

Oestrogens

It is indicated in the treatment of hormonal urinary incontinence in bitches, adenomata, excess libido and prostatic hyperplasia in males. Side effects are G.I. upsets and polyuria.

Trophovet Inj	**Indian Imunology**
Comp	Ethynyl estradiol 0.02mg
Adm.	Oral
@	1-3mg daily orally
Pres.	30

Progynon Depot	**German Remedies**
Comp	Oestradiol Valerate 10mg/ml
Adm.	IM
@	0.5-1mg
Pres.	1ml amp

Progestogens

Progesterone

It is indicated for the treatment of threatened or habitual abortion, induction of parturition and control of oestrous Hydroxy Progestron, and Medroxy Progesterone are used.

Curaprogen inj	**Carvet Pharma**
Comp	Hydroxyl Progesteron 250mg/ml
Adm.	IM
@	1-3mg/kg B.wt
Pres.	3ml

Duraprogen inj	**Unichem**
Comp	Hydroxyl Progesteron 250mg/ml
Adm.	IM
@	1-3mg/kg B.wt
Pres.	3ml

Hyprogen inj	Unichem
Comp	Hydroxyl Progesteron 250mg/ml
Adm.	IM
@	1-3mg/kg B.wt
Pres.	2ml

Polluton Depot	German Remedies
Comp	Hydroxyl Progesteron 250mg/ml
Adm.	IM
@	1-3mg/kg B.wt
Pres.	1ml

Provera Tab	Max
Comp	Medroxy progesterone acetate 10mg
Adm.	Oral
@	5mg daily upto 25kg and 10mg od above 25kg B.wt
Pres.	10

Testosterone

It is the main male androgenic steroid. It has prolonged action than hormone itself. It may increase libido and effects increased spermatogenesis. It has anabolic action of effecting erythropoesis.

Testoviron Depot inj	German Remedies
Comp	Testosterone 25mg Testosterone inanthate 110mg
	Total testosterone 110mg/ml
Adm.	IM/ SC
@	5-20mg
Pres.	1ml

Aquaviron	Nicholas
Comp	Testosterone 25mg/ml
Adm.	IM/SC
@	5-25mg
Pres.	1ml

Uterine Stimulant

Vetrabutine

It is uterine relaxant and musculo tropic stimulant. It is indicated in bitches to dilate the cervix and coordinate uterine contractions to ease and shorten parturition.

Vetrabutine inj	**Generic**
Comp	Vetrabutine clorhydrate 100mg
Adm.	IM
@	2mg/kg B.wt repeat after 30-60 minutes upto 3 times
Pres.	1ml

Thyroid Drugs

Levothyroxine

It is used to treat hypothyroidism. Side effects are osteoporosis, tremors, loss of weight and restlessness.

Lethyrox Tab	**Intas**
Comp	Levothyroxine sodium
Adm.	Oral
@	0.02-0.04mg/kg od
Pres.	Tab 25mcg, 50mcg, 100mg x30

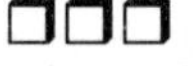

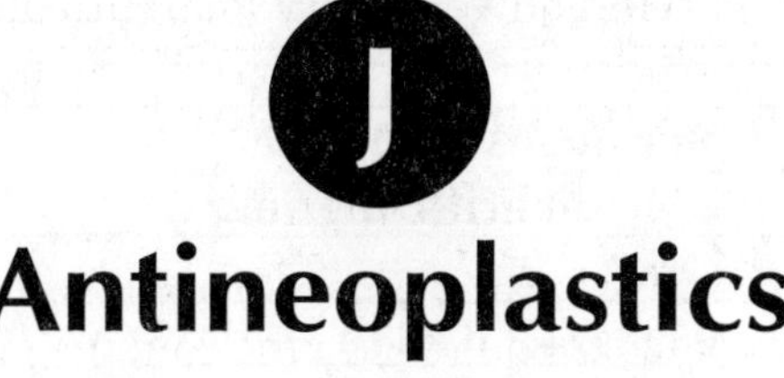

Antineoplastics

These are toxic and have narrow therapeutic indices. So the dosage rates are usually calculated based on body surface area for higher physiological accuracy. Clinical response to chemotherapy include palliation, partial or complete regression of neoplastic tissues and complete cellular cure. Cancer care is associated with clinical management of dose limiting toxicity along with control of nutritional support as well as comfort.

Fluorouracil

It interferes with DNA synthesis by blocking the methylation of mammary glands, GI tract, liver and lungs. Side effects of Neurotoxicity are seizures.

Fivoflo Inj	**Dabur**
Comp	5 fluorouracil 250mg, 500mg
Adm.	IV
@	150-200mg weekly or 5-10mg/kg B.wt weekly
Pres.	5ml, 10ml

Fluracil Inj	**Biochem**
Comp	5 fluorouracil 250mg, 500mg
Adm.	IV
@	150-200mg weekly or 5-10mg/kg B.wt weekly
Pres.	5ml, 10ml

Busulphan

It is alkylating antineoplastic drug. It arrests G2 premiotic stage of cell divisions breaking down DNA leading to their death. It can cause irreversible bone marrow depression. There can be diarrhea, hyper pigmentation.

Myleran Tab	**Burroughs Wellcome**
Comp	Busulphan
Adm.	Oral
@	3-4mg od or 0.1mg/kg B.wt
Pres.	100

Chlorambucil

Action is same as Busulphan. It is indicated in Lymphoreticular neoplasia. It may cause immunosuppression.

Leukeran Tab	**Burroughs Wellcome**
Comp	Chloramucil 25mg 5mg
Adm.	Oral
@	0.2mg/kg B.wt in 2-4 days/ weeks
Pres.	10's

Cyclophosphamide

As Busulphan. It is also indicated in Lymphorecticular neoplasia, mammary and pulmonary carcinoma. It is cytotoxic and may cause sterile necrotizing haemorrhagic cystitis. It is an immuno suppressant.

Cycloxan Tab/inj	**Biochem**
Comp	Tab 50mg, 100mg, Inj 200mg, 500mg, 1g of cyclophosphamine
Adm.	Tab oral, IM IV
@	2.2mg/kg B.wt in days/week orally
Pres.	Tab 10, inj 200mg, 500mg, 1g vial

Endoxan Asta Tab/Inj.	**German Remedies**
Comp	Tab 50mg Inj 200mg, 500mg 1g of cyclophosphamine
Adm.	Tab oral, IM IV
@	2.2mg/kg B.wt in days/week orally
Pres.	Tab 10, inj 200mg, 500mg, 1g vial

Ledoxan Tab/Inj	**Dabur**
Comp	Tab 50mg Inj 200mg, 500mg 1g of cyclophosphamine
Adm.	Tab oral, IM IV
@	2.2mg/kg B.wt in days/week orally
Pres.	Tab 10, inj 200mg, 500mg, 1g vial

Doxorubicin

It is a cytotoxic anthracyclin antineoplastic. It acts by binding to DNA and by inhibition of nucleic acid synthesis. It is indicated in nonfunctional thyroid carcinoma and lymphosarcoma. It may cause severe bone marrow suppression.

Adrim inj.	**Dabur**
Comp	2mg/ml of Doxorubicin
Adm.	IV
@	30mg in 150ml 5%. Dextrose or Normal saline solution
Pres.	2ml

Cardia inj	Zydus
Comp	2mg/ml of doxorubicin
Adm.	IV
@	30mg in 150ml 55 Dextrose or Normal saline sol
Pres.	10mg or 5ml

Doxorubicin inj	Biochem
Comp	2mg/ml of doxorubicin
Adm.	IV
@	30mg in 150ml 55 Dextrose or Normal saline sol
Pres.	10mg or 5ml

Melphalan

It is as Busulphan. It is indicated in multiple myeloma, lymphoreticular neoplasia.

Alkeran Tab	Burrogh's Wellcome
Comp	Melphalan 2mg, 5mg
Adm.	Oral
@	0.1mg/kg B.wt for 10 days followed by 0.05-0.1mg/kg B.wt daily
Pres.	25

Metacaptopurine

It is antineoplastic called Purine antineoplastic. It inhibits acid biosynthesis and interferes with several metabolic steps related to DNA and RNA functions of cell. It is indicated in the lympho sarcoma, acute lymphocytic leukemia, granulocytic leukemia. Its major toxic effect is bone marrow depression. It effects liver causing cholestatic Jaundice, vomiting and diarrhea.

Empurine Tab	Dabur
Comp	50mg tablet of Metacaptopurine
Adm.	Oral
@	2mg/kg B.wt od
Pres.	10

Purinethol Tab	Burrough's Wellcome
Comp	50mg tablet of Metacaptopurine
Adm.	Oral
@	2mg/kg B.wt od
Pres.	25

Methotrexate

It is a folic acid antagonist and inhibits enzyme dihydrofoliate reductase and interfers with DNA synthesis and cell replication and ultimately causing death. It is indicated in Lymphoreticular neoplasia, myeoproliferative disorder, transmissible veneral tumor, sertol cell tumor, osteosarcoma. Its side effects are myelo suppression, nausea, vomiting, diarrhea, alopecia, pyrexia, liver and Kidney damage.

Biotrexate Tab/inj	**Biochem**
Comp	Methotrexate 2.5mg, Tab. inj 5mg, 50mg/ml
Adm.	Oral, IV
@	0.3-0.8mg/kg B.wt IV and 2.5mg oral od
Pres.	10 inj 2ml in both

Methotrexate inj	**Ledrle**
Comp	5mg/ml methotrexate
Adm.	IV
@	0.3-0.8mg/kg B.wt
Pres.	1ml vial

Zexate Inj/Tab	**Dabur**
Comp	Methotrexate 2.5mg Tab Inj 5mg, 25mg/ml
Adm.	IV
@	0.3-0.8mg/kg B.wt
Pres.	Tab 10 Inj 25mg-2ml 5mg-3ml

Vincristine

It is a Vinca alkaloid and antineoplastic. It arrests the cell division at metaphase stage by inhibiting microtubule formation in the mitotic spindle. It also inhibit nucleic acid and protein synthesis in cells. It is indicated in Lymphosarcoma, immune thrombocytopenia. It is local irritant. Side effects are peripheral neuropathy, paresthesia, muscle weakness, constipation and alopecia.

Cytocristin inj	**Cipla**
Comp	Vincristine 1mg/ml
Adm.	IV
@	0.025mg/kg B.wt once weekly
Pres.	1ml

Vincristine inj or VCR inj	**Biochem**
Comp	Vincristine 1mg/ml
Adm.	IV
@	0.025mg/kg B.wt once weekly
Pres.	1ml

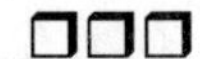

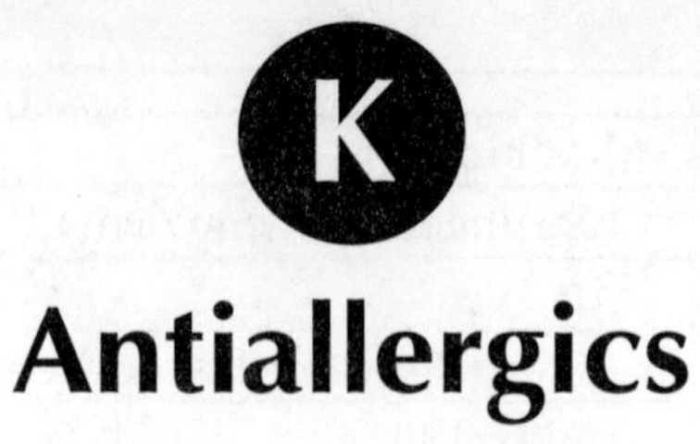

Antiallergics

Antihistamins

Anistamin	Intas
Comp	Chlorpheniramine maleate 10mg/ml
Adm.	IM
@	0.4-2mg/kg B.wt bid
Pres.	10ml

Cadistin inj	Sarabhai
Comp	Chlorpheniramine maleate 10mg/ml
Adm.	IM
@	0.4-2mg/kg B.wt bid
Pres.	10ml

Catalan inj	Cattle Remedies
Comp	Chlorpheniramine maleate 10mg/ml
Adm.	IM
@	0.4-2mg/kg B.wt bid
Pres.	30ml

Chlorazin inj	Ranbaxy
Comp	Chlorpheniramine maleate 10mg/ml
Adm.	IM
@	0.4-2mg/kg B.wt bid
Pres.	10ml

Chloril inj	TTK
Comp	Chlorpheniramine maleate 10mg/ml
Adm.	IM
@	0.4-2mg/kg B.wt bid
Pres.	10ml

Zeet inj	Alembic
Comp	Chlorpheniramine maleate 10mg/ml
Adm.	IM
@	0.4-2mg/kg B.wt bid
Pres.	10ml

Avil inj	Intervet
Comp	Pheniramine maleate 22.75mg/ml
Adm.	IM
@	0.5-1ml
Pres.	10ml

Hisloc inj	Cadila Pharma
Comp	Pheniramine maleate 22.75mg/ml
Adm.	IM
@	0.5-1ml
Pres.	10ml

Pheneramine maleate inj	Prima Vetcare
Comp	Pheniramine maleate 22.75mg/ml
Adm.	IM
@	0.5-1ml
Pres.	10ml

Phenrgan inj/ Tab/Syp	Rhone Poulnec
Comp	Promethazine Inj- 25mg/ml, Tab- 10mg,25mg, Syp- 5mg/ML
Adm.	Tab and Syp oral, inj IM IV
@	1.5mg-2.5mg/kg B.wt oral IM, IV
Pres.	Tab 10, inj 2ml, Syp 60ml

Cural inj	Wockhardt
Comp	Chlorpheniramine maleate 10mg/ml
Adm.	IM
@	0.4-2mg/kg B.wt bid
Pres.	10ml

Histal Inj	**Vetcare**
Comp	Chlorpheniramine maleate 10mg/ml
Adm.	IM
@	0.4-2mg/kg B.wt bid
Pres.	10ml

Synistamine Inj	**Sarabhai**
Comp	Halopyramine hydrochloride 10mg/ml
Adm.	IM, IV
@	0.5-1ml
Pres.	2ml

Larfen Inj	**Vets Farma**
Comp	Chlorpheniramine maleate 10mg/ml
Adm.	IM
@	0.4-2mg/kg B.wt bid
Pres.	30ml

Vetistin D S Inj	**Carevet Pharma**
Comp	Chlorpheniramine maleate 20mg/ml
Adm.	IM
@	0.4-2mg/kg B.wt bid
Pres.	30ml

Cistamin Inj	**Century**
Comp	Pheniramine maleate 22.75mg/ml
Adm.	IM
@	0.5-1ml
Pres.	10ml

Glucocorticoids

Brisone inj	**Brihans**
Comp	Dexamethasone Sodium phosphate 4mg/ml
Adm.	IM, IV
@	0.25-0.5ml
Pres.	2ml

Cadex inj	Cattle Remedies
Comp	Dexamethasone Sodium phosphate 4mg/ml
Adm.	IM, IV
@	0.25-0.5ml
Pres.	5ml

Curadex inj	Concept
Comp	Dexamethasone Sodium phosphate 4mg/ml
Adm.	IM, IV
@	0.25-0.5ml
Pres.	2ml

Dexavet Inj	Wockhardt
Comp	Dexamethasone Sodium phosphate 4mg/ml
Adm.	IM, IV
@	0.25-0.5ml
Pres.	5ml

Dexona Inj	Sarabhai
Comp	Dexamethasone Sodium phosphate 4mg/ml
Adm.	IM, IV
@	0.25-0.5ml
Pres.	5ml

Ketocart Inj	Intas
Comp	Dexamethasone Sodium phosphate 4mg/ml
Adm.	IM, IV
@	0.25-0.5ml
Pres.	2ml

Vector Inj	Alembic
Comp	Dexamethasone Sodium phosphate 4mg/ml
Adm.	IM, IV
@	0.25-0.5ml
Pres.	5ml

Vetalog Inj	Sarabhai
Comp	Triamcinolone acetomide 6mg/ml
Adm.	IM or SC
@	0.2mg/kg B.wt
Pres.	1ml, 5ml

Prednisolone inj	**Wockhardt / Intervet**
Comp	Prednisolone 10mg/ml
Adm.	IM
@	1-3ml
Pres.	10ml

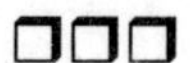

L

Antidotes

Toxicity of Chemicals

Toxic	Source	Treatment
Acids	Direct drinking	Orally 2% Sodium bicarbonate
Alkalies	Direct drinking	Orally 5% Acetic acid (vinegar)
Arsenic	Insecticide	B.A.L inj 4.-5mg/kg IM
Carbamates	Pesticide	Atropine sulphate 0.2-2mg/kg B.wt IM
Atropine	Plant	Gastric lavage with Potassium Permanganate Saline purgative
Chlorinate hydrocarbons	Pesticide	Saline purgative Activated charcoal
Cyanide	Fertilizers, Rodenticide	IV slow inj of Sodium thiosulphate 20% sol
Formaline	Fumigant/ Disinfectant	Oxygen therapy, wash eyes orally sodium bicarbonate
Fluoride	Insecticide Ectoparasiticides	Gastric lavage Fluid therapy with Normal saline Aluminium sulphate 3g orally
Iron	Ingestion of Iron salt	Adrenaline and antihistamin orally milk of Magnesia
Lead	Paint	B.A.L inj 2mg/kg B.wt IM Thiamine 2mg/kg B.wt S/C
Mercury	Organo mercurial, industrial	Milk or raw eggs Dimercaprol 3mg/ kg B.wt
Ntrates or Nitrites	Pasture feed and water of fertilizer residue	Methylene blue 1% IV
Organo-phosphorous Compound	Insecticide/ Pesticide	Atropine sulphate 0.2-2mg/kg B.wt IM
Phosphorous	Rodenticide	Gastric lavage with 0.01% Potassium permanganate
Selenium	Insecticides	Saline purgatives
Urea	Urea treated feed or fertilizer	2% Acetic acid or Vinegar orally
Warfarin	Rodenticide	Oxygen therapy, Tranquilizer clotting factor & Vit K 0.5-1mg/kg B.Wt

Zinc phosphide	Rodenticide	Gastric lavage with 5% sodium bicarbonate

Toxicity of Plants

Green algae	With food or state food	Treatment
Onion	From food	Symptomatically, Liver stimulant
Poppy	Medicine or drug	Narcotic antagonist Naloxone 0.04mg/kg B.wt IV/IM
Potato	Food	Gastric lavage demuscents
Sweet pea	Vegetable	Symptomatic and calcium supplement
Tobacoo	Nicotine	Caffeine and oxygen therapy

Toxicity of Animal origin

Bee	Biting	Apply bicarbonate solution Locally and antihistamines
Centipede	Cyanogenic factors	Antihistamines, Analgesic
Scorpion	Neurotoxins	Pressure bandage, antitoxin, Symptomatic
Snake	Neurotoxins	Antivenom (Polyvalent) anti inflammatory, antitetanus, analgesic, Fluid therapy
Spider	Neurotoxins	Antivenin, calcium gluconate IV
Ticks	Neurotoxins	Ectoparasiticides, Anti-histamine, Supportive therapy
Wasp	Histamine	Apply vinegar locally

Toxicity of Moult Origin

Aflatoxin	Food	Aciviated charcoal orally Stanozolol 2mg/kg B.wt IM
Ergot alkaloid	Food contaminated with fungi	Antibiotic, antiseptic Purgative
Mouldy toxins	Corns	Treat symptomatically for GI disorder

❑❑❑

Eyes and Ear Leprations

Eye & Ear Disease

Asteroid hyalosis: Degenerative condition of eye involving small white opacities in vitreous humor.

Canine glaucoma: Increase of pressure within eye caused by abnormal development of drainage angle of eye.

Cataract: Opacity of the lens

Chalazion: Granuloma that forms in the eyelid due to blocked secretions from meibomian gland. It may result inflammation of eyelid

Cherry eye: The gland of third eyelid prolapses and becomes visible

Chronic superficial Keratitis: Inflammation of cornea

Conjunctivitis: Inflammation of conjunctiva caused by mechanical irritation, allergies or bacterial infection.

Corneal dystrophy: A condition characterised by bilateral non-inflammatory opacity of cornea. It appears as grayish white lines, circles or clouding of cornea.

Corneal ulcer or Ulcerative Keratitis: It is an inflammatory condition of cornea involving loss of its outer layer. It is caused by trauma, detergent, burns and infection

Distichia: An eyelash that arises from an abnormal spot on eyelash. These can irritate the eye causing tearing, squinting and inflammation and corneal ulcers.

Ear otitis media: Inflammation of middle ear canal

Ectropion: Eyelid folding outwards

Entropion: Eyelid folding inward

Eye proptosis: A condition resulting in forward displacement and entrapment of eye from behind by the eyelids.

Florida Keratopathy: Presence of multiple spots within both corneas

Fly strike dermatitis: Caused by bites of stable fly. It occurs at the tip and folds of ear

Horner's Syndrome: It results from damage to sympathetic innervation of the eye. Signs include sunken eye, small pupil elevated third eyelid and dropping of upper eyelid.

Iris cysts: Small hollow structures attached to the iris of eye or flouting free in anterior chamber

Kerato conjunctivitis sicca: There is eye redness, a yellow or greenish discharge, ulceration of cornea, pigmented cornea

Lens luxation: Displacement of lens from its normal position

Nuclear sclerosis: It appears as a bilateral bluish grey haziness at the centre of lens

Optic neuritis: Inflammation of optic nerve caused by granulomatous meningoencephelitis or infection.

Otitis media: Inflammation of middle ear canal

Retinal dysplasia: It is caused by viral infection, drugs or vitamin A deficiency. It is characterised by folds or rosettes (round clumps) of retinal tissue

SARD: Sudden acquired Retinal degeneration: It is caused by toxin, or cushing's disease or unknown reason. Symptoms include permanent blindness, dilated pupils and loss of pupillary light reflex

Trichiasis: It is in from the eyelid growing in wrong direction and rubbing on eye, causing irritation. Usually occurs at lateral upper eyelid

Uveitis: Inflammation within eye caused by trauma, cataract, infectious hepatitis, leptospirosis or fungal infections

Betnesol N Eye/Ear oint	**Intas**
Comp	Betamethasone sod Phos 0.1%
	Neomycin sulphate 0.5%
Adm.	Ear drop, Eye drop locally
@	1-2 drops in each eye/ ear
Pres.	5ml

Betnesol N Eye/Ear drops	**Glaxo**
Comp	Betamethasone sod Phos 0.1%
	Neomycin sulphate 0.5%
Adm.	Ear drop, Eye drop locally
@	1-2 drops in each eye/ ear
Pres.	5ml

Ciplox Eye Drop	**Cipla**
Comp	Ciprofloxacin hydrochloride 0.3%
	Benzalkonium chloride 0.0225%
Adm.	Eyes locally
@	1-2 drops in each eye qid
Pres.	5ml

Dexona Eye/Ear Sol	**Cadila Healthcare**
Comp	Dexamettsone sodium phosphate 0.1% Neomycin sulphate 0.5% Benzal- korium chloride 0.02%
Adm.	Eye – Ears locally
@	1-2 drops qid
Pres.	3ml

Neosporin H Ear drop	**Glaxo**
Comp	Polymyxin B sulph 10000 IU Neomycin sulphate 3400 IU Hydrocortisone 10mg per ml
Adm.	Ear locally
@	1-3 drops tid
Pres.	5ml

Otirel Ear drop	**Ranbaxy**
Comp	Gentamycin sulphate 0.3% Clotrimazole 1% Betamethasone dipropionate 0.025% Lignocain hydrochloride 2%
Adm.	Ear locally
@	1-3 drops tid
Pres.	15ml

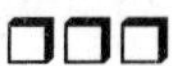

Nutrition and Metabolism

Nutrients

Vitamins

Biotin: Biotin deficiency in canine is very rare. But in cases of inappetence, weightloss, dermatitis and alopecia Biotin helps.

Choline: Indicated in weight gain, growth and hepatic lipidosis.

Folic acid: Indicated in decreased antibody resistance to infections Canine hepatitis virus and Canine distemper. Helpful in weight gain, as supportive in anemia, leu kopenia and glossitis.

Pantothenic acid: Indicated in inappetence weightloss, growth depression, lowered anti body response and hindleg spasticity.

Vitamin A: Used as Keratinization stabilizing. This reduces sebaceous gland size and inhibits its activity and decreases sebaceous secretion. Also used to treat Acne and sebaceous adenitis. To treat night blindess. It is useful for maintenance of spermato genesis & foetal development used in unhealthy Gastro intestinal mucosa, diarrhea and sterility, stunted growth debility and staggering growth.

Vitamin B_1: It is indicated for better metabolism of carbohydrate and protein. Also plays important role in neuromuscular transmission. Given prophylactically in young ones, pregnants, neurological and cardiovascular disorders, chronic anorexia and constipation.

Vitamin B_{12}: Cyanocobalamine is required by body cells for DNA synthesis. Indicated in anemia, skin lesions, hindleg paralysis and loss of voice.

Vitamin B_2: It acts as co-enzyme in various oxidation reduction reactions. It is indicated in anemia, muscular weakness, dermatitis, Eye sores as a supportive factor.

Vitamin B_3: It is essential for lipid synthesis and oxidative metabolism. Indicated in canine pellagra and black tongue disease with signs of anorexia, depression, loss of body weight, glossitits, gingintis and bloody diarrhea.

Vitamin B_6: Indicated in inappetence, weightloss, or growth depression ataxia, convulsive seizers, cardiomyopathy and microcytic hypochromic anemia.

Vitamin C: It plays important role in many oxidation and other metabolic reactions. Indicated in treatment of scurvy, postoperative anemia, common cold, asphyxia etc. to treat vit C deficiency and is antioxidant. Effective for preventing Cancer or Cardiovascular disease.

Vitamin D: Rickets, osteomalacia, and normal matrix biosynthesis. It also stimulates calcium and Phosphorus absorption by small intestine. It helps pathologic fracture and locomotory abnormalities.

Vitamin E: Antioxiolant and protective to cell membrane. It helps in healing process. As supportive in sterility, incoordination and disturbed gait.

Vitamin K: It is used to treat coagulopathies caused by anticoagulant toxicosis. Anti coagulants deplete vit K in the body which is essential for synthesis of clotting factor. Anemia due to any etiology or blood loss due to any factor.

Minerals

Calcium: Very essential for metabolism of fat and carbohydrate. So, indicated in depressed growth rate, weight gain, bone formation in conditions like ricket, bone deformities of limbs.

Chromium: essential for growth and immune functions requirement increases during infections.

Cobalt: Helps in reduced appetite, decreased growth rate and reproductive functions.

Copper: Essential for enzymic activities and hemoglobin formation. Indicated in anemia. Stiffles syndrome, with thriftiness and weight gain.

Fluorine: Prevents dental caries but should not be supplemented.

Iodine: Essential for hormone secretion by Thyroid glands. Added to enhance the metabolic activity of body and overall reproductive cycle. It strengthens muscle.

Iron: essential for hemoglobin formation & used as hematinic indicated in pregnants & growing animals in tonics for overall health.

Magnesium: Essential cofactor for many enzymes particularly involved in Protein & DNA synthesis. Good for muscular coordination & strength. Added in general tonics and immune modulations.

Manganese: Can be supplemented in newborn pups for better growth. Also controls growth of deformities specially of limbs. It helps in cartilage formation.

Molybodenun: No document for action.

Phosphorous: To maintain cell phosphorus ratio which results better weigth gain, growth and healthy adult.

Potassium: Indicated for growth and increasigns dietary protein intake of growing pups & kittens. For feed efficiency specially for growing pups it is good.

Selenium: Helps as immune modulator and treat myo-degenerative disorders.

Sodium: Generally not needed for supplementation. Food and feeds contain Sodium which is sufficient for body requirement.

Sulfur: Requirement is usually met by normal food. During stress/ fasting animal may need usually not supplemental.

Zinc: Helps in potentiating immunity & optimum growth. To control lymphocyte depletion. Also used as to control skin lesions characterised by parakeratosis hyperkeratosis, erosions, ulcerations, vesiculations, alopecia epidermititis.

Infusion Fluids

Borocalcinate inj	**Sarabhai**
Comp	Calcium barogluconate 25%
Adm.	IV, SC
@	2-5ml
Pres.	200ml

Boromag inj	**Zydus**
Comp	Calcium gluconate 18% Magnesium hypophosphite 4% Dextrose 18.1%
Adm.	IV, SC
@	3-5ml
Pres.	200ml

Calciboro inj	**Glaxo**
Comp	Calcium barogluconate 25%
Adm.	IV, SC
@	2-5ml
Pres.	450ml

Calvib inj	**Glaxo**
Comp	Calcium gluconate 20.75% (calcium 1.86%) Boric acid 4.25%
Adm.	IV / SC
@	2-5ml
Pres.	450ml

Calgonite inj	**Indian Immunologicals**
Comp	Calcium barogluconate 25%
Adm.	IV, SC
@	2-5ml
Pres.	450ml

Hiphocal inj	**Indian Immunologicals**
Comp	Calcium gluconate, Magnesium hypophosphite, Dextrose and Boric acid
Adm.	IV/ SC
@	3-5ml
Pres.	450ml

Intacal inj	**Intas**
Comp	Calcium gluconate 20.75% Proportiion of Boric acid 2.26%
Adm.	IV/ SC
@	25-50ml
Pres.	500ml

Lacrivet inj	**Brihans**	
Comp	100ml contains	
	Dextrose 20g	Sodium chloride 0.6g
	Potassium chloride 0.04g	Calcium chloride 0.027g
	Lactic acid 0.24g	Sodium hydroxide 0.116mg
Adm.	IV/ SC	
@	25-50ml	
Pres.	500ml	

Woktrose 25 inj	**Wockhardt**
Comp	Dextrose 25g per 100ml
Adm.	IV
@	25-50ml
Pres.	540ml

Thiacal inj	**Wockhardt**
Comp	Calcium gluconate 20%, Boric acid 5%, Dextrose 15%, B1 300mg
Adm.	IV/ SC
@	2-5ml
Pres.	450ml

Lactaid inj	**Intas**
Comp	Calcium 1.86% Proportion of Broric acid 2.26:1
Adm.	IV/ SC
@	3-5ml
Pres.	450ml

Lactomag inj	**Intas**
Comp	Calcium gluconate, Magnesium hypophosphite, Dextrose and Boric acid
Adm.	IV/ SC
@	3-5ml
Pres.	450ml

Mineral and Vitamins Prep.

Alvitone Liq	**Alembic**	
Comp	5ml contains	
	Vit A 250000 IU	D_3 25000 IU
	E 150 IU	C 500mg
Adm.	Oral	
@	3-5ml od	
Pres.	20ml, 500ml	

Ambiplex Liq	**Brihans**	
Comp	5ml contains	
	Vit B_1 7mg	B_2 2.5mg
	B_6 1mg	B_{12} 12.5mcg
	Biotin 25mcg	Calcium pantothenate 2.5mg
	Niacin 75mg	Choline chloride 10mg
	Methinonine 10mg	Lysine 20mg
Adm.	Oral	
@	2-3ml	
Pres.	30ml, 100ml	

Beekom L inj	**Wockhardt**	
Comp	Thiamine 25mg	Riboflavin 1.5mg
	Niacinamide 50mg	Vit B6 5mg
	B_{12} 50mcg	Choline chloride 25mg
	Crude liver extract with B_{12} activity 2mcg/ml	
Adm.	IM	
@	1-2ml thrice a week	
Pres.	10ml	

Belamyl inj	**Sarabhai**		
Comp	Each ml contains		
	Vit B_1 10mg	B_2 3mg	Niacinamide 100mg
	B_{12} 10mcg		Liver crude 0.60/ml
Adm.	IM		
@	0.5ml twice weekly		
Pres.	10ml		

Bicoral Forte Liq	**Intervet**	
Comp	Each ml contains	
	Vit B_1 50mg	B_2 5mg
	B_6 5mg	Pantothenol 10mg
	Inositol 2mg	Methionine 5mg
	Liver extract with B_{12} activity equal to 0.2mcg of B_{12}	
Adm.	IM	
@	1ml twice in a week	
Pres.	10ml	

Boiplex inj	**Sarabhai**	
Comp	Thiamine 10mg	B_2 5mg
	Niacinamide 100mg	B_{12} 10mcg
	Liver inject 0.66ml per ml	
Adm.	IM	
@	2-5ml three or more days in a week	
Pres.	30ml	

Brotone liq	**Glaxo**	
Comp	Liver 1.25g, from 31.25g Freshliver with B_{12} activity 7.5mcg of cyano cobalamine	
	Yeast extract 0.4g	Thiamine 2.5g
	Nicotinic acid 24mg/10ml	
Adm.	Oral	
@	5-10ml bid	
Pres.	120ml	

Cadisol Liq	**Cadila**
Comp	Vit A 100000 IU per ml
Adm.	Oral
@	1ml od x3 days
Pres.	100ml

Cadisol Plus inj	**Cadila**	
Comp	Calcium gluconate 833mg	Vit D 1600 IU
	B_{12} 16.7mcg	Iron 162 mg
	Stomach extract 3.3mg/10ml	
Adm.	Oral	
@	10ml bid	
Pres.	100ml, 500ml	

Cal –D Plus D 5 liq	**Sarabhai**
Comp	Calcium gluconate 416.5mg Cholecalciferol 800 IU Stomach extract 1.65mg Ferric ammonium citrate 8.3mg Vit B_{12} 8.35mcg/5ml
Adm.	Oral
@	10ml bid
Pres.	100ml

Cal –D Rubra liq	**Cadila**
Comp	Calcium gluconate 416.5mg Cholecalciferol 800 IU Stomach extract 1.65mg Ferric ammonium citrate 8.3mg Vit B_{12} 8.35mcg/5ml
Adm.	Oral
@	10ml bid
Pres.	100ml

Caldivet inj	**Ranbaxy**
Comp	5ml contains Calcium lactate 250mg Calcium gluconate 200mg Vit D_3 500 IU Cyano cobalamine 5mcg Cobalt 5mg
Adm.	Oral
@	5-10ml bid
Pres.	500ml

Caldee 12 inj	Wockhardt	
Comp	Calcium levulinate 76.4mg	Vit D_3 5000 IU
	B_{12} 50mcg/ml	
Adm.	IM	
@	1-3ml thrice a week	
Pres.	10ml	

Calovite C Paste	Ranbaxy	
Comp	1G contains	
	Vit A 3500Iu	B_1 30mg
	B_2 5mg	B_6 20mg
	B_{12} 15mcg	D_3 300 IU
	E 100 IU	Niacinamide 10mg
	Folic acid 0.5mg	Calcium pantothenate 15mg
	Manganese 3.5mg	Magnesium 1mg
	Iodine 0.75mg	Iron 1.0mg
Adm.	Oral	
@	1g/5kg B.wt	
Pres.	50g	

Capovit inj	Indian Immunology	
Comp	Each ml contains	
	Vit A 12000 IU	D_3 6000 IU
	E 48mg	B_{12} 20mcg
Adm.	Oral	
@	5-10ml od	
Pres.	30ml, 500ml	

Capsola pet inj	Ranbaxy	
Comp	20ml contains	
	Calcium 325.6mg	Phosphorous 167.7mg
	D_3 1600 IU	B_{12} 20mg
Adm.	Oral	
@	10-20ml bid	
Pres.	500ml	

Catasol 10% inj	**Bayer**
Comp	Butaphosphan 100mg Cyanocobalamin 50mg/ml
Adm.	IV/ IM/ SC
@	1-5ml
Pres.	30ml, 100ml

Cholymbi Pow	**Lyka**	
Comp	Choline chloride (50%) 10g DL Methinoine 10g Vit B_{12} 1.5mg/50g	Lysine 10g Biotin 1mg
Adm.	Oral	
@	5-10g od in milk/food	
Pres.	50g, 500g	

Cobacal D inj	**Unichem**		
Comp	Calcium	Vit D_3	B_{12} injection
Adm.	IM		
@	1-3ml thrice a week		
Pres.	10ml		

Cobaphos inj	**Glaxo**
Comp	Sodium salt of oxybenzylphosphinate 125mg Sodium dihydrogen phosphate 9mg Cyanocobalamin 50mcg/ml
Adm.	IM, IV, SC
@	2-5ml every 2nd day
Pres.	5ml, 10ml

Conciplex inj	**Concept**		
Comp	3ml contains Vit B1 100mg B_{12} 100mcg D Panthenol 5mg	 B_2 5mg Niacinamide 100mg	 B_6 10mg
Adm.	IM		
@	1ml od		
Pres.	10ml		

E care Se inj	Vetcare	
Comp	Tocopherol 50mg	Selenium 1.5mg/ml
Adm.	IM	
@	1ml per 25kg B.wt	
Pres.	10ml	

Hivit inj	Ranbaxy	
Comp	Each ml contains	
Vit A 2000 IU	Vit A 2000 IU	D_3 32000 IU
	E 4 IU	Niacinamide 10mg
	Thiamine hydrochloride 5mg	
	Pyridoxine hydrochloride 5mg	
	Riboflavin 1mg	D Panthenol 1mg
	B_{12} 10mg	Biotine 10mcg
	Calcium glycerophosphate 10mg/ml	
Adm.	IM/ IV/ SC	
@	2ml on alternate day	
Pres.	30ml	

Livaplax inj	Pranav	
Comp	1ml contains	
	Vit B_1 25mg	B_2 1.37mg
	B_6 5mg	B_{12} 30mcg
	Choline chloride 15mg	D panthenol 5mg
	Niacinamide 100mg	
Adm.	IM	
@	1-2ml od	
Pres.	30ml	

Liverjet inj	Sarabhai
Comp	liver extract containing B_{12} not lessthan 2mcg/ml
Adm.	IM
@	1-2ml od
Pres.	10ml

Livobex inj	**TTK**
Comp	1ml contains B_1 10mg B_2 3mg B_6 5mg Niacinamide 100mg B_{12} 25mcg Crude liver 0.66ml
Adm.	IM
@	1ml od
Pres.	10ml

Merical Pet BrisKit	**Wockhardt**
Comp	Each brisket contains Calcium 350mg Phosphorous 175mg D_3 1600 IU B_{12} 20mcg Iron 3mg
Adm.	Oral
@	1-2 briskit od
Pres.	12's pack

Merical Pet liq	**Wockhardt**
Comp	20ml contains Calcium 350mg Phosphorous 170mg D_3 1600 IU B_{12} 20mcg
Adm.	Oral
@	20ml od
Pres.	360ml

Meritone inj	**Wockhardt**
Comp	Vit B_1 25mg B_2 1.37mg Nicotinamide 100mg D Panthenol 5mg B_6 5mg Choline chloride 15mg Liver extract 8g B_{12} 2mcg/ml
Adm.	IM
@	1-2ml od
Pres.	10ml

Neuroxin inj 12	**Sarabhai**
Comp	Each ml contains Vit B_1 30mg B_6 13.75mg B_{12} 800mcg

Adm.	IM
@	2-3ml od
Pres.	10ml

Nutribix Economy	**Petcare**	
Comp	Each briskit contains	
	Protein 20%	Fat 10%
	Crude fibre 4.0%	Calcium 1.0%
	Moisture 10%	Phosphorus 0.8%
	Energy 3100 Kcal/ kg	
Adm.	Oral	
@	As often as you like	
Pres.	250g	

Nutribix Dog Rolls	**Petcare**	
Comp	Vit A 5000 IU	B_2 9mcg
	B_{12} 500mcg	D_3 1000 IU
	Niacin 14mcg	Pantothenic acid 40mcg
	Lysine 50mg	Methionine 19mg
	Other amino acids 250mg	Choline 100mg
	Protein 160mg	Fat 250mg
	Fibre 150mg per 10	
Adm.	Oral	
@	5-10gm	
Pres.	400g	

Nutricoat Tonic	**Petcare**	
Comp	5g contains	
	Linoleic acid 1000mg	Linolenic acid 1000mg
	Oleic acid 1000mg	Lecithin 50mg
	Vit B_6 400mcg	A 1000 IU
	E 10 IU	D_3 100 IU
	Zinc 4.5mg	Selenium 0.2mcg
	Biotin 45mcg	
Adm.	Oral	
@	2.5g od, 10g for pregnant od	
Pres.	150g, 400g	

Nutripet junior	**Petcare**	
Comp	Protein 30%	Fat 9%
	Energy 3540Kcal	Calcium 1.5%
	Phosphorous 0.8%	Fiber 1.18%
	Vitamins, trace minerals and antioxidant	
Adm.	Oral	
@	Balance food to be given as per body weight	
Pres.	1kg	

Nutripet Food Booster	**Petcare**
Comp	Formulated food supplement with complete nutritional spectrum
Adm.	Oral
@	20g/kg B.wt
Pres.	150g, 200g, 1kg

Nutrisam 365 Briskit	**Wockhardt**
Comp	Not given
Adm.	Oral
@	1-2 briskit od
Pres.	Bottle of 50

Orcalmin susp	**TTK**
Comp	Extract of bone providing 33mg Calcium 15mg Phosphorous in 5ml
Adm.	Oral
@	5-10ml od
Pres.	200ml

Ossopan granules	**TTK**
Comp	Bone extract containing Calcium 165mg Phosphorus 75mg/g
Adm.	Oral
@	5g od
Pres.	100g

Ostocalcium Pet	**Glaxo**	
Comp	20ml contains	
	Calcium 325.6mg	Phosphorus 176.7mg
	Vit D_3 1600 IU	B_{12} 20mcg
Adm.	Oral	
@	10ml bid	
Pres.	150ml	

Preplin Forte inj	**Glaxo**
Comp	Vit A 600000 IU per 2ml
Adm.	IM
@	0.5ml weekly
Pres.	2ml

Promix Y Tab	**Alembic**	
Comp	Protein 35%	Carbohydrate 30%
	Mineral salt 8%	Vit B_1 0.03mg
	B_2 0.012mg	
	Nicotinic acid 0.09mg per tab	
Adm.	Oral	
@	3 tab bid	
Pres.	150 tab	

Recovit liq	**Brihans**	
Comp	Each ml contains	
	Vit A 50000 IU	D_3 5000 IU
	E 50mg	C 100mg
	B_{12} 25mcg	
Adm.	Oral	
@	1ml od	
Pres.	30ml, 100ml	

Rubraplex Elixir	**Sarabhai**	
Comp	Elemental Iron (As ferric ammonium citrate 39.45mg and Ferric chloride hydrate 144mg) 114mg	
	Vit B_1 4.5mg	B_2 4.5mg
	B_6 1.5mg	B_{12} 7.5mcg
	D-Panthenol 24mg	Niacinamide 48mg

Adm.	Oral
@	15ml od
Pres.	120ml, 240ml

Stronic inj	**Ranbaxy**	
Comp	Each ml contain	
	Vit B_1 250mg	B_2 5mg
	B_{12} 50mcg	Niacinamide 50mg
	Pyridoxine 5mg	Liver crude
	B_{12} equivalent to 2mcg	
Adm.		IM
@	2-5ml od	
Pres.	10ml, 30ml	

Tribivet inj	**Intas**		
Comp	Each ml contain		
	Vit B_1 50mg	B_{12} 500mcg	B_6 50mg
Adm.	IM		
@	1ml		
Pres.	10ml, 30ml		

Vadeb liq	**Zydus**		
Comp	Vit A 12000 IU	D_3 6000 IU	E 48mg
	B_{12} 20mcg		
Adm.		Oral	
@	2-5ml od		
Pres.	30ml, 500ml		

Veta A inj	**TTK**
Comp	Vit A 6 Lac IU per 2ml
Adm.	IM
@	0.5ml weekly
Pres.	2ml

Vetade inj	Sarabhai
Comp	Vit A 25000 IU, D_3 100 IU E, 48mg
Adm.	IM
@	2-3ml od
Pres.	10ml

Vibelan inj	Glaxo
Comp	Each ml contain B_1 25mg B_2 4.1mg B_6 25mg Nicotinamide 100mg D panthenol 15mg Lignocaine 5mg
Adm.	IM
@	3.5ml od
Pres.	30ml

Vinueral liq	Glaxo
Comp	Each ml contain Vit A 12000 IU D_3 6000 IU E 48mg B_{12} 20mcg
Adm.	Oral
@	1ml od
Pres.	30ml, 60ml, 120ml, 300ml

Viselam liq	Brihans
Comp	Vit A 60000 IU D_3 30000 IU E 150mg B_{12} 25mcg Folic acid 2.5mg C 100mg L lysine 25mg DL methionine 25mg Tryptophan 5mg Selenium 100mcg
Adm.	Oral
@	5ml od
Pres.	100ml

Vitacept inj	Concept
Comp	Vit A 2.5 Lac IU D_3 25000 IU E 100mg per ml
Adm.	IM
@	1-2ml od
Pres.	5ml

Vitapet liq	**Glaxo**	
Comp	Codliver oil 50%	Refined soya oil 50%
Adm.	1.5-2 tsp od	
Pres.	150ml	

Wokantol inj	**Wockhardt**		
Comp	Each ml contains		
	Vit A 600000 IU	D_3 60000 IU	E 200mg
Adm.	IM		
@	2ml		
Pres.	2ml		

Limcee Tab	**Sarabhai**
Comp	Ascorbic acid (Vit C) 500mg
Adm.	Oral
@	100-500mg od
Pres.	10

Calci Royal Sol Pow	**Concept**
Comp	5g contains Calcium 174mg Elemental phosphorus 50mg Vit C 30mg Vit B_{12} 50mcg Vit D 1000 IU Citric acid 1g
Adm.	Oral
@	5g od
Pres.	100g

Ostophos FS liq	**Neospark**	
Comp	5ml contains	
	Calcium 104mg	Phosphorus 52mg
	D_3 500 IU	B_{12} 7.5mcg
	Predigested protein 75mg	Iron 15mg
Adm.	Oral	
@	10-20ml bid	
Pres.	IL	

Orcal P granules	**TTK**	
Comp	Microcrystalline hydroxy apatite complex equivalent to	
	Calcium 165mg	Phosphorus 75mg
	Vit D_3 500 IU per g	
Adm.	Oral	
@	5g od	
Pres.	500g	

Lyvim liq	**Cadila Pharma**	
Comp	5ml contains	
	Vit A 250000 IU	D_3 25000 IU
	C 500mg	E 150mg
	Lysine 25mg	Methionine 10mg
Adm.	Oral	
@	5-10ml od	
Pres.	100ml, 500ml	

Amnovit Pow	**Glaxo**	
Intervet	100g contains	
	Vit A 5lac IU	E 200 IUB6 60mg
	K 40mg	D3 29000 IU
	B2 300mg	B12 400mcg
	Choline chloride 150mg	Pantothenate 440mg
	Niacinaminde 1.32g	Folic acid 10mg
	L Lysine 1g	L methionine 2g
	L Tryptophan 200mg	
Adm.	Oral	
@	1.2-5g od	
Pres.	200g	

Urimin inj	**Virbac**
Comp	Sodium acid phosphate 40.3% equal to Elemental Phosphorous 8% per ml
Adm.	IV
@	1-2ml od
Pres.	10ml, 30ml

Calcium Sandoz Tab	**Novartis**
Comp	Tab 625mg of calcium carbonate
Adm.	Oral
@	1-2 tab od
Pres.	250 tab

Sandocal Tab	**Novartis**
Comp	Tab calcium carbonate 1.25g
Adm.	Oral
@	1 tab od
Pres.	500

Anabolic Steroid

It is also a testosterone derivative with anabolic and anticatabolic action. It is indicated for repairs and stimulating bone marrows.

Decaneurabol inj	**Cadila Healthcare**
Comp	Nandrolone Decanoate 25mg/ml
Adm.	IM
@	1-5mg/kg B.wt
Pres.	1ml

Nandrilone inj	**Generic**
Comp	Nandrolone Decanoate 25mg/ml
Adm.	IM
@	1-5mg/kg B.wt
Pres.	1ml

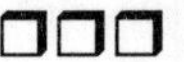

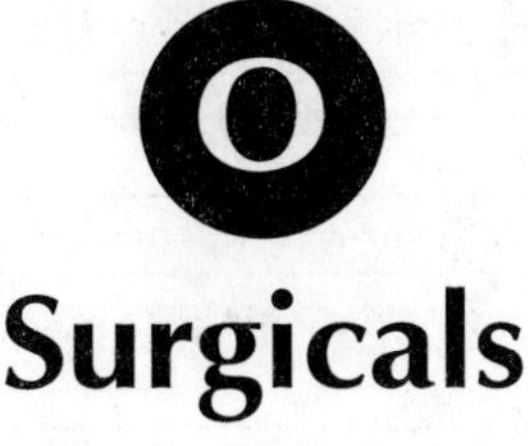

Surgicals

Antiseptics

Wokadine Sol	Wockhardt
Comp	Povidone Iodine 5%
Adm.	Topical
@	As per need
Pres.	100ml

Wokadine scrub	Wockhardt
Comp	Povidone Iodine 5%
Adm.	Local application
@	As per need
Pres.	100ml, 500ml

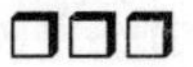

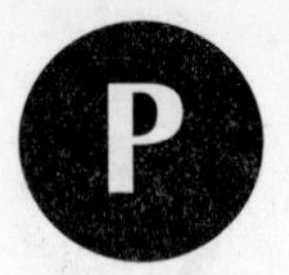

Vaccines

Antirabic Vaccines

Antirabic vaccine	**HVVI Hisar**
Comp	20% in activated ARV
Adm.	S/C
@	5ml above 3 months
Pres.	5ml vial

Candur R	**Intervet**
Comp	Inactivated ARV
Adm.	S/C/ IM
@	1ml I dose of 7 weeks of age Booster 4-6 weeks then annually

ARV 20%	**IAHVB Delhi**
Comp	Carboliseed ARV
Adm.	SC
@	5ml at 3 months age then annual

Megavac R	**Indian Immunology**
Comp	Cell cultured inactivated ARV
Adm.	SC or IM
@	1ml after 3 months then annually

Nobivac R or Rabivac	**Intervet**
Comp	Not given
Adm.	IM/ SC
@	Single dose 1ml at age of 3 months then after 3 years
Pres.	1ml single dose

Rabdomum	**Sarabhai**
Comp	Not given
Adm.	IM/ SC
@	Single dose 1ml at age of 3 months then after 3 years
Pres.	1ml single dose

Rabguard Rabies vaccine	**Pfizer**
Comp	Tissue culture Rabies vaccine
Adm.	IM/ SC
@	1ml at 3 months then annual
Pres.	10 dose vial 10ml

Rabigen Mono	**Ranbaxy**
Comp	Tissue culture Rabies vaccine
Adm.	SC/IM
@	1ml at age 3 month then annual
Pres.	1ml single dose

Rabies Vaccine	**BPDIVRI Izet nagar**
Comp	Living flurry strain LEP
Adm.	IM
@	2ml
Pres.	10ml

Rabies Vaccine	**IVPM Ranipet** **OBPI Bhubneshwar**	**IAHBP Mhow** **Biomed Gaziabad**	**BPS Calcutta** **IAHVB Delhi**
Comp	Living flurry strain LEP		
Adm.	IM		
@	2ml		
Pres.	10ml		

Rabies Vaccine	**IAHVBP Mhow** **BPS Calcutta**	**APVBRI Hydrabad** **IVB Guwahati**	**PVVI Ludhiana**
Comp	Inactivated 20% ARV		
Adm.	IM or SC		
@	1ml		
Pres.	Single dose 1ml		

Rabisin	**Glaxo**
Comp	Not given
Adm.	IM/ SC
@	Single dose 1ml at age of 3 months then after 3 years
Pres.	1ml single tose

Rabisin	**Serum Institute**
Comp	Not given
Adm.	SC/ IM
@	1ml in all age or size of animals. 4 weeks, Booster dose, 3-4 weeks after 1st than annually
Pres.	1ml, 10ml

Raksha Rab	**Indian Immunology**
Comp	Not given
Adm.	IM/ SC
@	1ml at 3 month then annually. For treatment course of 6 Inj 0,3,7,14,28,90th days
Pres.	5ml, 10ml,30ml, single dose with disposable syringe

Canine Distemper

Canine distemper vaccine	**BPDIVIRI Izatnagar**
Comp	Modified live virus
Adm.	SC/ IM
@	1ml at 9 week, 12 week, 16 week
Pres.	1ml single dose

Canine distemper vaccine	**Biomed**
Comp	Not given
Adm.	IM
@	2ml at 10-12 week of age then annually
Pres.	Single dose vial

Megavac D	**Indian Immunology**
Comp	Not given
Adm.	SC/ IM
@	1ml 1st dose 6 week then annually
Pres.	1ml single dose

Corona Vaccine

Canine Corona vaccine	**Pfizer**
Comp	Corona vaccine
Adm.	IM/ SC
@	1ml
Pres.	Single dose

Galaxy Corona virus vaccine	Pfizer
Comp	Corona vaccine
Adm.	IM/ SC
@	1ml
Pres.	Single dose

Megavac CC	Indian Immunology
Comp	Canine Corona Virus
Adm.	IM/ SC
@	1ml 1st at 8-9 week Booster 12 week then annually
Pres.	Single dose vial

Leptospirosis Vaccine

Novibac L vaccine	Intervet
Comp	Inactivated Leptospira
Adm.	IM/ SC
@	1ml at 6 week of age then at 12 week then annually
Pres.	Single dose

Vanguard Lepto	Pfizer
Comp	Inactivated Leptospira
Adm.	IM/ SC
@	1ml 2 injection with interval of 2 week then annual
Pres.	25ml 25 dose

Parvovirus

Candur P	Intervet
Comp	Not given
Adm.	IM/ SC
@	1ml
Pres.	1ml Single dose

Megavac P	Indian Immunology
Comp	Inactivated
Adm.	IM/ SC
@	1ml 1st 8-9 weeks. Yearly booster dose
Pres.	Single dose 1ml

Megavac P2 Live	**Indian immunology**
Comp	Vaccine
Adm.	IM/ SC
@	1ml primary at 6 weeks then annually
Pres.	Single dose 1ml

Nobivac Parvo C	**Intervet**
Comp	Freezed dried
Adm.	IM/ SC
@	1ml at 6 weeks then 10-12 weeks then annual
Pres.	Single dose

Vanguard CVP	**Pfizer**
Comp	Not given
Adm.	IM/ SC
@	1ml before 16 week. Second dose after 14 days interval then annually
Pres.	10ml

Parvocine or Parvodog	**Serum Institute of India**
Comp	Not given
Adm.	IM/ SC
@	1ml 1st dose 9-12 week 2nd 15-16 week then annually
Pres.	1ml, 10ml

Combined Vaccine

Candur DH	**Intervet**
Comp	Distemper and Hepatitis vaccine
Adm.	SC/ IM
@	2ml at 7-9 week then 12-14 week then annually
Pres.	2ml Single dose vial

Nobivac DH	Intervet
Comp	Distemper and Hepatitis Freezed dried vaccine
Adm.	IM/ SC
@	At 6 week of age
Pres.	Single dose with solvent

Novibac Puppy DP	**Intervet**
Comp	Distemper and Parvovirus vaccine
Adm.	SC
@	1ml 1st 6-7 weeks 2nd 9-12 week
Pres.	Single dose with solvent

Novivac RL	**Intervet**
Comp	Distemper and Rabies vaccine
Adm.	SC/ IM
@	1ml at 9-12 week
Pres.	Single dose with solvent

Vanguard CVPL	**Pfizer**
Comp	Parvovirus, Leptospirosis
Adm.	IM/ SC
@	1ml
Pres.	25ml

Nobivac DHP or Puppy DP	**Intervet**
Comp	Distemper, hepatitis and Parvovirus vaccine
Adm.	IM/ SC
@	1ml I dose 6 week then II dose 9 week after it annual
Pres.	Single dose

Vanguard DMLP	**Pfizer**
Comp	Distemper, Leptospirosis and Parvovirus
Adm.	IM/ SC
@	1ml I dose 7 week then II dose 11 week III annual
Pres.	25 dose vial (not for Pregnants)

Penta dog	**Serum institute of India**
Comp	Distemper, Rabies, Hepatitis and Leptospirosis
Adm.	SC
@	1ml I 7 week then II 11 week then annual
Pres.	Single dose

Commander 7L	**Bayer**
Comp	Distemper, Adenovirus, Parainfluenza, Parvovirus and Leptospirosis
Adm.	SC/ IM
@	1ml I 12 week and II 2-3 week later then annually
Pres.	Single dose

Canigen	**Ranbaxy**
Comp	Distemper, Hepatitis, Parainfluenza, Parvovirus, Adenovirus and Leptospirosis
Adm.	SC/ IM
@	1ml
Pres.	Single dose

Vanguard 6	**Pfizer**
Comp	Distemper, Adenovirus, Hepatitis,Parainfluenza and Leptospirosis
Adm.	SC
@	1ml
Pres.	Single dose

Virbagen C Vaccine	**Ranbaxy**
Comp	Distemper, Rabies, Hepatitis and Leptospirosis
Adm.	SC
@	1ml
Pres.	Single dose

Caniffa	**Serum Institute of India**
Comp	Distemper, Hepatitis and Leptospirosis
Adm.	SC/ IM
@	1ml I 7 week and II 11 week then annually
Pres.	Single dose

Megavac DHL	**Indian Immunology**
Comp	Distemper, Hepatitis and Leptospirosis
Adm.	SC/ IM
@	1ml of 8-9 week Booster 12 week revaccinate annually
Pres.	Single dose

Novivac DHL	Intervet
Comp	Distemper, Hepatitis and Leptospirosis
Adm.	SC/ IM
@	1ml I at 7-9 week and II 12-14 week then annually
Pres.	1ml + solvent

Candor DHLP	Intervet
Comp	Distemper, Hepatitis, Parvovirus, Leptospirosis
Adm.	SC/ IM
@	1ml I 7-9 week and II 12-14 week then annually
Pres.	Single dose

Canilep DHLP	Glaxo
Comp	Distemper, Hepatitis, Parvovirus and Leptospira
Adm.	SC
@	2ml I 6-8 week and II 12 week then annually
Pres.	Single dose with syringe

Megavac C	Indian Immunology
Comp	Freeze dried component Distemper, Parvovirus, Hepatitis, 2 containers of Inactivated Letospira Canicola and Leptospira Ichterhaemorrhagia
Adm.	IM/SC
@	1ml
Pres.	Single dose 1ml with syringe and needle or single dose packed in PVC containing 30 doses

Antigen DHLR	Ranbaxy
Comp	Distemper, Rabies, Hepatitis and Leptospirosis
Adm.	IM/SC
@	1ml I 7 week and II 12 week then annually
Pres.	Single dose

Megavac DH+LR	**Intervet**
Comp	Distemper, Rabies, Hepatitis and Leptospirosis
Adm.	IM/SC
@	1ml I 8-9 week and II 12 week then annually
Pres.	Single dose

Novivac DH+LR	**Intervet**
Comp	Distemper, Rabies, Hepatitis and Leptospirosis
Adm.	IM/SC
@	1ml I 8-9 week and II 12 week then annually
Pres.	Single dose

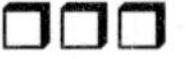

IMPORTANT TERMS-GLOSSARY

ACUTE: Having severe symptoms and short course.

ADJUVANT: Any substance used in conjunction with another to enhance its activity.

ADSORBANT: A substance which has property of adsorbing gases or toxic substances from intestine etc.

AEROBIC BACTERIA: Bacteria, which can live only in presence of air or oxygen.

AFFINITY: tendency of a drug to bind.

AFLATOXIN: Refers to the toxins which are elaborated by moulds and contaminate the food or other material.

ALLERGENS: Refers to substances that can elicit antibody formation.

AMPOULE: A glass container which is sealed after filling and contents are withdrawn after breaking it.

ANABOLIC: These tends to increase protein anabolism or decrease amino acid catabolism which causes weight gain and muscular development.

ANAEROBIC BACTERIA: Bacteria, which can live without air or oxygen.

ANAESTHESIA: Refers to a state of reversible unconciousness induced by a general or local anesthetic drug.

ANALEPTICS: Drugs controlling depression produced by epilepsy or overdose of depressant.

ANALGESICS: A drug having the property of relieving pain.

ANAPHRODISIAC: Refers to drugs that diminishes sexual desire.

ANAPHYLAXIS: An increased sensitivity to the action of a normally nontoxic protein when injected with it for second time. It may cause a severe or even a fatal reaction.

ANIMAL: A living being which cannot manufacture its own food with all characteristics of a living being.

ANODYNE: Soothing medicines that relieves pain.

ANTACID: Drug death neutralizes gastric acid.

ANTAGONISM: Reduction of the effect of one drug by another drug.

ANTHELMINTIC: Or Anti helmintic drug having the property of killing parasite helminthes (worms).

ANTIALLERGIC: Drugs having property of suppressing some symptoms to check allergens.

ANTIBIOTIC: A chemical substance produced by micro-organisms, which is used to kill or inhibit the growth of another micro-organisms.

ANTIBODY: Term used for a protein which is having the properties of immunoglobulin and are produced in the body.

ANTICOAGULANT: Drug having the property of delaying or preventing the process of blood coagulation.

ANTICONVULSANT: Drug having the property of reducing convulsions and its severity.

ANTIDIARRHOEAL: Drug which can control diarrhea.

ANTIDOTE: Drug to counter the action of any other drug or poison.

ANTIEMETIC: Drug which is used to control vomiting.

ANTIFLATULANT: Or Antizymotics/ Antibloat – product to treat impaction and emptying stomach with gas.

ANTIGEN: A substance that is able to elicit a specific immune response when introduced into the body.

ANTIHISTAMINE: Drug having the property of antagonizing histamine.

ANTI-INFLAMMATORY: A drug used to suppress signs and symptoms of inflammation.

ANTIMYCOTIC: A drug active against fungi.

ANTINEOPLASTIC: Drug used to control cancer.

ANTIOXIDANT: Agent that control oxidants proced by oxidation.

ANTIPYRETIC: A drug used to lower down body temperature up to normal Body temperature.

ANTIPRURITIC: A drug used to relieve itching (Pruritis).

ANTIRHEUMATIC: Drug used to relieve the symptom of rheumatism like swelling of joint.

ANTISEPTIC: Agent that is able to counter sepsis by killing or inhibiting multiplication of micro-organisms.

ANTISPASMODIC: Drug which can control spasm of muscular or intestinal origin.

ANTISTRESS: Agent used to control the effect of stress on the animal body.

ANTITUSSIVE: Drugs having properties of reducing anxiety, agitation or tension. Also called anti-anxiety.

APHRODIXIC: Drug that is able to stimulate sexual desire.

APPETIZER: Or Appetite stimulant are drugs used to increase the desire to eat.

ASTRINGENT: Substance that brings a protective coagulated layer on membrane or inflamed skin.

AURAL PREPARATION: Related to ears/

B.P.vet.: British pharmacopeia veterinary.

BACTERIA: It is a unicellular micro-organism surrounded by rigid cell wall. Some bacteria are useful and some are harmful to plants and animals.

BIOAVAILABILAITY: When dosage form is meant for systemic action, its efficacy depends upon how completely and rapidly its active ingredient is absorbed in to the blood or availability of active drug in the blood for action.

BIOEQUIVALEMCE: Comparison made between generic formulation of a drug or product in which a change has been made.

BIOPSY: Removal and examination of tissue from living individual.

BITTERS: Terms used for non- toxic substances used to stimulate flow of saliva and gastric juice that promotes appetite.

BOLUS: (or Bol) The bigger sized tablets.

BOTTLE: A small container with a cork or a seal for storing liquid preparations

BRONCHOCONSTRICTOR: Drug able to produce constriction of bronchi (Lungs).

BRONCHODILATOR: Drug able to produce dilation of bronchi (Lungs).

CAPSULE: These are shells of gelatin containing active drug and may be hard or soft.

CARCINOGENICITY: Property to cause carcinoma or cancer.

CARMINATIVE: Substance having property of assisting Expulsion of gas from stomach and intestines.

CATHARTIC: Drug that is able to produce emptying of bowels by increasing G.I. motility.

CHEMOTHERAPY: Branch of Pharmacology dealing with drugs that selectively inhibit or destroy specific agents of disease such as bacteria, virus, fungus and other parasites.

CHOLAGOGUE: Stimulate bile flow from gall bladder to intestine.

CHOLERETIC: Substances that increase secretion of bile of hepatocytes.

CHRONIC: Any state continuing for a very long period.

CLINICAL: Referring to a clinic or patient, observation or treatment.

COCCIDIOSTAT: Agent that is able to control Coccidiosis.

COLD BLOODED ANIMALS: Those animals whose temperature varies directly with environment like reptiles.

COLLAPSIBLE TUBE: A container for ointment/ gel preparations which are sealed and capped.

CONTAGIOUS DISEASE: These spread to other animals through air, water, food, contact in cohabitation, etc.

CONVULSANT: Drug that produces convulsions i.e. contraction of voluntary muscles.

CORTICOSTEROIDS: Steroid hormones which are synthesized and secreted by adrenal cortex.

COUNTER-IRRITANTS: Substance that relieve a troublesome irritation by producing less unpleasant sensation.

CREAM: Semisolid pasty preparation with non-greasy water miscible base.

DEBILITY: Weakness of whole body.

DEMULCENT: Substance used to coat mucous membrane which effectively protect it from irritation.

DEODRANTS: Preparations intended to reduce body odour.

DERMATOLOGICAL: Agents related to skin.

DETOXIFICATION: Chemical transformation of drug usually in liver and converted to water soluble products eliminated in urine.

DIAGNOSTIC AGENTS: Agents used to aid in diagnosis of a disease.

DIAPHORETICS: Drug able to promote excessive sweating whether or not body temperature is raised.

DILUENT: (Also Solvent) An agent used to dilute or make powder form of drug to liquid form.

DISCHARGE: An excretion or substance evacuated.

DISEASE: The deviation from normal state of health. Disease in animals adversely affect the economic production and in turn profit. The losses due to diseases can be permanent or temporary, complete or partial.

DISINEFCTANTS: Germicides used to destroy bacteria or other infective organisms.

DIURETIC: Increase the rate of production of urine specially excretion of Sodium.

DOMESTIC ANIMAL: Animal which is reared for some benefit like milk, meat and draught.

DOSE: Amount of drug necessary that will produce a therapeutic effect for a certain period.

DOUGHY: When structure pits on pressure like in oedema.

DRAINAGE: Systemic withdrawal of fluids and discharge from a wound.

DRESSING: Any material used for covering or protecting a wound.

DRIP: The slow drop by drop infusion of liquid.

DROP: Minute sphere of liquid as it hangs or falls.

DROPPER: A pipe or tube for dispensing liquid in drops.

DRUG: It is a chemical agent that affects living processes and is used for diagnosis, precaution or treatment.

DRUG METABOLISM: Chemical transformation of drug along with its action and excretion.

DRUG RESISTANCE: When a drug becomes inactive or unable to achieve desired action, it is called drug resistance.

DUSTING POWDER: Drugs in powder form used for spreading over a part or whole body.

ECBOLICS: Produce the cleansing and contraction of uterus.

ECTOPARASITICIDE: Agent that can kill external parasite.

EFFICACY: Capacity of a drug to initiate a response.

ELECTROLYTE: important nutrients required for the body including minerals.

ELECTUARY: A semisolid material prepared for oral administration having drug and jaggery or flour.

ELIXIRS: Alcohol containing mixture/ syrups.

EMACIATED: Excessively thin condition of body.

EMOLLIENTS: Agent that softens or soothes the skin.

ENDECTOPARASITICIDE: Agent that can kill internal and external parasites.

ENDEMIC: a disease that is constantly present in certain animal population.

ENDOPARASITICIDE: Agent that can kill internal parasites.

ENEMAS: Fluid medications given rectally either for washing out the colon or for local action in colon.

ENZOOTIC: Outbreak of a disease among animals in an area.

EPIDEMIC: When many animals in a region are attacked by same disease at same time.

EPIDURAL: The space between vertebrae i.e. spinal dural space is filled with a product which travels through nerves. Route is used for anaesthetizing lower portion of animal.

EUTHANASIA: Product to produce quiet painless death in animal for humane.

EXPECTORANT: Term used for a drug which increases the secretion of mucous in dry cough.

EXTRACTS: Solids obtained by evaporating the solvent from fluids or tinctures.

FEED ADDITIVES: Nutrients added to feed to increase its nutritive value.

FEED SUPPLEMENTS: Products used for supplementation of nutritive value of food.

FERTILITY: Ability to reproduce.

FEVER OR PYREXIA: A syndrome in which there is rise in body temperature.

FORMULATION: A formula or preparation of one or more than one drug to produce a desirable result. Can be of any form tablet, capsule, liquid or injectable.

GAIT: Movement of limbs.

GALACTOGOGUE: Agents effecting letting down of milk.

GASTROINTESTINAL: Term related to stomach and intestine combined.

GOITEROGENIC: Refers to agents that induce goiter or enlargement of thyroid gland.

GRAM NEGATIVE: AND GRAM POSITIVE- In medicinal chemistry bacteria are mainly divided into two types depending upon their staining characteristics. Those bacteria which retain violet stain of Gram's reagent are called Gram +ve and which do not retain stain are called Gram –ve bacteria.

GROWTH PROMOTER: Products used to promote the growth of animals.

HALF LIFE: Rate of elimination of a drug expressed in terms of half life. Period when half of drug is excreted from body.

HEALTH: State of an individual living in complete harmony with his environment.

HEMATINICS: Agent helps in formation of blood.

HEMOSTATICS: Drug able to control the bleeding.

HEPATICS: Drugs supporting the liver action.

HEPATOTOXICITY: Toxicity which get manifested in the liver.

HEPATOTROPIC: Agents having special effect on liver.

HERBAL: Product that contains herb or any part or material related.

HISTAMINE: Product of amino acids produced in body or can be synthesized involved in physiological and pathological processes.

HORMONE: Chemical messenger (Steroids, or derivatives of amino acids or simple protein) which is synthesized stored and secreted by ductless gland.

HYDROCHLORETIC: Substances that stimulate liver to increase the output of bile.

HYPERCALCAEMIA: When there is excess of calcium.

HYPERSENSITIVITY: Also known as allergy. Adverse reaction related to dose. It may be local anaphylaxis with urticaria and oedema or systemic anaphylaxis like shock.

HYPERTHERMIA: Temperature above the normal body temperature.

HYPNOTICS: Drug that promotes sleep.

HYPOCALCAEMIA: Where there is shortage of calcium.

HYPODERMIC NEEDLE: Needle (hollow) administered beneath skin.

HYPOTHERMIA: Temperature below the normal body temperature.

I.P.Vet: Indian Pharmacopeia veterinary.

IDIOSYNCRASY: Individually a qualitatively different response to the drug. In most of cases it is due to genetic bio-chemical defect.

ILLNESS: It is a condition marked by pronounced deviation from normal health state or sickness.

IMMUNOPOTENTIATING Or IMMUNOMODULATOR: Agent that enhances immune mechanism.

IMPLANT OF DRUG: Method of placing drugs in pellet form under the skin to achieve a prolonged action.

INCUBATION PERIOD: The time that elapses between infection and appearance of symptoms of a disease.

INFECTIOUS DISEASE: disease caused by micro-organisms i.e. bacteria, virus, protozoa, fungi or parasites.

INFUSION: Continuous intravenous injection (usually) of a solution of drug for a period of minutes, hours or even day.

INHALENTS: volatile anaesthetic such as ether, nitrous oxide and Halothanes.

INJECTION: Introduction of a solution or suspension through a hypodermic needle by various routes.

INJURY: Hurt, damage or harm.

INTRA-ARTERIAL: Injection into an artery.

INTRA-DERMAL: Injection between the skin layers.

INTRAMAMMARY: Inside the mammary gland.

INTRAMUSCULAR: Injection is made into fleshy muscle. Muscles provide rapid absorption and can tolerate large volumes of drugs and reasonable degree of irritation. Suspension can form a depot in muscle for sustained release which becomes long acting.

INTRANASAL: Inside the nose.

INTRAOCCULAR: Inside the eye.

INTRAPERITONEAL: Injection into peritoneal cavity.

INTRATHECAL: Injection into cerebrospinal fluid.

INTRAUTERINE: Inside the uterus.

INTRAVAGINAL: Inside the vagina.

INTRAVENOUS: Direct into the vein and only solution is injected in blood. Drug effect is immediate. Large volumes of fluid are given. Intravenous must be given slowly.

ITCHING: Unpleasant cutaneous sensation provoking desire to scratch or rub the skin.

LACTATION: Milking period i.e. immediately after delivery till the milk is secreted by animal, varies from animal to animal and breed to breed of same type of animal.

LAXATIVE: Drug that produces emptying of bowels by increasing frequency of defecation or fecal volume or consistency.

LETHAL DOSE: A particular dose of drug able to kill.

LINIMENTS: These have an oil, alcoholic or hydro-alcoholic base and are applied locally to skin with friction or rubbing. Their ingredients usually are counter-irritants i.e. cause mild stimulation of superficial nerves which reflexly relieve pain in underlying deeper structure.

LIPOTROPIC: Agents that hasten the removal of fat and reduce its deposition in liver.

LIQUID ORAL FORM: A liquid medication to be taken orally is called mixture. Physically mixture may be a solution or suspension or emulsion.

LIVABILITY: Ability to live longer.

LOTION: These are aqueous solutions or suspensions meant for local application. Ingredients have soothing, cleansing, or antiseptic properties.

LUTEOLYTIC: Agent that is able to inhibit the corpus luteum's action to secrete progesterone.

MAMMALS: Those animals which can rear youngones and suckle them through mammary glands.

MANGER: Feeding trough for animals.

MIC: Minimum inhibitory concentration.

MORTALITY: Death rate

MULTIVITAMIN: Combination of more than one vitamin.

MUSCLE RELAXANT: Drug that produces relaxation of non-cardial muscles.

NARCOTIC DRUG: Drug that produces reversible unsensibility or stupor.

NON-CONTAGIOUS DISEASE: Disease when these are stick to one animal and do not pass to even animals living aside.

NON-INFECTIOUS DISEASE: Disease when cause is other than micro-organism.

NSAID (Non Steroidal Anti-Inflammatory drug): A drug used to control inflammation, without steroid base.

OBESITY: Fatness in animals.

OESTROGEN: Oestrus producing steroids.

OINTMENTS: These are semisolid pasty preparation in which active drug is dispersed or dissolved in a greasy or non-greasy base.

ONCOGEN: substance that produce cancer.

OPTHALMIC: Related to eyes.

ORAL ADMINISTRATION: Given by mouth.

ORAL CONTRACEPTIVE: Contraceptive agents active after oral administration.

OVULATORY STIMULANT: That stimulates ovulation in female.

OXYTOCIC AGENTS: Agents that hasten evacuation of uterus by stimulating contraction of myometrium.

PANACEA: A cure all.

PARASITICIDE: Agent that can kill parasites.

PARENTERAL ADMINISTRATION: Administration other than by gut usually with injection.

PENICILLIN RESISTANCE: Resistance of normally sensitive strains of bacteria to killing effect of penicillin.

PENICILLINASE: Enzyme produced by some organisms induced by drug making it the organism resistant.

PESSARY: Dosage form, a medicated suppository for insertion into the vagina.

PHOTOSENSITIZATION: Some drugs induce sensitivity to suns' ray so that exposed area of skin develop sunburns in fair person.

PHOTOPHOBIA: Fear of light

PILLS: For all tablet form.

PLACEBO: An inactive substance or preparation given to satisfy patients symbolic need for drug therapy.

POISON: A substance which on ingestion, inhalation, absorption, application, injection or development within body in small amount may cause structural damage or functional disturbance.

POTENTIATE: To make more potent.

POTENTIATION: If two drugs produce a given effect through different action their combined effect is usually greater than the sum of their individual effect i.e. 2+2=6 or to make more potent.

POUCH: Pocket like space or sac.

POWDER: Active drug is diluted in inert substance such as starch or lactose. Powder may be for oral use or for local application.

PRECURSOR: A compound used by body to form another compound.

PRESCRIPTION: An order to a pharmacist by a vet to prepare the written medicine and to affix the directions.

PRESERVATIVES: Agents added for the preservation of a formulation.

PURGATIVE: Drug used to produce vigorous emptying of bowel could be used to remove poison from alimentary canal.

PYREXIA: Also known as fever. A syndrome in which there is rise in body temperature.

REAGENT: Substance used to produce a chemical reaction so as to detect or measure.

RELAPSE: Recurrence.

RUMENOTORIC: Act by stimulating the rumen and ruminal activity.

SACHET: a small sealed envelope with medicine for storing powder form of drugs.

SEDATIVE: Drugs used to sedate i.e. to calm, anxious or restless patient without sleep.

SEPSIS: Presence of unwanted bacteria/ virus.

SHAMPOOS: Preparations used to cleanse and nourish the hair or body coat.

SPERMICIDAL: Agent able to kill sperm or hasten their degeneration.

SPORADIC: A disease that occurs occasionally in animal population.

STERILIZATION: A process of freeing a commodity of living organisms.

STEROIDS: Steroid harmones include all gonadal and adrenal cortical hormone.

STETHOSCOPE: An instrument for performing mediate auscultation.

STILLBIRTH: Expulsion of dead foetus at full term.

STRESS: Forcibly exerted influence, pressure, a physical, chemical or emotional or management error.

STUNTED: Arrest in growth or development.

SUBCONJUNCTIVAL: Inside the conjunctiva of eye.

SUBCUTANEOUS: Drugs injected into loose subcutaneous tissue. Irritant drugs should not be injected because they induce severe local inflammation leading to necrosis and sloughing.

SUBLINGUAL ADMINISTRATION: Usually a tablet form put under the tongue. Absorption is through surrounding mucous membrane.

SUPPORTIVE THERAPY: When a treatment is added to support the principal treatment of disease.

SUPPOSITORIES: Bullet shaped solid dosage form meant for insertion in rectum or vagina. These are solid at room temperature but melt at body temperature. Mostly for local action.

SURFACTANTS: Agents that are able to reduce surface tension e.g. in skin cleansing agents.

SUSTAINED RELEASE: when the action of drug is for a longer period or is sustained for a period more than its normal time.

SYMPTOM: A change in body function felt by a patient as a result of disease.

SYNDROME: A set of symptoms occurring together symptom complex.

SYNERGISM: The effect of two drugs are complementary in a therapeutic sense 2+2=6.

SYRINGE: a device of plastic, glass or steel used for injecting the drug with measurement.

SYRUPS: Sweet mixtures are known syrups.

TABLETS: A sugar coated, film coated of different size and shape of drug mixed with inert substance. Inert substance helps in disintegration and dissolution of active drug.

TERATOGENICITY: Potential of drug causing development abnormalities in the foetus when drug given to mother during pregnancy.

THERAPEUTIC: Describing treatment of the disease in general, includes use of drug, surgery, radiation etc.

TOPICAL ADMINISTRATION: Local application of drug where there is problem i.e. skin, uterus, eyes, ears etc.

TOXIC: When an unwanted effect is severe in intensity and potentially harmful.

TRANQUILLIZER: Drug having sedative and anti-anxiety action.

U.S.P.: Pharmacopeia of United States.

UROGENITAL: Urinary and genital organs combined.

UROLITHOLYTICS: Medicines used to help excretion of stones from urinary tract.

VASOCONSTRICTOR: Drugs able to increase the caliber of blood vessels.

VIAL: A drug put in a small container usually of glass which is capped in such a way that drug can be withdrawn with the help of a syringe and needle. Usually injections are contained.

VICE: Bad habits.

VIRUS: Virus are also very small micro-organism. Virus have only one kind of nucleic acid either DNA OR RNA. These cannot produce energy or synthesize protein. Viruses do not reproduce by binary fission. These can multiply in living tissue or tissue culture.

WARM-BLOODED ANIMALS: Whose temperature does not vary with environment like mammals and birds.

WEBWING: In birds the web of the wing is used for vaccination the drug is put here by scratch method.

WITHDRAWL PERIOD: Time period taken to excrete the drug from the body of animal/ bird.

Manufacturers and Marketeers

Alembic Ltd. 2nd Floor, Prime Corporate Park, Andheri-Sahar Road, Andheri (East) Mumbai-400099
Alivira Animal Health Ltd. Unit No. 301, Dosti Pinnacle Plot No. E/7, Road No. 2,, Wagle Estate Thane (W), Mumbai-400604
Animax Health Care www.animaxhealthcare.com
Animax Pharma Pvt. Ltd. B-173, Nehru Vihar, New Delhi-110054
Anmarks Pharmaceuticals Pvt. Ltd. Regd. Off : P.O. 196, Madar Gate, Ajmer
Argano Organic Ltd. Ind. Estate, Delhi Road, Saharanpur-247001
Arosol Pharmaceuticals Pvt. Ltd. 1st Floor, Opp. Hotel Valley Plaza, Behind Raj Plaza Complex, Rajpur A21Road Dehradun-248001 (U.K.)
Avivet Pharma Pvt. Ltd. avivetpharma@gmail.com
Bayer Animal Health Business Bayer House Central Avenue Hiranandani Garden Powai Mumbai-400076
Biomedica (P) Ltd. 736-Industrial Area B, 28-D Sarabha Nagar, Ludhiana-141001 (Pb.)

Boehringer Ingelheim India Pvt. Ltd. 1102, Hallmark Business Plaza, Near Guru Nanak Hospital, Bandra (E), Mumbai-400 051.
Bovian Healthcare Pvt. Ltd. 501, SSR Corporate Park, 13/6 NH-2, Mathura Road, Faridabad-121003 (Haryana)
Brihans Laboratories Animal Health Division of the B.M.S.S. Ltd. Plot No. T 51-55, M.I.D.C. Bhosari, Pune-411 026, Maharashtra
Burroughs Wellcome & Co. (India) Private Limited 16, Bank Street, P.O. Box No. 290, Bombay-1
Cadila Healthcare Ltd. - Agrovet A37Division Post Box No. 12, Ahmedabad-380052
Cadila Pharmaceuticals Limited B.O. Patel House, Near Sardar Patel Colony, Naranpura, Ahmedabad-380017
Cadila Veterinary, Maninagar 244, Ghodasar, Ahmedabad-380050 (India)
Care Vet Pharma 314-AZ, Model Town, Extn. II Ludhiana-141002

Provimi Animal Nutrition India Pvt. Ltd.
IS-40, KHB Industrial Area,
Yelahanka New Town,
Bengaluru-560 064, Karnataka
T + 91-80-3368-0002

Carus
95/3, HSIDC
Karnal

Cattle Remedies India Limited (CRIL)
F-12, Adrshni Plaza, 91,
Adchini, Sri Aurobindo Marg,
New Delhi-1100617

Century Pharmaceuticals Limited
406, World Trade Centre, Sayajigunj
Vadodara-390005

Cipla Ltd.
Mumbai Central, Mumbai-400 008

Concept Pharmaceuticals Limited
167, C.S.T. Road, Santacruz (East),
Mumbai-400 098.

Dosch Animal Health
Dosch Pharmaceuticals Pvt. Ltd.
15-C, Laxmi Industrial Estate,
New Link Road,
Andheri (West), Mumbai-400053

G. Loucatos & Co.
Mercantile Chamber
12, J.N. Heredia Road,
Bellard Estate Mumbai-400001

Glaxo India Ltd.
Agrivet Farm Care
Dr. A.B. Road - 252
Worli Mumbai-400025

Hester Biosciences Limited
Pushpak, Level One, Panchvati Circle,
Motilal Hirabhai Road, Ahmedabad,
Gujarat 380006

Hindustan Antibiotics Ltd.
Agrivet Division,
Pimpri, Pune-411018

Hoechst Pharmaceuticals Limited
(Agrovet Division)
Backbay Reclamation,
Post Box No. 273, Bombay-1

Indian Drugs and Pharmaceuticals Ltd.
25 Gopala Tower, Rajendra Place,
New Delhi-110008

Indian Immunologicals Ltd.
Road No. 44, Jubilee Hills,
Hyderabad-500033

Intas Pharmaceutical Ltd.
2 Floor Chinubhai Centre
Abraham Road,
Ahmedabad-380009

Intercare Ltd. (Intervet Division)
Suneja House, 3rd Floor, Community
Centre, Gulmohar Enclave,
New Delhi-110049

Intervet International B.V. Boxmeer
Holland
P.O. Box 31 5830 AA

Karnataka Antibiotics Pvt. Ltd.
Dr. Raj Kumar Road, Ist Block Rajori
Nagar, Bangalore-560010

Kepler
Corp. Off: Paras 7, Vidhyanagar A78Society,
Part-3 Opp. Vidhyanagar School,
Usmanpura, Ahmedabad-380013

Lyka Labs Limited
Animal Health Division
77, Nehru Road, Vile Parle-East,
Bombay-400 099

Macnor Life Sciences Pvt.Ltd.
3 Floor, Neelkanth Building Bishan
Sarup Colony, Panipat-132103

Macwell Pharmaceuticals Pvt. Ltd. website : www.macwellpharma.com E-mail : macwellpharma@gmail.com Customer care : +91 88262-71502
Marc Laboratories Pvt. Ltd. 3, Vidhan Sabha Marg, Lucknow.
Merial Animal Health 54/A, Sir M.V. Road, Andheri (E) Mumbai-400093
Neospark Drugs & Chemicals Pvt. Ltd. Corporate Centre 241 B.L. Bagh Panju gutta Hyderabad-500082
Novartis India Limited Business Unit – Animal Health 14, J. Tata Road, Church Gate, Mumbai-400 020.
Pail Pharma (P) Ltd DSK Akash Ganga, 504, New D.P. Road, Pune-07
Pfizer Ltd. (Animal Health Div.) Express Towers, Nariman Point, Bombay-400021
Pharma Vision e-mail: pharmavision433@gmail.com Phoenix Life Sciences Pvt. Ltd. Phoenix Tower D-83 Ext. II 2nd Floor, Delhi-110041.
Piramal Health Care Ltd. Vitamins and Fine Chemical Division Balkum, Bombay Agra Road, P.O.B. No. 33, Thane - 400608
Polchem Hygiene Laboratories Pvt. Ltd. 6, Gandharva, 28, Erandwane, Near Mehendale Garage, Pune-411004
Pranav Agro Industries Ltd Nav Maharashtra House, 43, Shaniwar Peth, Pune-411030 (M.S.)

Prima Vet Care Pvt. Ltd. G 12/14, Creative Industrial Estate, N.M. Joshi Marg, Mumbai-400011
Rakesh Pharmaceuticals C-1/158, GIDC, Kalol (NG), Ahmedabad-382725
Ranbaxy Animal Health Care Division – 11th Floor, Ansal Tower, 38 Nehru Place, New Delhi-110019 Devika Tower, 12th Floor 6 Nehru Place, New Delhi-110019
Relife Pharmaceuticals Opc Pvt. Ltd. Juhu Church Road, Juhu, Mumbai-49 (www.relifepharma.com)
Rhone Poulenc (India) Ltd. Rhone Poulenc House, Worli Bombay-400025
RR Animal Health Care Ltd. Plot No. 49 & 50, Adarsh Nagar Colony, Road No. 2, Nagole, Hyderabad- 500068
Sarabhai Chemicals A Division of Ambalal Sarabhai Enterprises Ltd. Wadi Wadi Baroda-390007
Smith Kline & French (India) Limited 25-31, Ropewalk Lane, P. Box No. 1953, Bombay-1
Stallen South Asia Pvt. Ltd. 101, Shyam Kamal 'D' Bldg., Vile Parle (East), Mumbai-400057
Sterling Lab. 203 Swiss Complex, 33, Race Course Road, Bangalore-560001
Sushima Pharmaceuticals Pvt. Ltd. S.O. 132/13, Radhey Shyam Palace, Nai Basti, Ghaziabad-201001 (U.P.) Regd. Off. A-40, New Krishana Park, Vikas Puri, New Delhi.

T.T.K. Pharma Pvt. Ltd. 66, Luz Church Road, Madras-600004 91 Santhome High Road, Chennai-600028
Tineta Pharma Pvt. Ltd. A/8, Sahyog, Anand Nagar, Vasai Road (West), Mumbai-401202
Torrent Veterinary Products (P) Ltd. 'Sanskrut' High Court Road, Ahmedabad-380003
Unjha Formulations Khali Char Rasta, State Highway, Ta. Sidhpur-384151 (N.Guj.)
Venky's Livestock B.V. Bio-Corp Pvt. Ltd. Unit No. 3/303, 3rd Floor, Sharada Center, 11/1-Erandwane, Pune-411004 (Maharashtra)
Ventri Chemicals Pvt. Ltd. AHPD, 13/6, Milestone, P.O. Girinagar, Pune-411025
Vest Pharma Pvt. Ltd. Jalandhar-144 003
Vet Avenue K-2 Textile Colony, Industrial Area A Ludhiana-141003

Vetcure Pharma S.P.O. : Plot No. 44/C, Near Education Point, Badli, Delhi-110042
Vetmankind 236, Okhla Industrial Estate 3 New Delhi.
Vets Farma Pvt. Ltd. Gurmit Building, Police Line Road, Jalandhar-144001
Virbac Animal Health India Pvt. Ltd. 604, 6 Floor, Western Edge I Magathane, Western Express Highway Borivali (East) Mumbai-400066
Wellcon Animal Health 201, Sai Prasad Building, Plot No. E17C, Sector-3, Belpada, Kharghar, Navi Mumbai-410210
Wockhardt Limited Wockhardt Towers Barvila Kurla Complex, Bandra East, Mumbai-400051
Zoetis India Limited Pfizer Centre, Patel Estate, Off S.V. Road, Jogeshwari (West), Mumbai-400 102

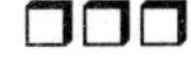

Index Product